REDUCING
UNDERAGE DRINKING
A COLLECTIVE RESPONSIBILITY

Committee on Developing a Strategy to Reduce and
Prevent Underage Drinking

Richard J. Bonnie and Mary Ellen O'Connell, Editors

Board on Children, Youth, and Families
Division of Behavioral and Social Sciences and Education

NATIONAL RESEARCH COUNCIL
INSTITUTE OF MEDICINE
OF THE NATIONAL ACADEMIES

THE NATIONAL ACADEMIES PRESS
Washington, D.C.
www.nap.edu

THE NATIONAL ACADEMIES PRESS   500 Fifth Street, N.W.   Washington, DC 20418

NOTICE: The project that is the subject of this report was approved by the Governing Board of the National Research Council, whose members are drawn from the councils of the National Academy of Sciences, the National Academy of Engineering, and the Institute of Medicine. The members of the committee responsible for the report were chosen for their special competences and with regard for appropriate balance.

This project, N01-OD-4-2139, Task Order No. 109, received support from the evaluation set-aside Section 513, Public Health Service Act, of the U.S. Department of Health and Human Services. The content of this publication does not necessarily reflect the views or policies of the U.S. Department of Health and Human Services, nor does mention of trade names, commercial products, or organizations imply endorsement by the U.S. government.

Library of Congress Cataloging-in-Publication Data

Reducing underage drinking : a collective responsibility / Committee on Developing a Strategy to Reduce and Prevent Underage Drinking ; Richard J. Bonnie and Mary Ellen O'Connell, editors.

    p. ; cm.
Includes bibliographical references.
  ISBN 0-309-08935-2 (hardback with CD-ROM)
  1. Teenagers—Alcohol use—Prevention. 2. Youth—Alcohol use—Prevention. 3. Alcoholism—Prevention. 4. Drinking of alcoholic beverages—Prevention. 5. Community organization.
  [DNLM: 1. Alcohol Drinking—prevention & control—Adolescent—United States. 2. Alcohol Drinking—epidemiology—Adolescent—United States. 3. Alcohol-Related Disorders—prevention & control—Adolescent—United States. 4. Mass Media—United States. WM 274 R321 2003] I. Bonnie, Richard J. II. O'Connell, Mary Ellen, 1960- III. National Research Council (U.S.). Committee on Developing a Strategy to Reduce and Prevent Underage Drinking.
  RJ506.D78R43 2003
  362.292'7'08350973—dc22
                       2003018014

Additional copies of this report are available from the National Academies Press, 500 Fifth Street, N.W., Lockbox 285, Washington, DC 20055; (800) 624-6242 or (202) 334-3313 (in the Washington metropolitan area); Internet, http://www.nap.edu.

Printed in the United States of America.

Cover: First Night celebrations are meant to recapture the symbolic significance of the passage from the old year to the new; to unite the community through a shared cultural celebration; to deepen and broaden the public appreciation of the visual and performing arts; to help revitalize the urban core of a community; and to offer a family-friendly, alcohol-free alternative to traditional New Year's Eve revelry. For more information or to find a First Night Celebration near you go to www.firstnight.com.

Suggested citation: National Research Council and Institute of Medicine (2004). *Reducing Underage Drinking: A Collective Responsibility*. Committee on Developing a Strategy to Reduce and Prevent Underage Drinking, Richard J. Bonnie and Mary Ellen O'Connell, Editors. Board on Children, Youth, and Families, Division of Behavioral and Social Sciences and Education. Washington, DC: The National Academies Press.

THE NATIONAL ACADEMIES
Advisers to the Nation on Science, Engineering, and Medicine

The **National Academy of Sciences** is a private, nonprofit, self-perpetuating society of distinguished scholars engaged in scientific and engineering research, dedicated to the furtherance of science and technology and to their use for the general welfare. Upon the authority of the charter granted to it by the Congress in 1863, the Academy has a mandate that requires it to advise the federal government on scientific and technical matters. Dr. Bruce M. Alberts is president of the National Academy of Sciences.

The **National Academy of Engineering** was established in 1964, under the charter of the National Academy of Sciences, as a parallel organization of outstanding engineers. It is autonomous in its administration and in the selection of its members, sharing with the National Academy of Sciences the responsibility for advising the federal government. The National Academy of Engineering also sponsors engineering programs aimed at meeting national needs, encourages education and research, and recognizes the superior achievements of engineers. Dr. Wm. A. Wulf is president of the National Academy of Engineering.

The **Institute of Medicine** was established in 1970 by the National Academy of Sciences to secure the services of eminent members of appropriate professions in the examination of policy matters pertaining to the health of the public. The Institute acts under the responsibility given to the National Academy of Sciences by its congressional charter to be an adviser to the federal government and, upon its own initiative, to identify issues of medical care, research, and education. Dr. Harvey V. Fineberg is president of the Institute of Medicine.

The **National Research Council** was organized by the National Academy of Sciences in 1916 to associate the broad community of science and technology with the Academy's purposes of furthering knowledge and advising the federal government. Functioning in accordance with general policies determined by the Academy, the Council has become the principal operating agency of both the National Academy of Sciences and the National Academy of Engineering in providing services to the government, the public, and the scientific and engineering communities. The Council is administered jointly by both Academies and the Institute of Medicine. Dr. Bruce M. Alberts and Dr. Wm. A. Wulf are chair and vice chair, respectively, of the National Research Council.

www.national-academies.org

COMMITTEE ON DEVELOPING A STRATEGY TO REDUCE AND PREVENT UNDERAGE DRINKING

RICHARD J. BONNIE (*Chair*), School of Law, University of Virginia

MARILYN AGUIRRE-MOLINA, Mailman School of Public Health, Columbia University

PHILIP J. COOK, Department of Public Policy Studies, Duke University

JUDITH A. CUSHING, The Oregon Partnership, Portland

JOEL W. GRUBE, Prevention Research Center, Berkeley, California

BONNIE L. HALPERN-FELSHER, Department of Pediatrics, University of California, San Francisco

WILLIAM B. HANSEN, Tanglewood Research Inc., Greensboro, North Carolina

DENISE HERD, School of Public Health, University of California, Berkeley

ROBERT HORNIK, Annenberg School for Communication, University of Pennsylvania, Philadelphia

JANIS JACOBS, Undergraduate Education and International Programs, Pennsylvania State University

MARK H. MOORE, John F. Kennedy School of Government, Harvard University

DANIEL A. TRUJILLO, Department of Community Development and Substance Abuse Programs, Massachusetts Institute of Technology

MARY ELLEN O'CONNELL, *Study Director*

JOAH IANNOTTA, *Research Associate*

SUSAN McCUTCHEN, *Research Associate*

ANTHONY MANN, *Senior Project Assistant*

MICHAEL BIEHL, *Consultant*

Acknowledgments

In addition to the expertise and hard work of the committee members, we benefited from the expertise and intellectual insights of a range of leaders in the field who enthusiastically contributed to the project. Numerous leading researchers wrote papers on a range of topics that helped to inform the work of the committee; see Appendix D for a list of their names.

Most of these papers were presented by the lead author and discussed at an October 2002 workshop, and many of the papers are on the CD-ROM attached to the inside back cover. The many participants at this workshop (see Appendix B) helped to enrich the discussion. The committee is grateful for their insights. The committee would also like to acknowledge contributions of Robert Pandina, Rutgers University, who shared his extensive expertise as a respondent at the workshop.

In November 2002 numerous individuals and organizations concerned with underage drinking provided written and verbal comments to the committee on their research findings, priorities, and concerns. We are thankful for the tireless, continued efforts of these groups; see Appendix C for the meeting agenda and participants. The committee also thanks Jeff Arnett, University of Maryland, for his insightful comments on youth perspectives at the November meeting.

Dozens of stakeholders and scientists provided program materials, literature, and other written materials or responded to requests for information from the committee; see Appendix D.

This report has been reviewed in draft form by individuals chosen for their diverse perspectives and technical expertise, in accordance with procedures approved by the Report Review Committee of the National Research Council (NRC). The purpose of this independent review is to provide candid and critical comments that will assist the institution in making its published report as sound as possible and to ensure that the report meets institutional standards for objectivity, evidence, and responsiveness to the study charge. The review comments and draft manuscript remain confidential to protect the integrity of the deliberative process.

We thank the following individuals for their review of this report: David S. Anderson, Center for the Advancement of Public Health, George Mason University; Johnnetta Davis-Joyce, Pacific Institute for Research and Evaluation, Calverton, MD; Mary Jane England, Regis College; Susan Ennett, Department of Health Behavior and Health Education, University of North Carolina; Rob MacCoun, Goldman School of Public Policy and Boalt Hall School of Law, University of California at Berkeley; Michael Moore, Darden School of Business, University of Virginia; Rosalie Pacula, RAND, Santa Monica, CA; Seth J. Schwartz, Center for Family Studies, Department of Psychiatry and Behavioral Sciences, University of Miami School of Medicine; Jose Szapocznik, Center for Family Studies, Department of Psychiatry and Behavioral Sciences, University of Miami School of Medicine; Larry Wallack, School of Community Health, Portland State University; and Henry Wechsler, Harvard School of Public Health.

Although the reviewers listed above have provided many constructive comments and suggestions, they were not asked to endorse the conclusions or recommendations nor did they see the final draft of the report before its release. The review of this report was overseen by David S. Cordray, Institute for Public Policy Studies, Vanderbilt University, and John E. Dowling, The Biological Laboratories, Harvard University. Appointed by the National Research Council, they were responsible for making certain that an independent examination of this report was carried out in accordance with institutional procedures and that all review comments were carefully considered. Responsibility for the final content of this report rests entirely with the authoring committee and the institution.

Several people reviewed specific papers to add to the assessment of committee members and staff and the comments on them from workshop participants. The committee thanks the following people for their review of one or more papers: George Balch, Balch Associates; Maxine Hayes, Washington State Department of Health; Ralph Hingson, Department of Social and Behavioral Sciences, Boston University; Bernard Murphy, Center for Policy Analysis and Training, Pacific Institute for Research and Evaluation; Robert Pandina, Center for Alcohol Studies, Rutgers University; Cheryl Perry, Division of Epidemiology, School of Public Health,

University of Minnesota; Henry Saffer, National Bureau of Economic Research; and Susan Tapert, Department of Psychiatry, University of California, San Diego.

The committee recognizes the support provided by members of the Board on Children, Youth, and Families under the leadership of Michael Cohen. We are grateful for the leadership and support of Susanne Stoiber, executive officer of the Institute of Medicine; Michael Feuer, executive director of the NRC's Division of Behavioral and Social Sciences and Education; his predecessor, Barbara Torrey; Jane Ross, director of the Center for Economic and Social Sciences; and Susan Cummins, former director of the Board on Children, Youth, and Families.

Finally, the committee benefited from the support and assistance of several members of The National Academies staff. Joah Iannotta and Susan McCutchen provided valuable assistance in collecting, summarizing, and organizing materials and helping draft sections of the report. The research needs of the project were greatly aided by the able assistance of Georgeann Higgins of the NRC library. Anthony Mann managed numerous and sometimes complicated administrative responsibilities. We are indebted to Eugenia Grohman, who worked with us on several revisions and provided superb editorial guidance; and Yvonne Wise, who helped prepare the report for publication.

We also acknowledge Michael Biehl, University of California, San Francisco, who tirelessly prepared analyses of National Household Survey on Drug Abuse data and provided invaluable assistance to the committee.

Richard J. Bonnie, *Chair*
Mary Ellen O'Connell, *Study Director*
Committee on Developing a Strategy
to Reduce and Prevent Underage
Drinking

Contents

BACKGROUND PAPERS*

*The background papers are not printed in this book but are on the CD-ROM attached to the inside back cover.

Preface

By the time children are seniors in high school, about 30 percent are drinking heavily at least once a month. And 40 percent of full-time college students and more than 36 percent of other young adults (ages 18-22) report heavy drinking.

The consequences and costs of youthful alcohol use are enormous. Many of these harmful consequences are immediate and all too evident—injuries due to impaired driving or violence, sexual assault and unwanted pregnancies, and educational failure. The best available estimate places the annual social cost of underage drinking at $53 billion, far exceeding the costs of youthful use of illegal drugs. In recognition of the enormity of the problem, Congress asked the National Academies to develop a strategy for reducing and preventing underage drinking.

This is a daunting challenge. To what extent can public policy really affect underage drinking when alcohol is so widely used and approved by adults and when youthful indulgence is so often overlooked or condoned? After all, "kids will be kids." Presumably, the answer depends on whether instruments of public policy can affect the main determinants of underage drinking, particularly the factors associated with the most harmful features of underage alcohol use.

Some people believe that the dangers of underage drinking are at least partly attributable to the very fact that it is "underage" (i.e., illegal) conduct. Obviously, lowering the minimum drinking age would (by definition) reduce the amount of "underage" drinking. More importantly, according to some experts, at least some of the harmful drinking practices of underage drinkers would not occur if their drinking were lawful. People who hold this view often point to European countries with lower drinking ages where, they claim, young people learn to drink under the supervision of adults and are not as inclined to drink heavily. The facts do not support this view, however. As the committee demonstrates in this report, countries with lower drinking ages are not better off than the United States in terms of the harmful consequences of youths' drinking. And one thing we do know for sure is that raising the drinking age to 21 in the United States has saved many thousands of lives. That is why Congress enacted the National Minimum Drinking Age Act of 1984, using the leverage of federal highway funds to induce every state to raise the drinking age to 21.

It turns out that the patterns and consequences of youthful drinking are closely related to the overall extent and patterns of drinking in the society, and they are affected by the same factors that affect the patterns of adult consumption. From this standpoint, it is possible that the most effective way to reduce the extent and adverse consequences of youthful drinking would be to reduce the extent and consequences of adult drinking. It is clear, however, that Congress intended for the committee to focus on youth drinking, rather than developing a strategy targeting adult drinking as well as youth drinking. This is what the committee has done.

The report outlines the committee's proposed strategy in detail. Substance abuse prevention is typically targeted on young people themselves—to persuade them to abstain and try to keep the dangerous substance out of their hands. At the center of the committee's strategy, however, is the judgment that parents and adults must be the main target of a strategy to reduce and prevent underage drinking. In requesting this report, Congress was specifically seeking advice about the message that should be conveyed to young people, especially in a national media campaign. However, in the committee's view, if we do no more than pepper kids with anti-drinking messages, things are not likely to get any better. We have to do more. We have to resolve, as a national community, to reduce underage drinking and the problems associated with it and to take comprehensive measures to achieve this goal. If we do this without equivocation, there is a reasonable prospect of success. And success—measured in many thousands of young lives and futures saved—is well worth the investment.

Richard J. Bonnie, *Chair*
Committee on Developing a
Strategy to Reduce and Prevent
Underage Drinking

REDUCING
UNDERAGE DRINKING

Executive Summary

A lcohol use by young people is dangerous, not only because of the risks associated with acute impairment, but also because of the threat to their long-term development and well-being. Traffic crashes are perhaps the most visible of these dangers, with alcohol being implicated in nearly one-third of youth traffic fatalities. Underage alcohol use is also associated with violence, suicide, educational failure, and other problem behaviors. All of these problems are magnified by early onset of teen drinking: the younger the drinker, the worse the problem. Moreover, frequent heavy drinking by young adolescents can lead to mild brain damage. The social cost of underage drinking has been estimated at $53 billion including $19 billion from traffic crashes and $29 billion from violent crime.

More youth drink than smoke tobacco or use other illegal drugs. Yet federal investments in preventing underage drinking pale in comparison with resources targeted (mostly to youths) at preventing illicit drug use. In fiscal 2000, $71.1 million was targeted at preventing underage alcohol use by the U.S. Departments of Health and Human Services (HHS), Justice, and Transportation. In contrast, the fiscal 2000 federal budget authority for drug abuse prevention (including prevention research) was 25 times higher, $1.8 billion; for tobacco prevention, funding for the Office of Smoking and Health, only one of several HHS agencies involved with smoking prevention, was approximately $100 million, with states spending a great deal more with resources from the states' Medicaid reimbursement suits against the tobacco companies.

Although it is illegal to sell or give alcohol to youths under age 21, they do not have a hard time getting it, and they often get it from adults. More than 90 percent of twelfth graders report that alcohol is "very easy" or "fairly easy" to get. And when underage youths drink, they drink more heavily and recklessly than adults. They report that they "usually" drink an average of four and a half drinks, an amount very close to the threshold of five drinks typically used to define heavy drinking (also referred to as binge drinking). In contrast, adult drinkers report usually drinking fewer than three drinks.

In response to a congressional request in the HHS fiscal 2002 appropriations act, the Board on Children, Youth, and Families of the National Research Council and the Institute of Medicine formed the Committee on Developing a Strategy to Reduce and Prevent Underage Drinking. The committee was directed to review a broad range of federal, state, and nongovernmental programs, from environmental interventions to programs focusing directly on youth attitudes and behaviors, and to develop a cost-effective strategy to reduce and prevent underage drinking. In conducting this review, the committee relied on the available scientific literature, including a series of papers written for the committee, public input, and its expertise.

The committee conducted its work within the framework of the current national policy establishing 21 as the minimum legal drinking age in every state. We concentrated more on population-based primary prevention approaches rather than on individually oriented approaches.

STRATEGY OVERVIEW

The committee reached the fundamental conclusion that underage drinking cannot be successfully addressed by focusing on youth alone. Youth drink within the context of a society in which alcohol use is normative behavior and images about alcohol are pervasive. They usually obtain alcohol—either directly or indirectly—from adults. Efforts to reduce underage drinking, therefore, need to focus on adults and must engage the society at large.

The preeminent goal of the recommended strategy is to create and sustain a broad societal commitment to reduce underage drinking. Such a commitment will require participation by multiple individuals and organizations at the national, state, local, and community levels who are in a position to affect youth decisions—including parents and other adults, alcohol producers, wholesalers and retail outlets, restaurants and bars, entertainment media, schools, colleges and universities, the military, landlords, community organizations, and youths themselves. The nation must collectively pursue opportunities to reduce the availability of alcohol to underage drinkers, the occasions for underage drinking, and the demand for alcohol among young people.

THE STRATEGY

The committee's proposed strategy for broad societal commitment to reduce underage drinking has ten main components.

National Adult-Oriented Media Campaign

Most adults express concern about youth drinking and support public policy actions to reduce youth access to alcohol. Nonetheless, youth obtain alcohol from adults. Parents tend to dramatically underestimate underage drinking generally and their own children's drinking in particular. The first component in the strategy calls for the development of a media campaign, including rigorous formative research on effective messages, aimed at increasing specific actions by adults meant to reduce underage drinking and decreasing adult conduct that facilitates underage drinking.

Recommendation 6-1: The federal government should fund and actively support the development of a national media effort, as a major component of an adult-oriented campaign to reduce underage drinking.

Partnership to Prevent Underage Drinking

Despite laws that aim to preclude drinking by those under the age of 21, a significant amount of underage drinking occurs, generating revenues for producers, wholesalers, and retailers of alcoholic beverages, especially beer. The alcohol industry has declared its commitment to reducing underage drinking and has invested in programs with that aim. However, the outcomes of these efforts are not always apparent, and the motives are sometimes questioned. A partnership between the alcohol industry, government, and other private partners would facilitate a coordinated, evidence-based approach to reduce and prevent underage drinking.

Recommendation 7-1: All segments of the alcohol industry that profit from underage drinking, inadvertently or otherwise, should join with other private and public partners to establish and fund an independent nonprofit foundation with the sole mission of reducing and preventing underage drinking.

Alcohol Advertising

A substantial proportion of alcohol advertising reaches an underage audience and is presented in a style that is attractive to youths. For example, television alcohol advertisements routinely appear on programs for which the percentage of underage viewers is greater than the percentage of underage youths in the population. Although a clear causal link between advertising and youth consumption has not been established, youth exposure to advertising and marketing of products with particular appeal to youths should be reduced. Strengthened self-regulation would be in keeping with the industry's stated commitment to avoid sale to minors and with recommendations by the Federal Trade Commission (FTC) in 1999 regarding industry advertising standards. Only one company has adopted the FTC's 1999 recommendation that the industry create independent external review boards to address complaints regarding violations of advertising codes. In light of constitutional constraints on direct advertising restrictions, and to enable the industry to be responsive to public concerns about advertising, the most fruitful governmental response would be to facilitate public awareness of advertising practices.

Recommendation 7-2: Alcohol companies, advertising companies, and commercial media should refrain from marketing practices (including product design, advertising, and promotional techniques) that have substantial underage appeal and should take reasonable precautions in the time, place, and manner of placement and promotion to reduce youthful exposure to other alcohol advertising and marketing activity.

Recommendation 7-3: The alcohol industry trade associations, as well as individual companies, should strengthen their advertising codes to preclude placement of commercial messages in venues where a significant proportion of the expected audience is underage, to prohibit the use of commercial messages that have substantial underage appeal, and to establish independent external review boards to investigate complaints and enforce the codes.

Recommendation 7-4: Congress should appropriate the necessary funding for the U.S. Department of Health and Human Services to monitor underage exposure to alcohol advertising on a continuing basis and to report periodically to Congress and the public. The report should include information on the underage percentage of the exposed audience and estimated number of underage viewers of print and broadcasting alcohol advertising in national markets and, for television and radio broadcasting, in a selection of large local or regional markets.

Entertainment Media

Since artistic expression inevitably reflects the culture in which it is embedded, it is hardly surprising that alcohol use and alcohol products are frequently displayed or mentioned in prime-time television, movies, and music. Although the viewing or listening audiences for most of these media products are predominantly adult, some of them are disproportionately underage, and even the predominantly adult audiences inevitably include large numbers of young people. As in the case of commercial alcohol advertising, the entertainment media have a social responsibility to eschew displays or lyrics that portray underage drinking in a favorable light or that glamorize or promote alcohol consumption in products that are targeted toward or likely to be heard or viewed by large underage audiences. Labeling and notice requirements have been voluntarily adopted in analogous contexts. Although the industry restrictions should be undertaken on a voluntary basis, some independent oversight and public awareness of these standards is warranted.

Recommendation 8-1: The entertainment industries should use rating systems and marketing codes to reduce the likelihood that underage audiences will be exposed to movies, recordings, or television programs with unsuitable alcohol content, even if adults are expected to predominate in the viewing or listening audiences

Recommendation 8-2: The film rating board of the Motion Picture Association of America should consider alcohol content in rating films, avoiding G or PG ratings for films with unsuitable alcohol content, and assigning mature ratings for films that portray underage drinking in a favorable light.

Recommendation 8-3: The music recording industry should not market recordings that promote or glamorize alcohol use to young people; should include alcohol content in a comprehensive rating system, similar to those used by the television, film, and video game industries; and should establish an independent body to assign ratings and oversee the industry code.

Recommendation 8-4: Television broadcasters and producers should take appropriate precautions to ensure that programs do not portray underage drinking in a favorable light, and that unsuitable alcohol content is included in the category of mature content for purposes of parental warnings.

Recommendation 8-5: Congress should appropriate the necessary funds to enable the U.S. Department of Health and Human Services to conduct a periodic review of a representative sample of movies, television programs, and music recordings and videos that are offered at times or in venues likely to have a significant youth audience (e.g., 15 percent) to ascertain the nature and frequency of lyrics or images pertaining to alcohol. The results of these reviews should be reported to Congress and the public.

Limiting Access

Limiting youth access to alcohol has been shown to be effective in reducing and preventing underage drinking and drinking-related problems. Since 21 became the nationwide legal drinking age, there have been significant decreases in drinking, fatal traffic crashes, alcohol-related crashes, and arrests for "driving under the influence" (DUI) among young people. Given the widespread availability of alcohol and easy access by underage drinkers, minimum drinking age laws must be enforced more effectively, along with social sanctions. The effectiveness of underage drinking laws could be enhanced through such approaches as compliance checks, server training, zero tolerance laws, and graduated driver licensing laws.

Recommendation 9-1: The minimum drinking age laws of each state should prohibit

- purchase or attempted purchase, possession, and consumption of alcoholic beverages by persons under 21;
- possession of and use of falsified or fraudulent identification to purchase or attempt to purchase alcoholic beverages;
- provision of any alcohol to minors by adults, except to their own children in their own residences; and
- underage drinking in private clubs and establishments.

Recommendation 9-2: States should strengthen their compliance check programs in retail outlets, using media campaigns and license revocation to increase deterrence.

- Communities and states should undertake regular and comprehensive compliance check programs, including notification of retailers concerning the program and follow-up communication to them about the outcome (sale/no sale) for their outlet.
- Enforcement agencies should issue citations for violations of underage sales laws, with substantial fines and temporary suspension of license for first offenses and increasingly stronger penalties thereafter, leading to permanent revocation of license after three offenses.
- Communities and states should implement media campaigns in conjunction with compliance check programs detailing the program, its purpose, and outcomes.

Recommendation 9-3: The federal government should require states to achieve designated rates of retailer compliance with youth access prohibitions as a condition of receiving relevant block grant funding, similar to the Synar Amendment's requirements for youth tobacco sales.

Recommendation 9-4: States should require all sellers and servers of alcohol to complete state-approved training as a condition of employment.

Recommendation 9-5: States should enact or strengthen dram shop liability statutes to authorize negligence-based civil actions against commercial providers of alcohol for serving or selling alcohol to a minor who subsequently causes injury to others, while allowing a defense for sellers who have demonstrated compliance with responsible business practices. States should include in their dram shop statutes key portions of the Model Alcoholic Beverage Retail Licensee Liability Act of 1985, including the responsible business practices defense.

Recommendation 9-6: States that allow Internet sales and home delivery of alcohol should regulate these activities to reduce the likelihood of sales to underage purchasers. States should

- require all packages for delivery containing alcohol to be clearly labeled as such;
- require persons who deliver alcohol to record the recipient's age identification information from a valid government-issued document (such as a driver's license or ID card); and
- require recipients of home delivery of alcohol to sign a statement verifying receipt of alcohol and attesting that he or she is of legal age to purchase alcohol.

Recommendation 9-7: States and localities should implement enforcement programs to deter adults from purchasing alcohol for minors. States and communities should

- routinely undertake shoulder tap or other prevention programs targeting adults who purchase alcohol for minors, using warnings, rather than citations, for the first offense;
- enact and enforce laws to hold retailers responsible, as a condition of licensing, for allowing minors to loiter and solicit adults to purchase alcohol for them on outlet property; and
- use nuisance and loitering ordinances as a means of discouraging youth from congregating outside of alcohol outlets in order to solicit adults to purchase alcohol.

Recommendation 9-8: States and communities should establish and implement a system requiring registration of beer kegs that records information on the identity of purchasers.

Recommendation 9-9: States should facilitate enforcement of zero tolerance laws in order to increase their deterrent effect. States should

- modify existing laws to allow passive breath testing, streamlined administrative procedures, and administrative penalties and
- implement media campaigns to increase young peoples' awareness of reduced blood alcohol content (BAC) limits and of enforcement efforts.

Recommendation 9-10: States should enact and enforce graduated driver licensing laws.

Recommendation 9-11: States and localities should routinely implement sobriety checkpoints.

Recommendation 9-12: Local police, working with community leaders, should adopt and announce policies for detecting and terminating underage drinking parties, including:

- routinely responding to complaints from the public about noisy teenage parties and entering the premises when there is probable cause to suspect underage drinking is taking place;
- routinely checking, as a part of regular weekend patrols, open areas where teenage drinking parties are known to occur; and
- routinely citing underage drinkers and, if possible, the person who supplied the alcohol when underage drinking is observed at parties.

Recommendation 9-13: States should strengthen efforts to prevent and detect use of false identification by minors to make alcohol purchases. States should

- prohibit the production, sale, distribution, possession, and use of false identification for attempted alcohol purchase;
- issue driver's licenses and state identification cards that can be electronically scanned;
- allow retailers to confiscate apparently false identification for law enforcement inspection; and
- implement administrative penalties (e.g., immediate confiscation of a driver's license and issuance of a citation resulting in a substantial fine) for attempted use of false identification by minors for alcohol purchases.

Recommendation 9-14: States should establish administrative procedures and noncriminal penalties, such as fines or community service, for alcohol infractions by minors.

Youth-Oriented Interventions

Although the proposed strategy focuses mainly on adult attitudes and behavior toward underage drinking and on reducing the availability of alcohol to underage youth, approaches that directly target youth are also needed. A national youth-oriented media campaign to reduce and prevent underage drinking would be premature in the absence of more evidence supporting this approach. However, effective education-oriented approaches in schools and other settings aimed at preventing alcohol use by youths, as well as interventions with youths who have already developed alcohol problems, play a role. Interventions that rely on provision of information alone, or that focus on increasing self-esteem or resisting peer pressure, have not been demonstrated to be effective.

Residential colleges and universities have witnessed serious drinking problems among students under 21. Despite efforts by nearly all campuses to address this problem, heavy drinking has not declined over the past decade. Residential colleges and universities are in a unique position to develop and evaluate comprehensive approaches that address both individual and population-level issues.

Recommendation 10-1: Intensive research and development for a youth-focused national media campaign relating to underage drinking should be initiated. If this work yields promising results, the inclusion of a youth-focused campaign in the strategy should be reconsidered.

Recommendation 10-2: The U.S. Department of Health and Human Services and the U.S. Department of Education should fund only evidence-based education interventions, with priority given both to those that incorporate elements known to be effective and those that are part of comprehensive community programs.

Recommendation 10-3: Residential colleges and universities should adopt comprehensive prevention approaches, including evidence-based screening, brief intervention strategies, consistent policy enforcement, and environmental changes that limit underage access to alcohol. They should use universal education interventions, as well as selective and indicated approaches with relevant populations.

Recommendation 10-4: The National Institute on Alcohol Abuse and Alcoholism and the Substance Abuse and Mental Health Services Administration should continue to fund evaluations of college-based interventions, with a particular emphasis on targeting of interventions to specific college characteristics, and should maintain a list of evidence-based programs.

Recommendation 10-5: The U.S. Department of Health and Human Services and states should expand the availability of effective clinical services for treating alcohol abuse among underage populations and for following up on treatment. The U.S. Department of Education, the U.S. Department of Health and Human Services, and the U.S. Department of Justice should establish policies that facilitate diagnosing and referring underage alcohol abusers and those who are alcohol dependent for clinical treatment.

Community Interventions

Community mobilization can be a powerful vehicle to implement and support interventions, especially those that target community-level policies and practices. Communities can design multipronged comprehensive initiatives that rely on scientifically based strategies and are responsive to the specific problems of their communities. College campuses and local communities have a reciprocal influence on one another in relation to student alcohol use and the need to develop complementary strategies.

Recommendation 11-1: Community leaders should assess the underage drinking problem in their communities and consider effective approaches—such as community organizing, coalition building, and the strategic use of the mass media—to reduce drinking among underage youth.

Recommendation 11-2: Public and private funders should support community mobilization to reduce underage drinking. Federal funding for reducing and preventing underage drinking should be available under a national program dedicated to community-level approaches to reducing underage drinking, similar to the Drug Free Communities Act, which supports communities in addressing substance abuse with targeted, evidence-based prevention strategies.

Government Assistance and Coordination

The ultimate responsibility for preventing and reducing underage drinking lies with the entire national community, not with government alone.

However, the federal and state governments have important responsibilities in addition to enforcing the law. These responsibilities include funding media campaigns, supporting community efforts, monitoring alcohol and entertainment industry portrayals of drinking, monitoring trends in underage drinking and the effectiveness of efforts to reduce it, coordinating multiple agency activities, and supporting continued research and evaluation.

Recommendation 12-1: A federal interagency coordinating committee on prevention of underage drinking should be established, chaired by the secretary of the U.S. Department of Health and Human Services.

Recommendation 12-2: A National Training and Research Center on Underage Drinking should be established in the U.S. Department of Health and Human Services. This body would provide technical assistance, training, and evaluation support and would monitor progress in implementing national goals.

Recommendation 12-3: The secretary of the U.S. Department of Health and Human Services should issue an annual report on underage drinking to Congress summarizing all federal agency activities, progress in reducing underage drinking, and key surveillance data.

Recommendation 12-4: Each state should designate a lead agency to coordinate and spearhead its activities and programs to reduce and prevent underage drinking.

Recommendation 12-5: The annual report of the secretary of the U.S. Department of Health and Human Services on underage drinking should include key indicators of underage drinking.

Recommendation 12-6: The Monitoring the Future Survey and the National Survey on Drug Use and Health should be revised to elicit more precise information on the quantity of alcohol consumed and to ascertain brand preferences of underage drinkers.

Alcohol Excise Taxes

Alcoholic beverages are far cheaper (after adjusting for overall inflation) today than they were in the 1960s and 1970s. While raising excise taxes, and therefore prices, would have some effect on alcohol use by adults, price has been documented to have a differential effect on youth alcohol consumption patterns. Taxes can also be a source of revenue for funding strategies aimed at reducing underage drinking and its associated harms.

Recommendation 12-7: Congress and state legislatures should raise excise taxes to reduce underage consumption and to raise additional revenues for this purpose. Top priority should be given to raising beer taxes, and excise tax rates for all alcoholic beverages should be indexed to the consumer price index so that they keep pace with inflation without the necessity of further legislative action.

Research and Evaluation

Rigorous research and evaluation are needed to assess the effectiveness of specific interventions and to ensure that future refinements of the strategy are grounded in evidence-based approaches. Research related to prototype development for the proposed adult media campaign is a core component of the strategy outlined in this report. In addition, continued research and evaluation are necessary to develop new approaches aimed at reaching all segments of the underage population.

Recommendation 12-8: All interventions, including media messages and education programs, whether funded by public or private sources, should be rigorously evaluated, and a portion of all federal grant funds for alcohol-related programs should be designated for evaluation.

Recommendation 12-9: States and the federal government—particularly the U.S. Department of Health and Human Services and the U.S. Department of Education—should fund the development and evaluation of programs to cover all underage populations.

In sum, our proposed strategy calls for development of a national campaign to engage adults in a concerted effort to stop enabling or ignoring youth drinking. The proposed strategy calls on the alcohol industry to enter a partnership with government and other private funders to implement a coordinated, evidence-based approach to reducing underage drinking. It proposes steps to increase compliance with laws against selling or providing alcohol to minors. It calls for reducing youth exposure to alcohol advertising or music and other entertainment with products and ads that glorify drinking. It recognizes the potential importance of school-based education approaches and the need for residential colleges and universities to implement comprehensive approaches. It calls on local leaders to apply the multiple tools available to address underage drinking within the context of their communities. And it challenges federal and state governments to coordinate their efforts and to raise excise taxes to reduce underage consumption and raise revenues for the proposed strategy. Finally, it recommends ongoing monitoring and continued research and evaluation to facilitate continued refinement of the strategy and its implementation.

1

Introduction: The Challenge

A lcohol use by children, adolescents, and young adults under the legal drinking age of 21 produces human tragedies with alarming regularity. Motor vehicle crashes, homicides, suicides, and other unintentional injuries are the four leading causes of death of 15- to 20-year-olds, and alcohol is a factor in many of these deaths. Indeed, so many underage drinkers die in car crashes that this problem, by itself, is a major national concern. In relation to the number of licensed drivers, young people under age 21 who have been drinking are involved in fatal crashes at twice the rate of adult drivers (National Highway Traffic Safety Administration, 2002a).

Car crashes are the most visible and most numbing consequences of underage drinking, but they represent only a small proportion of the social toll that underage drinking takes on the present and future welfare of society. Other damaging problems include dangerous sexual practices that lead to both serious disease and unwanted pregnancies, unintentional injuries, fights, and school failures that lead to expulsions or withdrawals. Levy et al. (1999) estimated that in 1996 underage drinking led to 3,500 deaths, 2 million nonfatal injuries, 1,200 cases of fetal alcohol syndrome, and 57,000 cases of treatment for alcohol dependence. Worse yet, underage drinking reaches into the future by impeding normal development and constricting future opportunities. Conservatively estimated, the social cost of underage drinking in the United States in 1996 was $52.8 billion (Pacific Institute for Research and Evaluation, 1999).

For many children, alcohol use begins early, during a critical developmental period: in 2002, 19.6 percent of eighth graders were current users of alcohol (use within the past 30 days), which can be compared with 10.7 percent who smoked cigarettes and 8.3 percent who used marijuana. Among each older age cohort of high school students, the prevalence, frequency, and intensity of drinking increase, contributing to increasing rates of educational failure, injury, and death as children move from grade to grade. By the time young people are seniors in high school, almost three-quarters (71.5 percent) report having drunk in the past year, almost half (48.6 percent) are current drinkers, and more than one-quarter (28.6 percent) report having had five or more drinks in a row in the past 2 weeks (Johnston et al., 2003). Among 18- to 22-year-olds, 41.4 percent of full-time college students and 35.9 percent of other young adults report heavy drinking (Substance Abuse and Mental Health Services Administration, 2002). Heavy childhood and teenage drinking injures the developing brain and otherwise interferes with important developmental tasks. In addition, children and adolescents who begin drinking early are more likely than others to wind up with alcohol problems throughout their adult lives.

The public is certainly aware of these problems, especially drunk driving by teens. However, recent surveys demonstrate that parents underestimate the prevalence and intensity of alcohol use by their own children and by the underage population (see Chapter 6). Moreover, as measured by media attention and government expenditures, public concern about teenage alcohol use has not been remotely commensurate with the magnitude of the problem. A telling measure of the current societal response is the large gap in the federal government's investment in discouraging illicit drug use among teenagers and in discouraging underage drinking, given that the social damage from underage alcohol use far exceeds the harms caused by illicit drug use. In fiscal 2000, the nation spent approximately $1.8 billion on preventing illicit drug use (Office of National Drug Control Policy, 2003), which was 25 times the amount, $71.1 million, targeted at preventing underage alcohol use (U.S. General Accounting Office, 2001). The amount spent on preventing underage drinking also appears to be less than the amount spent on preventing tobacco use: in fiscal 2000, the Office of Smoking and Health, only one of many agencies in the Department of Health and Human Services concerned with smoking prevention, spent approximately $100 million. In addition, the states spent a great deal more, including funds generated by the agreement that settled the states' Medicaid reimbursement suits against the tobacco companies.

There are signs that public attention to underage drinking is increasing and that the public recognizes the need to address the problem more aggressively than has thus far occurred. A recent study on public attitudes toward underage drinking (Wagenaar et al., 2002) shows almost universal recognition of this problem. In fact, 98 percent of adults polled said they were concerned about teen drinking and 66 percent said they were "very concerned." Moreover, a majority of respondents favored strong regulatory actions, such as additional controls on alcohol sales and advertising that would "make it harder for teenagers to get alcoholic beverages." In 1999, Mothers Against Drunk Driving (MADD) added the goal of reducing underage drinking to its mission statement, and its activities and public statements increasingly reflect this focus (e.g., Mothers Against Drunk Driving, 2002). Underage drinking has also won the attention of the spouses of the nation's governors, many of whom have come together to form the Leadership to Keep Children Alcohol Free, in collaboration with the Robert Wood Johnson Foundation (RWJF) and the National Institute on Alcohol Abuse and Alcoholism (NIAAA, part of the National Institutes of Health). In collaboration with the American Medical Association (AMA), the RWJF has also provided long-term support to 12 community and 10 university-based coalitions with the specific mission of reducing and preventing underage drinking. The AMA has itself also become increasingly active on the issue of underage drinking, calling for tighter regulation of alcohol availability, higher excise taxes, and restrictions on alcohol advertising. Members of the alcohol industry also have continued their efforts to discourage underage drinking through responsible drinking campaigns and approaches such as server, parent, and youth-oriented education and involvement in prevention efforts on college campuses.

Underage drinking has also begun to attract increased government attention in Washington. The U.S. Federal Trade Commission (FTC), at the request of Congress, recently reviewed the alcohol industry's advertising and marketing practices. Its report (U.S. Federal Trade Commission, 1999) called on alcohol companies to move toward the "best practices" in the industry "to reduce underage alcohol ad exposure." In 2003 Congress called on the FTC to revisit its inquiry into alcohol advertising and youth and to investigate if and how the recommendations issued in its 1999 report have been implemented by the alcohol industry. Advocacy groups have also urged Congress to include underage alcohol use in the major media campaign being waged against illegal drug use under the auspices of the Office of National Drug Control Policy.

THE COMMITTEE STUDY

In 2001 Congress responded to the increasing level of public concern about underage alcohol consumption by appropriating funds for a study by The National Academies. Acting through the NIAAA and the Substance

Abuse and Mental Health Services Administration of the U.S. Department of Health and Human Services (HHS), Congress requested[1] The National Academies to undertake an examination of the pertinent literature, to "review existing federal, state, and nongovernmental programs, including media-based programs, designed to change the attitudes and health behaviors of youth," and to "develop a cost effective strategy for reducing and preventing underage drinking." Based on consultations with several of the Academies' standing advisory boards, members of the Academies, and the Academies' governing bodies, the final statement of task directs the committee to examine programs ranging from environmental interventions (e.g., taxation, access restrictions) to programs focusing directly on the attitudes and behavior of young people (see Appendix A for the full statement of task).

In response, the Board on Children, Youth, and Families (BCYF) of the National Research Council and the Institute of Medicine of the National Academies established a committee of 12 members with special expertise in key domains relating to underage drinking. To supplement the expertise of its members, the committee commissioned a set of papers to provide systematic reviews of the scientific literature on determinants of underage drinking and effective ways of reducing it. Topics explored in these papers include the demographics of underage drinking; its economic and social costs; adolescent decision making and risk and protective factors; and the effectiveness of various prevention programs and approaches, including media campaigns, school-based education, pricing, and access. Draft papers were presented at public meetings in October and November 2002 (see Appendixes B and C) and subsequently reviewed and revised.[2]

Numerous programs with the common goal of reducing underage drinking have been implemented at the national, state, and local levels, by governments and nonprofit and grassroots organizations. At the federal level, the Departments of Health and Human Services (HHS), Justice, and Transportation operate several programs that specifically target underage drinking. Seven other federal agencies fund efforts that include underage alcohol use within a broader mandate (U.S. General Accounting Office, 2001). Similarly, numerous state-level agencies administer programs to reduce underage drinking. In most states, the health, human service, transportation, criminal justice, and education departments play some role. State alcohol beverage control bodies also play a role. Many communities, colleges and universities, and grassroots organizations across the country have initiated

---

[1]Department of Labor, Health and Human Services, and Education, and Related Agencies Appropriations Act, 2002, H.R. 3061.
[2]A select compilation of these papers is available as a CD-ROM attached to the inside back cover.

efforts to reduce underage drinking and its associated problems in their communities. The alcohol industry also has implemented a range of efforts with the goal of reducing underage drinking.

The committee reviewed the 2001 report of the General Accounting Office on federal programs. This report focused on federal funding that targets underage drinking or includes underage drinking within a broader mandate. It does not include evidence on the effectiveness of specific programs. For the programs operated by the Departments of Transportation and Justice, the report provides general information on the types of activities funded—traffic safety and enforcement of underage drinking laws, respectively. No information is provided on the HHS-funded programs or activities, the largest overall funder of targeted underage drinking activities (see Chapter 12), probably because the funds generally do not represent a national program but, rather, funding for select state or local programs or research aimed at specific aspects of the problem. Although HHS has funded evaluations of specific state and community-level programs, the committee is not aware of any national-level HHS evaluations, or national evaluations of the Department of Transportation program. Each of the federal agencies have initiatives to highlight promising practices, based on varying levels of evidence. Evaluations of state or local programs that receive federal funding that are available in the literature, are reflected in the papers prepared for the committee's study.

The largest single federal program that targets underage drinking is the Enforcing the Underage Drinking Laws (EUDL) Program, operated by the Department of Justice's Office of Juvenile Justice and Delinquency Prevention (OJJDP). A national evaluation of this program is in its fourth year, with only very preliminary outcomes information now available (see Chapter 9). The training and technical assistance center funded by the EUDL program produces a variety of materials that highlight best practices, many of which were reviewed by the committee.

The committee also reviewed written materials submitted by numerous organizations and individuals and considered both written and oral information presented at a public meeting held on November 21, 2002, by a wide range of organizations and people (see Appendix C). This input highlighted programs or approaches considered effective by diverse communities and provided insights into their attitudes and experiences. The judgments provided through this process regarding effectiveness of particular programs or interventions were primarily subjective or based on informal evaluations.

Industry representatives provided extensive materials that were reviewed by the committee on the multiple activities they fund to reduce underage drinking. Included were descriptive materials such as summaries, brochures, pamphlets, videos, and guidebooks; testimonials from community representatives on the utility of specific activities, and an evaluation of Alcohol 101, an industry-funded college-based intervention (see Chapter 7 for further discussion of these activities).

The committee's basic charge is to provide science-based recommendations about how best to prevent and reduce underage drinking. Based on its expertise, consideration of public input, and review of the available scientific literature, including the papers written for the committee, the committee identified eight categories of programs or interventions and presents the evidence for each in the relevant chapter:

- media campaigns designed to discourage underage drinking directly, to affect the behavior of adults, and to build a broader public awareness of the nature and magnitude of the problem (Chapter 6 for adult-oriented campaigns and Chapter 10 for youth-oriented campaigns);
- measures to curtail or counteract activities by individuals or businesses, including alcohol marketing practices, that tend to encourage or facilitate underage drinking (Chapters 7 and 8);
- measures restricting youth access to alcohol in both commercial and noncommercial settings, together with programs enforcing these laws (Chapter 9);
- measures to reduce alcohol-related social harms by enforcing compliance with underage drinking restrictions, such as zero tolerance laws and other programs to reduce alcohol-related traffic injuries and criminal behavior (Chapter 9);
- educational activities undertaken by schools, colleges and universities, faith-based institutions, healthcare organizations, alcohol companies, parent associations, and other entities designed to discourage underage drinking (Chapter 10);
- community-based initiatives designed to tailor comprehensive approaches to the specific underage drinking problems of local communities (Chapter 11);
- screening, counseling, and treatment programs to assist underage drinkers who have developed alcohol problems (Chapter 11); and
- methods of increasing the price of alcohol to underage purchasers, including increases in excise taxes (Chapter 12).

It is important to recognize that implementation of any national "strategy" will depend on the cooperative actions of thousands of organizations and millions of individuals who have their own ideas about what is likely to be effective and valuable. These organizations include agencies at all levels of government (federal, state, and local) with an interest in underage drinking (e.g., alcoholic beverage control commissions, schools, and agencies responsible for law enforcement, substance abuse prevention, social services, and public health). It also includes all the companies and establishments involved in producing, distributing, and selling alcohol—including distillers, vintners, breweries, package stores, and bars—as well as the advertising agencies that advise companies about how to position their products in different segments of the markets they seek to reach. It includes entertainment companies and other organizations that shape popular culture and affect young people's attitudes about alcohol. A key role in any national response to the problem is played by parents who set models of drinking behavior for their children and who can affect the conditions under which their children have access to alcohol products. Of course, youths themselves make important decisions—not only about their own drinking, but also about how they view the drinking of their friends and peers.

The scope of the current efforts of many national, state, local, and nongovernmental group initiatives to prevent underage drinking or the consequences of drinking, particularly drinking and driving, is impressive. These programs include educational interventions, media campaigns, and activities to support enforcement of minimum drinking age laws. Young people themselves have organized efforts to discourage drinking among their peers. While few of these activities have been evaluated in any formal way, a successful national strategy will require the continued involvement, wisdom, and experience of the range of people and organizations that have been committed to preventing and controlling underage drinking.

A CHALLENGING TASK

The committee was charged with "developing a cost-effective strategy for preventing and reducing underage drinking." As we set about this important task, it soon became evident that preventing and reducing underage alcohol use poses unusual challenges. Four of those challenges are the pervasiveness of drinking in the United States, the need for a broad consensus for a national strategy, ambivalence about goals and means, and commercial factors.

Pervasiveness of Drinking

Alcohol is readily available to adults (those over 21) through a large number of outlets for on-premise or off-premise consumption. About half of U.S. adults currently drink alcohol; among drinkers, the mean number of drinking days per month in 1999 was approximately eight.[3]

---

[3]Based on the committee's analysis of 2000 data from the National Household Survey on Drug Abuse.

Notwithstanding the legal ban, alcohol is also readily available to underage drinkers. In recent surveys of high school students, 94.7 percent of twelfth graders and 67.9 percent of eighth graders reported that alcohol is "fairly" or "very" easy to get (Johnston et al., 2003). Purchase surveys reveal that from 30 to 70 percent of outlets may sell to underage buyers, depending in part on their geographic location (Forster et al., 1994, 1995; Preusser and Williams, 1992; Grube, 1997). Focus groups have also indicated that underage youths typically procure alcohol from commercial sources and adults or at parties where parents and other adults have left the youths unchaperoned (Jones-Webb et al., 1997; Wagenaar et al., 1993). Wagenaar et al. (1996) reported that 46 percent of ninth graders, 60 percent of twelfth graders, and 68 percent of 18- to 20-year-olds obtained alcohol from an adult on their last drinking occasion. Commercial outlets were the second most prevalent alcohol source for youths 18 to 20. For younger adolescents, the primary sources of alcohol are older siblings, friends and acquaintances, adults (through third-party transactions), and at parties (Harrison et al., 2000; Jones-Webb et al., 1997; Schwartz et al., 1998; Wagenaar et al., 1993). National surveys of college student drinking find that a large percentage of college youth report they do not have to pay anything for alcohol, presumably because they are at a party where someone else is supplying the alcohol (Wechsler et al., 2000).

American culture is also replete with messages touting the attractions of alcohol use, which often imply that drinking is acceptable even for people under 21. Recent content analyses of television showed that alcohol use was depicted, typically in a positive light, in more than 70 percent of episodes sampled from prime-time programs shown in 1999 (Christensen et al., 2000), and in more than 90 percent of the 200 most popular movie rentals for 1996-1997 (Roberts et al., 1999b). Roberts et al. (1999b) also found that 17 percent of 1,000 of the most popular songs in 1996-1997 across five genres of music that are popular with youth contained alcohol references, including almost one-half of the rap music recordings. Positive images are also disseminated by the alcohol industry, which spent $1.6 billion on advertising in 2001 and at least twice that amount in other promotional activity. Thus, overall, young people are exposed to a steady stream of images and lyrics presenting alcohol use in an attractive light.

Need for Consensus

An effective strategy to reduce a behavior as pervasive and widely facilitated as underage drinking will depend on a public consensus about both goals and means, which will require an unequivocal commitment from a broad array of public and private institutions. If the nation is to succeed in promoting abstention or reduced consumption by minors in a country that has more than 120 million drinkers, the need to do so has to be understood and embraced by many people in a position to reduce drinking opportunities for minors. An effective strategy will depend on adoption of public policies by authoritative decision makers about how to use tax money and public authority—for example, whether to use federal dollars to fund a national media campaign, how to enforce existing state laws banning sales to underage drinkers, or how local school boards should discipline students who drink. The process of enacting such policies will require some degree of public consensus, but this is only the start.

Ultimately, the effectiveness of government policies will depend on how enthusiastically a great many public and private agencies join in the effort to implement them. If parents, animated by a national media campaign, join local police and school boards in concerted efforts to discourage underage drinking and if alcohol distributors join with regulatory agencies to find means to deny underage drinkers easy access to alcohol, then the impact of government policies will be increased. In short, a public consensus to deal determinedly and effectively with underage drinking is needed not only to generate support for adopting strong policies, but also to make them effective. Conversely, both enactment and implementation will be seriously impeded if the public is divided or ambivalent about the importance of reducing underage drinking.

It is here that the greatest challenge lies. In the nation's diverse society, communities have differing beliefs and sensibilities about the consumption and social meaning of alcohol use in general, as well as about what should be expected and demanded of young people during the transition between childhood and adulthood. These differences contribute to varying beliefs, varying public policies, and varying individual practices regarding underage access to alcohol. Although the vast majority of families would agree that the nation as a whole has a powerful interest in reducing the negative consequences of underage drinking on society and on the youths themselves, individuals, families, groups, and communities all have different views on the wisdom and propriety of various approaches to the problem.

In this respect, surveys that show that certain steps by governments (e.g., increasing alcohol excise taxes or restricting advertising) are widely supported obscures disagreements about whether young people should be severely punished for using alcohol, whether parents should be punished for allowing parties with alcohol for youth in their homes, or whether the legal drinking age should be 21.

Ambivalence About Goals and Means

The problem of mustering a societal consensus to achieve an objective as subtle, complex, and contested as reducing underage drinking can be seen most sharply when one compares underage drinking with illegal drug use and underage smoking. The goal of the nation's policy toward illegal drugs and tobacco—abstention by everyone—is both unambiguous and widely, if not universally, embraced. Thus, the nation aims to discourage and suppress nonmedical use of marijuana, cocaine, and other controlled substances by everyone (whatever their age) through a comprehensive legal regime prohibiting the manufacture, distribution, and possession of these drugs for nonmedical purposes. Even though tobacco products, by contrast, are lawfully available to adults, the nation's clearly expressed goal is to discourage tobacco use by everyone, by preventing initiation and promoting cessation. The messages to young people and adults in these two contexts are identical: indeed, because few people take up smoking as adults, the overall success of the nation's anti-tobacco policy depends substantially on the success of its efforts to prevent initiation among young people.

The task of developing a strategy for preventing and reducing alcohol use among young people, in contrast, faces an uncertain policy goal. A strong cultural, political, economic, and institutional base supports certain forms of drinking in the society. Unlike the goals for illegal drugs and tobacco, the nation does not aim to discourage or eliminate alcohol consumption by adults. It is probably a fair characterization to say that the implicit aims of the nation's current alcohol policy are to discourage excessive or irresponsible consumption that puts others at risk, while being tolerant of moderate consumption (at appropriate places and times) by adults (especially in light of the possible health benefits of moderate use for some populations over 40). For example, as long as others are not endangered or offended, attitudes toward intoxication (per se) vary according to religious beliefs and personal moral standards. In short, current alcohol policy rests on a collective judgment, rooted in the Prohibition experience, that the wisdom and propriety of alcohol use among adults should be left to the diverse moral judgments of the American people. This is not to say that everyone supports this stance of government neutrality. Many public health experts would like to take steps (short of prohibition) to suppress alcohol consumption as a way of reducing alcohol problems, and some conservative religious groups would take a more aggressive public stance against intoxication itself. However, the current stance of tempered neutrality seems to be widely accepted and therefore fairly stable.

In this policy context, the message to young people as well as adults about alcohol use is both subtle and confusing. The message to young people is "wait" or "abstain now," rather than "abstain always," as it is with tobacco and illegal drugs. Unlike the policies for those other products, the ban on underage alcohol use explicitly represents a youth-only rule, and its violation is often viewed as a rite of passage to adulthood. The problem is exacerbated because the age of majority is higher for alcohol than it is for any other right or privilege defined by adulthood (e.g., voting, executing binding contracts). Explaining convincingly—to young people as well as adults—why alcohol use is permissible for 21-year-olds but not for anyone younger is a difficult but essential task for reducing or preventing underage drinking.

There is also confusion about whether messages to young people should emphasize abstention, perhaps drawing together alcohol, tobacco, and illegal drugs, or whether messages should focus on the dangers of intoxication and heavy drinking. Many people believe that abstention messages are more appropriate (and more likely to be effective) for younger teens than for older teens and college students.

This overall debate raises the same question posed by all wait rules: What is the age of demarcation between childhood and adulthood (see, generally, Zimring, 1982; Kett, 1977). The argument has been given a raw edge by the trend, in recent years, to curtail the jurisdiction of juvenile courts and to prescribe severe punishments, including the death penalty, for teenagers who commit crimes (Fagan and Zimring, 2000).

Commercial Factors

Alcohol is a $116 billion-per-year industry in the United States, catering to the tastes and needs of the more than 120 million Americans who drink. All states generate revenue from the sale of alcohol, either through excise taxes or product mark-ups, and 18 states participate in the alcohol market through retail and/or wholesale monopolies over distribution of certain alcoholic beverages. A strategy to suppress underage alcohol use must somehow be implemented in the very midst of a society replete with practices and messages promoting its use, and with a strong sector of deeply vested economic interests and the accompanying political and economic power. A significant level of underage use is inevitable under these circumstances—as an inevitable spillover effect, even if unintended by the industry—no matter what strategy is implemented. Foster et al. (2003) recently estimated that underage drinkers account for 19.7 percent of all drinks consumed and 19.4 percent of the revenues of the alcohol industry (about $22.5 billion). On the basis of the committee's independent calculations, we conclude that youth consumption falls somewhere between 10 and 20 percent of all drinks and accounts for a somewhat lower, although still significant, percentage of total expenditures (see Chapter 2).

Although a similar challenge confronts tobacco control policy makers in the effort to prevent youthful use of tobacco products, the potency and impact of tobacco industry activity are gradually being lessened by the growing consensus that tobacco is a deadly and disapproved product, that the industry has misled its customers for decades, and that aggressive regulation is needed to prevent young people from using tobacco and otherwise to protect the public health. It is generally believed that the tobacco industry has targeted young people to maintain demand for tobacco products as older consumers quit or die, notwithstanding the industry's professed efforts, in the wake of the Master Settlement Agreement, to discourage underage use of their products. In short, public health officials and the major tobacco companies are not on the same side, and "big tobacco" is regarded as the enemy of the public's health.

In contrast, the alcohol industry is diverse and uniformly acknowledges the dangers of underage drinking. Alcohol experts generally assume that the level of adult demand for alcohol products will not be substantially affected, over the long term, by reducing underage consumption—although getting young people to wait will obviously reduce the overall level of consumption. Thus, while the commercial interests of the alcohol industry are not perfectly aligned with the public health, they are not as antagonistic to the public health as the interests of the tobacco industry. In any case, a strategy for preventing and reducing underage drinking will have a much better chance for success if it attracts the active cooperation, and at least the acquiescence, of various segments of the alcohol industry.

The effectiveness of any policy focused explicitly on reducing underage drinking will be limited by the existence of a large legitimate practice of drinking and by the power of a large industry responding to legitimate consumer demand. When alcohol is available in many home liquor cabinets, the success of strategies to discourage young people from buying at package stores will be much different than in a world where relatively few parents have stocks of alcohol. The widespread legal use of alcohol in the society affects not only cultural and individual attitudes toward drinking, but also the extent to which any youth-oriented control regime can be effective in reducing opportunities for youths' access to alcohol and drinking opportunities. One can establish a clear-cut boundary between acceptable drinking and unacceptable drinking at conceptual, policy, and legal levels, but it must be understood not only that different communities will construct that boundary differently as a matter of policy but also that the scope created for legal drinking has a profound, practical effect on the effectiveness of other policy instruments in discouraging unwanted, underage drinking.

In sum, the committee set about its task of developing a strategy for preventing and reducing underage drinking while being fully aware of the complexity of defining the public interest in this area and mindful of the severe constraints within which the strategy must be framed and implemented.

UNDERLYING ASSUMPTIONS

In conducting its work, the committee did not begin with a blank slate. Instead, we were asked to develop a national strategy given the basic framework of the nation's current policy toward underage drinking. That policy aims to delay drinking by young people as long as possible and forbids lawful access to alcohol for people under 21.

Some people argue that the delay strategy is misguided and that the legal drinking age should be lower than 21 (typically 18). According to this view, allowing drinking at younger ages would mitigate youthful desire for alcohol as a "forbidden fruit"; would provide opportunities to "learn" to drink, thereby reducing harms; and would bring the age at which youth are allowed to drink into alignment with the age at which they can join the military, vote, and participate in other aspects of adult life. Whatever the merits of this view, the committee believes that Congress intended us to work within the framework of current law, anchored in the National Minimum Drinking Age Act of 1984, and that reconsideration of the 21-year-old drinking age, and of the premises on which it is predicated, is beyond our mandate. Moreover, as a practical matter, the current policy framework, though disputed by some, rests on a strong scientific foundation, is widely accepted, and is certain to be preserved for the foreseeable future.

Because the current policy framework provides the foundation for the committee's work, and for the strategy recommended in this report, it is useful to summarize it here and to highlight its basic rationale.

Evolution of Current Policy

Until the last decades of the 19th century, society relied largely on nonlegal mechanisms of social control to constrain youthful drinking. However, in the wake of urbanization, immigration, and industrialization, alcohol came under tighter control, including bans against selling it to people under the legal age (Mosher et al., 2002). After the repeal of Prohibition in 1933, it became settled that decisions about alcohol control rested with the states, and the structure of modern alcohol regulation took shape.

Until 1970, the minimum drinking age in most states was 21. Between 1970 and 1976, 21 states reduced the minimum drinking age to 18, and another 8 states reduced it to 19 or 20 (usually as part of a more general statutory reform reducing the age of majority to 18) (Wagenaar, 1981). Proposals to restore a higher age were soon introduced, however, largely because alcohol-related automobile crashes had significantly increased among teenagers and young adults. Of the 29 states that lowered their drinking age, 24 raised the age again between 1976 and 1984. By that time, only three states allowed 18-year-olds to drink all types of alcoholic beverages, while five others (including the District of Columbia) allowed 18-year-olds to drink beer and light wine while setting the age limit for distilled spirits and wine with high alcohol content at 21. Thirteen states set a uniform age of 19, and four others allowed 19-year-olds to drink beer and set the limit at 21 for other alcoholic beverages. Four states set the age at 20 for all alcohol, and the remaining 22 states set a uniform age of 21 (Bonnie, 1985).

In 1984 Congress enacted the National Minimum Drinking Age Act, as recommended by the Presidential Commission on Drunk Driving, using the threat of withholding 10 percent of federal highway funds to induce states to set the minimum drinking age at 21 for all alcoholic beverages. All states eventually complied and have a variety of mechanisms in place to enforce this restriction

The Goal of Delay

The explicit aim of existing policy is to delay underage alcohol use as long as possible and, even if use begins, to reduce its frequency and quantity as much as possible. Most people recognize that drinking itself is not the issue. Rather, the underlying challenge is protecting young people while they are growing up. Children and adolescents need to be protected in the first instance from the immediate harms that can occur when they are drinking. But they also need to be protected from the possibility that they will mortgage their own future prospects by initiating practices that could cause them permanent harm during a critical developmental period and that could lead to patterns of drinking that will worsen as they grow older.

The question is how best to go about that protective task. As indicated, some people argue that the most sensible approach is to permit drinking by young people (at least older teens) rather than trying to suppress it. In their view, a "wait" rule is not the best way to reduce the problems associated with underage drinking—at least in a society in which it is bound to occur with considerable frequency anyway. They would allow youthful drinking and focus on supervision rather than drinking per se (at least for older adolescents). In their view, a "learner's permit" for drinking is preferable to a prohibition that drives underage drinking into the shadows and sacrifices the opportunity for supervision. A learner's permit approach could be implemented in a variety of ways, such as by permitting youth access to only certain kinds of alcohol during the learning period (analogous to a graduated driving license) and by prescribing particular requirements for adult supervision.

If the drinking age were lowered, the critical question is whether the intensity of youthful drinking, and the accompanying problems, would decrease, as contended by proponents of the learner's permit approach.

Admittedly, the current approach may create incentives for heavy unsupervised drinking on the occasions where alcohol is available. However, as discussed in Chapter 9, young people who drink tend to do so heavily even in societies with a learner's permit approach.

In addition, a substantial body of scientific evidence shows that raising the minimum drinking age reduced alcohol-related crashes and fatalities among young people (Cook and Tauchen, 1984; U.S. General Accounting Office, 1987; Wagenaar and Toomey, 2002) as well as deaths from suicide, homicide, and nonvehicle unintentional injuries (Jones et al., 1992; Parker and Rebhun, 1995). Increasing the minimum drinking age to 21 is credited with having saved 18,220 lives on the nation's highways between 1975 and 1998 (National Highway Traffic Safety Administration, 1998). Voas, Tippetts, and Fell (1999), using data from all 50 states and the District of Columbia for 1982 through 1997, concluded that the enactment of the uniform 21-year-old minimum drinking age law was responsible for a 19 percent net decrease in fatal crashes involving young drivers who had been drinking, after controlling for driving exposure, beer consumption, enactment of zero tolerance laws, and other relevant changes in the laws during that time.

These findings reinforce the decision by Congress to act in 1984. In short, current national policy rests on the view, supported by substantial evidence, that delaying drinking reduces problem drinking and its consequences. The nation's legislators and public health leaders have reached the nearly uniform judgment that the benefits of setting it at 21 far exceed the costs of doing so.

The Instrumental Role of the Law

Our earlier comparison among alcohol, tobacco, and illegal drugs raises another important preliminary question—about the role of the law in the prevention of underage drinking. It is possible to imagine an official policy aiming to delay and discourage underage drinking that does not rely in any way on the coercive authority of the state to implement this policy: instead of banning underage access to alcohol by law, society might rely entirely on parenting, education, community expectations, and other mechanisms of social control to suppress youthful drinking and, for older teens, to transmit the desired drinking-related norms and to encourage adults to refrain from supplying youths with alcohol or otherwise facilitating their drinking. Various forms of social disapproval, including social and economic sanctions (e.g., not patronizing stores or bars that serve minors) can be imagined.

In contrast, the United States has decided that there must be laws against supplying alcohol to young people and that it should also be illegal for young people to possess or use alcohol, at least in public. Thus, because the law plays such a central role in the nation's policy toward underage drinking, it is essential to clarify the functions that these laws should reasonably be expected to serve.

At the outset, it should be emphasized that a secular society seeks to delay underage drinking because it is dangerous to youths and others, not because it is inherently evil or wrong. The ban on underage drinking is an age-specific prohibition, implying that the aim is to delay alcohol use, not to condemn it or inoculate against it. For this reason, the prohibition is distinctly instrumental in nature and is not grounded in the moral disapproval that characterizes many legal prohibitions. To use a traditional legal classification, underage drinking is an example of a prohibition that is *malum prohibitum* (wrong because it is prohibited) rather than *malum in se* (wrong in itself). Punishment for an underage drinker, or even for an adult facilitator, is not an expression of public moral condemnation as is, for example, punishment for child sexual abuse or robbery.

Enforcement of prohibitions against immoral behavior serves the twin goals of reducing the harmful behavior and condemning and punishing the perpetrator for the transgression. The prohibition of underage drinking does not aim to serve this second (retributive) objective in any strong sense. Its aim is exclusively instrumental. Consequently, the measure of the prohibition's effectiveness, and of the social policy it implements, has to be whether it reduces or avoids the dangerous consequences associated with youthful drinking.

Law is a blunt instrument. It is not self-executing, and it requires the affirmative support of a substantial proportion of the population and of those who are expected to enforce it. These characteristics of a law are particularly important for instrumental prohibitions, such as the ban against underage drinking, because the level of compliance will depend heavily on the willingness of a large number of individuals to adhere to the law simply because they accept its moral authority to command their obedience. That is, a legal norm of this kind, which affects so many people in so many everyday social and economic contexts, cannot be successfully implemented based on deterrence (the threat of punishment) alone. It must rely heavily on the "declarative" or "expressive" function of the law: by forbidding the conduct, it aims to shape people's beliefs and attitudes about what is acceptable social behavior and thereby to draw on their disposition to obey.

Since the ultimate goal is to protect youths (and others within the zone of danger) from harmful consequences, one might wonder whether it is possible to implement an underage alcohol policy by focusing exclusively on the dangerous behavior rather than the drinking itself. In theory, it might be possible to define the prohibited conduct exclusively in relation to the magnitude of the risk: for example, "don't drive a car after having had alcohol" or "don't give alcohol to a youth who intends to drive a car or is otherwise likely to behave dangerously." However, any such dangerous drinking prohibitions are extremely difficult to implement successfully and would not exert a sufficient deterrent by themselves to prevent the risky behaviors associated with underage alcohol use. As the nation's lawmakers have concluded, only a categorical prohibition of underage access to alcohol has any realistic chance of doing that, especially in a large industrial society in which the risks are pervasive (and magnified by developmental vulnerability) and where young people have large periods of time outside parental supervision and outside the reach of formal social controls. It is also relevant to note that at least one of the risks associated with underage drinking is intrinsic to the drinking itself—the permanent damage of alcohol consumption on the adolescent brain (see Chapter 3).

Given an age-based categorical prohibition aiming to serve exclusively instrumental aims, other policy judgments are needed regarding the scope of the restrictions, the severity of the prescribed sanctions, and the resources and tools that should be used to enforce the law. Banning commercial distribution of alcohol to underage persons is an essential element of the prohibition, but what about noncommercial distribution? Even if noncommercial distribution is banned, what about parental distribution to their own children in their own home? (Many states do not prohibit this distribution.) Is it also necessary to penalize young people who purchase or consume alcohol? Even in their own homes? What enforcement strategies should be used? And how severe should the sanctions be? These issues are addressed in Chapter 9. The answers require careful assessment of the possible benefits (in reducing harms associated with underage drinking) and the costs of any particular strategy. The degree of public support and the difficulty of enforcement bear on both the potential effectiveness and on the possible costs.

A POPULATION PERSPECTIVE

In requesting the National Academies to develop a strategy for reducing and preventing underage drinking, Congress clearly anticipated that we would do so from a public health perspective, reviewing the etiology and consequences of alcohol use by the underage population and assessing the effectiveness of interventions that might be deployed to reduce the prevalence of drinking in this population, particularly the patterns of consumption most clearly associated with alcohol problems. (The outcomes of interest in assessing the effectiveness of interventions are discussed in Chapter 5.) Recognizing that underage drinking substantially increases the short-term risks of death, injury, and other harms, as well as long-term risks of alcoholism and other dysfunction, a population-oriented strategy aims to lower the mean level of risk in the underage population in order "to shift the whole distribution of exposure in a favorable direction," typically by "altering some of society's norms of behavior" (Rose, 1985, p. 371). Accordingly, we emphasize the population-oriented tools of primary prevention, rather than the individually oriented methods of secondary or tertiary prevention. Thus, identification and treatment of youths with drinking problems, or at high risk for developing such problems, and the challenge of instilling habits of responsible drinking as young people mature are addressed only incidentally in this report. These issues are important for improved policy and practice, but they are peripheral to our basic charge— delaying underage drinking and reducing its prevalence.

In developing a strategy to delay and reduce underage drinking, the committee has tried to understand the problem from two angles. First, we looked at the problem from the viewpoint of a young person deciding whether and under what circumstances to use alcohol. Our framework draws on the developing literature regarding adolescent decision making, especially in relation to health and risk behaviors. We pay particular attention to youthful decision-making abilities at various ages in the context of the changing social realities of teenage alcohol use. Some components of a comprehensive strategy must aim to help young people make the right decisions, depending on their age and developmental stage, taking account of the dangers of alcohol use at varying points in development.

It is not enough, however, to try to persuade young people to make the right choices. If the strategy relied exclusively on tools directed at changing the attitudes and behavior of underage youths, it would not have much chance of succeeding. To complement a youth-centered decision-making perspective, the committee also drew on the multidisciplinary perspective used by public policy analysts. This framework combines the disciplines of epidemiology, economics, health communications, law, and other social sciences to envision the array of policy instruments that can be brought to bear on the problem and to assess their probable effectiveness and costs, used alone or in combination.

OVERVIEW OF THE REPORT

Although the committee's recommended strategy responds to a congressional request, the report is intended for a broad audience, including parents, businesses, alcohol companies, educators, state and local policy makers and legislators, healthcare producers and retailers, practitioners, and community organizers. Our work is presented in two parts.

Part I, Chapters 2 through 4, provides important contextual information about underage drinking and its consequences and determinants. Chapter 2 discusses key definitions and presents pertinent demographic and epidemiological data regarding the scope of underage drinking and the characteristics of underage drinkers. It includes data on the prevalence of alcohol use and drinking behavior by gender, race, and ethnicity as well as comparisons of youth and adult drinking patterns. Chapter 3 provides an account of the social consequences and costs of underage drinking.

Chapter 4 offers a context for the underlying reasons, motivations, social influences, and risk factors that influence young people's decisions about drinking. The chapter explores the specific motivations and influences relevant to young people's drinking behavior and attempts to answer why some young people choose to drink and do so intensively while others choose to drink moderately or not at all. The chapter also discusses the social environment in which young people are immersed and the ways that community and social factors affect underage drinking.

Part II, Chapters 5 through 12, presents the committee's recommended strategy to prevent and reduce underage drinking. In each of these chapters, the committee summarizes what is known about the effectiveness of existing programs or interventions in the pertinent domain and presents its conclusions and recommendations. The committee has tried to be realistic in assessing the potential effectiveness of efforts to prevent and reduce underage drinking. The committee assumes that most adults in the United States will continue to use alcohol and that most drinkers will begin their alcohol use sometime before they are 21, despite laws and policies to the contrary. Within that constraint, however, there is substantial room for preventing and reducing underage drinking in the United States, and this part of the report explores various tools that can be used in this effort.

At the heart of the committee's proposed strategy is the effort to foster a collective societal acceptance of responsibility for reducing underage drinking. Although continued efforts to speak directly to young people about the dangers of alcohol use are an important component of the committee's proposed strategy, the committee believes that the highest priority should be given to changing the attitudes and behaviors of adults. Adults often facilitate or enable underage drinking directly by supplying alcohol to young people, by failing to take effective precautions to prevent it, or by sending the message that alcohol use is to be expected. Few programs currently seek to influence parents to alter their behaviors and attitudes toward youth drinking as a way of reducing youth access to alcohol, changing permissive social norms about underage drinking, and galvanizing community action.

In Chapter 5 we explain our interpretation of the committee's charge and some of the key assumptions underlying the strategy, including the criteria for assessing effectiveness and cost. This chapter is the foundation for the rest of the report. In Chapter 6 we discuss development of a national media effort as a major component of a campaign aimed at educating parents and other adults about underage drinking and ways adults can help reduce opportunities for youth drinking. In Chapter 7 we discuss how the alcoholic beverage industry can become a partner in the overall effort by helping to establish and fund an independent nonprofit organization charged with reducing underage drinking and by exercising greater self-restraint in advertising and promotional activity. Our messages to the alcohol industry (and other industries that benefit from a large alcohol market) are clear: Your efforts to satisfy and expand the legitimate adult market for alcohol inevitably spill over to a large underage market. Even if you do not intend to stimulate or satisfy underage demand, you derive financial benefits from it. As a society, we cannot have a substantial impact on underage drinking without your active engagement in this effort. Chapter 8 issues a similar challenge to the entertainment media, urging more attentive self-regulation to reduce exposure of children and adolescents to lyrics and images that portray drinking in an attractive way. The committee believes that market incentives can be used to reward companies, including entertainment media, who take meaningful steps to help reduce underage drinking, and to punish companies that do not. Chapter 9 explores ways to reduce youth access to alcohol through both commercial and noncommercial channels.

Chapter 10 explains why the committee does not recommend a youth-oriented national media campaign at this time, preferring instead a cautious program of research and development. It also addresses educational efforts in schools, colleges, and other settings designed to persuade young people to choose not to drink and to reduce alcohol problems. The chapter also briefly discusses programs for assisting youths with alcohol problems. Chapter 11 reviews the potential advantages of mobilizing communities to implement locally specific efforts to reduce underage drinking.

Chapter 12 identifies several ways in which the federal and state governments can help implement the proposed strategy, including through increases in excise taxes. Regulatory action by the government is not at the center of the committee's proposed strategy. The major priority, in the committee's view, is to galvanize the necessary societal commitment to prevent and reduce underage drinking. Thus, the committee focuses its attention on community action, business responsibility, public-private partnerships, and all the other institutional expressions of a genuine social movement. In this context, government has a supportive, but nonetheless indispensable, role—to provide funding (possibly through increased excise taxes on alcohol) and technical support to strengthen and enforce access restrictions, to keep regulatory pressure on the alcohol industry to act responsibly, and to monitor the effectiveness of the overall strategy.

PART I

UNDERAGE DRINKING IN THE UNITED STATES

2

Characteristics of Underage Drinking

A lcohol is the most commonly used drug among America's youth. More young people drink alcohol than smoke tobacco or use marijuana. And young people who drink tend to drink a lot. They have easy access to alcohol, largely from adults. Yet adults tend to underestimate the prevalence of underage drinking, fail to recognize the full range of negative consequences that can result, and assume that drinking is something that other children, not theirs, do (Institute of Medicine and National Research Council, 2001).

PATTERNS AND TRENDS

Despite minimum legal drinking age laws, actual drinking patterns in the United States suggest that almost all young people use alcohol before they are 21. Those who drink tend to drink much more heavily than adults. Biglan et al. (in press) estimate, based on the National Household Survey on Drug Abuse (NHSDA), that 91 percent of all drinks consumed by teenagers are consumed by those who drink heavily. In addition, the average age of first alcohol use has generally decreased since 1965, indicating that youth are starting to drink at a younger age (Substance Abuse and Mental Health Services Administration, 2003). This early onset and heavy use of alcohol poses serious concerns for healthy, unimpeded development.

According to 2002 Monitoring the Future (MTF) data, almost half (48.6 percent) of twelfth graders reported recent (within the past 30 days) alcohol use. Based on 2001 NHSDA data, more than one in four (28.5

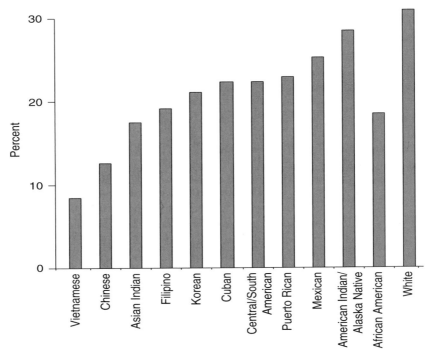

FIGURE 2-1 Past month alcohol use by 12- to 20-year-olds, by race or ethnicity: 1999-2000 annual averages.
SOURCE: NHSDA (2001).

percent) youth aged 12 to 20 have recently used alcohol. When disaggregated by racial and ethnic groups for that age group, whites reported the highest past month use of alcohol (30 percent), followed by American Indians and Alaska natives (28.4 percent), Mexican Americans (25.2 percent), and Puerto Ricans, Central and South Americans, and Cubans (22.9 percent, 22.3 percent, and 22.3 percent, respectively); see Figure 2-1.

Terminology

Multiple data sources—including the NHSDA, (now called the National Survey on Drug Use and Health), the Youth Risk Behavior Survey, and MTF—collect extensive information on the frequency and quantity of alcohol consumed (see Chapter 12 for additional discussion of these surveys). To provide consistency and allow comparisons with adult consumption patterns, the majority of data presented in this report are drawn from the NHSDA.[1] However, no measures of alcohol use or patterns of use have been universally accepted (Flewelling et al., 2004), and no common terminology is used to characterize different patterns of drinking (National Institute on Alcohol Abuse and Alcoholism, 2002). For example, having five or more drinks on the same occasion has been referred to as heavy drinking, heavy episodic drinking, and binge drinking. A report by the Substance Abuse and Mental Health Services Administration (SAMHSA, 2003) using NHSDA data, used binge drinking to refer to five or more drinks on one occasion and heavy drinking to refer to five or more drinks on at least 5 different days in the past 30 days. In the context of college drinking, binge drinking has been commonly used to refer to five or more drinks in a row for men and four or more drinks in a row for women. In other cases, binge drinking is referred to as 5 or more drinks in the last 30 days. Usage of other terms, such as heavy, frequent heavy, or heavy episodic drinking, are similarly inconsistent. For purposes of this report, the committee chose to use the terms "heavy drinking" and "frequent heavy drinking": heavy drinking refers to five or more drinks on the same occasion in the past 30 days; frequent heavy drinking refers to five or more drinks on at least five occasions in the last 30 days.

Long-Term Trends

MTF data, available for 1975-2002, document that the prevalence of drinking among high school seniors peaked in the late 1970s and then decreased throughout the 1980s. Drinking rates have been relatively stable since then, with 30-day prevalence rates hovering at approximately 50 percent throughout the 1990s. The proportion of high school seniors who reported drinking in the last 30 days was the same in 2002 as it was in 1993 (48.6 percent). The proportion of seniors who reported having five or more drinks in that past 2 weeks was higher in 2002 (28.6 percent) than it was in 1993 (27.5 percent). Rates of annual drinking show a similar pattern, but the 2003 rates are slightly lower than they were in 1993; see Figure 2-2. Although there have been modest reductions in the 30-day and annual prevalence rates for the past 5 years, current rates are not significantly different than they were in 1993, and they remain high. Nearly half (48.6

---

[1]Unless cited otherwise, reported NHSDA data are based either on a paper commissioned by the committee (Flewelling et al., 2004) or additional analyses conducted for the committee.

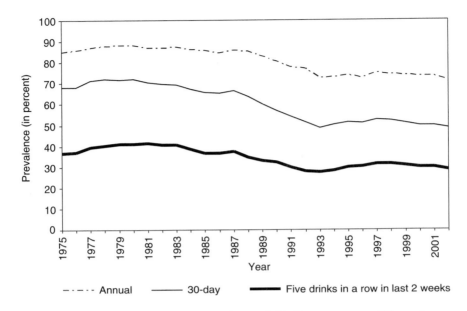

FIGURE 2-2 Long-term trends in prevalence of drinking among twelfth graders.
SOURCE: Data from the MTF online data tables.

percent) of high school seniors report drinking in the last 30 days—significantly more than the proportion of youth that report either using marijuana
(21.5 percent) or smoking (26.7 percent) in the last 30 days.

NHSDA data indicate that the average age of self-reported first use of
alcohol among individuals of all ages reporting any alcohol use decreased
from 17.6 years to 15.9 years between 1965 and 1999. Recent studies also
suggest that gender and some racial and ethnic differences are diminishing
and that these groups with historically low drinking rates are moving toward the higher rates of non-Hispanic white males. Finally, while college
surveys have indicated a decrease in overall drinking on college campuses
over the past decade, there has been little change in heavy drinking
(Wechsler et al., 2002a).

Overall Patterns

In 2000, about 9.7 million young people aged 12 to 20 had used
alcohol in the past 30 days. Of these recent users, almost 6.6 million were
heavy drinkers, and about 2.1 million were frequent heavy drinkers

(SAMHSA, 2003). Non-Hispanic white youth consistently report the highest prevalence of all types of drinking.

As shown in Table 2-1, underage drinkers of all ages are much more likely to drink heavily than are adults. Although drinking is very uncommon among 12- to 14-year-olds, even those in this group who drink are more likely to engage in heavy drinking than adults. With increasing age, more youth drink and more drinkers are heavy drinkers. By the ages of 18 to 20, the rate of any alcohol use in the last 30 days is identical with the rate for adults over 26, but among those who drink, the proportion of 18- to 20-year-olds who drink heavily is significantly higher than that of adults over 26. Rates of both any drinking and heavy drinking peak between ages 21 and 25, shortly after drinking has become legal.

Different patterns of adolescent alcohol use have been identified. Schulenberg and his colleagues used ten cohorts from the MTF study to identify six different trajectories for frequent drinking during late adolescence (Schulenberg et al., 1996). These included "chronic drinkers," who drank heavily in high school and continued this pattern into young adulthood (12 percent of males and 3 percent of females); the "decreased" group, who drank heavily in high school, but reduced their amount of heavy drinking as they moved into adulthood (14 percent of males and 7 percent of females); the "fling" group, who had a low rate of heavy drinking in high school, a substantial increase between the ages of 21 and 22, and a low frequency by age 23 to 34 (9 percent of males and 10 percent of females); the "rare" group, who maintained a low level of heavy drinking in

TABLE 2-1 Drinking Patterns Among Adults and Youths (in percent)

Drinking Pattern	Age				
	12-14	15-17	18-20	21-25	26+
Nondrinkers	93	74	51	38	51
Drinkers					
Alcohol use but no heavy drinking in past 30 days	51	32	29	36	61
Heavy drinking in past 30 days	42	49	45	44	29
Frequent heavy drinking in past 30 days	8	19	26	21	10

SOURCE: Data from the 2000 NHSDA.

high school and in young adulthood (15 percent of males and 18 percent of females); and the group who reported never drinking alcohol (24 percent of males and 45 percent of females). These data suggest that not all adolescents drink and that many who do drink in high school or college choose to drink less as they enter young adulthood, suggesting that both developmental and contextual factors contribute to alcohol consumption during adolescence.

Drinking Initiation

According to the most recent year that public NHSDA data on this topic are available, the average age of first use of alcohol among individuals of all ages reporting any alcohol use, based on the respondents' recall of this information, has decreased from 17.6 years in 1965 to 15.9 years in 1999 (SAMHSA 2003).[2] For 12- to 20-year-olds only, the average age of first use in 2000 is even younger—14 (Foster et al., 2003). According to Youth Risk Behavior Surveillance, United States, 2001 (Grunbaum et al., 2002), 33.7 percent of Latino youth were more likely to report drinking before age 13 than their white (28.4 percent) and African American (28.2 percent) counterparts; see Figure 2-3.

As discussed in Chapter 3, early onset is associated with a number of problematic consequences. For instance, individuals who begin drinking before the age of 15 are more likely to have substance abuse problems in their lifetimes, to engage in risky sexual behavior, and to suffer other negative consequences in comparison with those who begin drinking at a later age. However, we recognize that age of "first drink" may not be a good measure of age of onset of drinking.

How Youth Drink

Looking at data for youths, rather than just those who are drinkers, reveals similar patterns to those discussed above (see Figure 2-4): any recent use and heavy use progressively increases as youths approach the legal drinking age. Figure 2-4 also shows steady increases in frequent heavy drinking from ages 12 to 20.

Over 40 percent of 18-year-olds and a majority (56 percent) of 20-year-olds report having recently drunk alcohol. Although overall alcohol use is low for the youngest age group, almost one-half of the 12-year-olds who reported alcohol use reported having drunk heavily in the past 30 days. The

---

[2]"Age of first use" refers to the age respondents report having consumed at least one drink (e.g., a bottle of beer, glass of wine, shot glass of liquor, or a mixed drink), not having had "a sip or two from a drink."

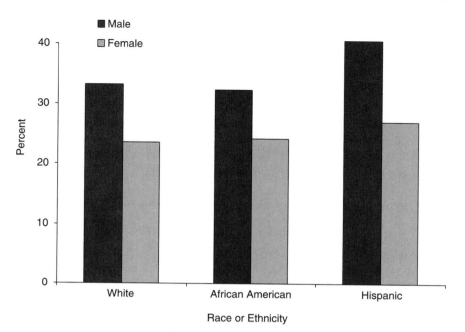

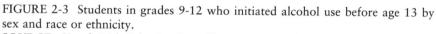

FIGURE 2-3 Students in grades 9-12 who initiated alcohol use before age 13 by sex and race or ethnicity.
SOURCE: Youth Risk Behavior Surveillance (2001, Table 26).

rate of heavy drinking doubles from age 14 (about 6 percent) to age 15 (about 12 percent) and continues to increase steadily. By age 18, more than 30 percent report heavy drinking, and at age 20 nearly 40 percent report heavy drinking. By ages 19 and 20 a full 70 percent of recent alcohol users engaged in heavy drinking.

Frequent heavy drinking also steadily increases for each age between 12 and 20. More than 10 percent of 18-year-olds and nearly 15 percent of 20-year-olds report frequent heavy drinking (Flewelling et al., 2004). When reported by race or ethnicity, white youths aged 12-20 have the highest reported rates of heavy drinking (21.4 percent), followed by American Indians and Alaska Natives (20.3 percent), Latinos (17.2 percent), African Americans (10.3 percent), and Asian Americans (7.9 percent) (SAMHSA, 2002). Data from MTF show somewhat different prevalence rates, but a similar pattern (see Table 2-2). Drinking prevalence increases as youth age, for lifetime use, use in the last 30 days, and five or more drinks in the past 2 weeks. As mentioned above, though MTF reports multiyear decreases in underage drinking (see Table 2-3) the rates remain disturbingly high. For

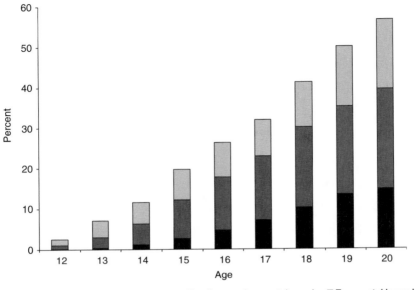

FIGURE 2-4 Prevalence of any use, heavy use, and frequent, heavy use of alcohol in the past 30 days, for youths aged 12 to 20, 2000.
SOURCE: Flewelling et al. (2004, Fig. 1).

example, despite continual decreases between 1996 and 2002 in lifetime use among junior high students (eighth graders), nearly one-half (47 percent) still report drinking in their lifetimes. Similarly, while the proportion of high school seniors who report having had five or more drinks in the past 2 weeks has decreased every year since 1998, nearly 30 percent (28.6) still report such use.

As drinking becomes legal, with the exception of 21- to 25-year-olds, the rate of heavy drinking and frequent, heavy drinking decreases substantially with increasing age (see Figure 2-5). In contrast, alcohol use that is not heavy (i.e., having fewer than five drinks on one occasion) increases and remains higher than that of underage drinkers until the age of 55. After their early 20s, adults begin to drink in a far more moderate manner than underage drinkers (SAMHSA, 2003).

TABLE 2-2 Drinking Prevalence Among Eighth, Tenth, and Twelfth
Graders (in percent)

Prevalence	8th Graders	10th Graders	12th Graders
Lifetime	47.0	66.9	78.4
Last 30 days	19.6	35.4	48.6
Heavy Drinking*	12.4	22.4	28.6

*Defined as five or more drinks in a row in the previous 2 weeks.
SOURCE: Data from Johnston et al. (2003).

Overall Drinking Frequency

Although underage drinkers tend to consume alcohol more heavily than the majority of adults, they drink less frequently: 12- to 20-year-olds averaged about 6 drinking days per month, compared with slightly more than 8 days for adults (see Table 2-4). However, while adults drank less than three drinks in a day, young people reported that when they drink, they "usually" consume about four-and-a-half drinks. Again, the evidence shows that adults tend to drink fewer drinks per occasion than young people.

To examine differences more closely, the committee analyzed the same data by the number of days that current drinkers reported drinking heavily in the past month for different age groups (see Table 2-5). This more detailed analysis confirms the similar findings discussed above that drinking patterns for underage drinkers are notably different than those for the adult population. The number of drinks usually consumed on a single occasion is higher for 15- to 20-year-olds than for 21- to 25-year-olds, and is nearly double that of drinkers aged 26 and older. Underage drinkers do have far fewer drinking days than those aged 26 and older: 15- to 17-year-olds have 61 percent as many drinking days, and 18- to 20-year-olds have 80 percent as many drinking days as adults older than 26.

College Drinking Patterns

Much attention has been devoted to drinking on college campuses. A recent report from the National Institute on Alcohol Abuse and Alcoholism (NIAAA, 2002) cited data that about four in five college students drink and that, among these drinkers, about half engage in heavy drinking. A recent

TABLE 2-3 Prevalence Rates for Eighth, Tenth, and Twelfth Graders:
1993-2002 (in percent)

	1993	1994	1995	1996
Lifetime				
8th Grade	55.7	_55.8_	54.5	_55.3_
10th Grade	71.6	71.1	70.5	_71.8_
12th Grade	80.0	_80.4_	_80.7_	79.2
Annual				
8th Grade	45.4	46.8	45.3	46.5
10th Grade	63.4	63.9	63.5	65.0
12th Grade	72.7	_73.0_	_73.7_	72.5
Last 30 Days				
8th Grade	24.3	_25.5_	24.6	_26.2_
10th Grade	38.2	_39.2_	38.8	_40.4_
12th Grade	48.6	_50.1_	_51.3_	50.8
Five or More Drinks in a Row in the Previous 2 Weeks				
8th Grade	13.5	_14.5_	_14.5_	_15.6_
10th Grade	23.0	_23.6_	_24.0_	_24.8_
12th Grade	27.5	_28.2_	29.8	_30.2_

NOTE: Underline indicates an increase from the previous year.
SOURCE: Data from Johnston et al. (2003).

Harvard School of Public Health survey (Wechsler et al., 2002b) indicated
that while the percentage of abstainers increased between 1993 and 2001,
both frequent heavy drinking (defined as three or more times in the past
two weeks) and drinking to intoxication also increased. Trends in college
drinking over the last decade have found that the rate of self-reported heavy
drinking has remained at approximately 44 percent (Wechsler et al., 2002a).
Nearly half (48 percent) of all the alcohol consumed by students attending
4-year colleges is consumed by underage students (Wechsler et al., 2002b).

Multiple studies have indicated that the most likely individuals to report participation in heavy drinking are white, male, fraternity members,
under the age of 24, involved in athletics, who do not hold strong religious
beliefs and have a tendency to socialize a great deal (for example, cf.
Wechsler et al., 2002a; Kellogg, 1999; Presley et al., 2002). However,
clearly not all students fitting this profile drink, and not all drinkers share
these characteristics.

Alcohol consumption rates increase significantly during the first year of
college: this increased use has been attributed by some to adjustment

1997	1998	1999	2000	2001	2002
53.8	52.5	52.1	51.7	50.5	47.0
72.0	69.8	70.6	71.4	70.1	66.9
81.7	81.4	80.0	80.3	79.7	78.4
45.5	43.7	43.5	43.1	41.9	38.7
65.2	62.7	63.7	65.3	63.5	60.0
74.8	74.3	73.8	73.2	73.3	71.5
24.5	23.0	24.0	22.4	21.5	19.6
40.1	38.8	40.0	41.0	39.0	35.4
52.7	52.0	51.0	50.0	49.8	48.6
14.5	13.7	15.2	14.1	13.2	12.4
25.1	24.3	25.6	26.2	24.9	22.4
31.3	31.5	30.8	30.0	29.7	28.6

experiences that adolescents report during that first year (Kenny and Donaldson, 1991; Rice, 1992; Brooks and DuBois, 1995). The first 6 weeks of the school year have been cited as the most dangerous with respect to drinking behavior due to the increased stress levels associated with a new environment and the pressure to be accepted by a peer group (Prendergast, 1994; Werch et al., 2000; Carlson et al., 2001).

According to data from the 2000 NHSDA, 41 percent of full-time college students aged 18 to 22 engaged in heavy drinking, compared with 36 percent of young adults who were attending college part time or not at all (see Table 2-6). This difference in drinking behavior by college enroll-ment status was greatest among 19- and 20-year-olds. The highest rates of heavy drinking occurred for both groups at age 21, and the gap between full-time students and other young adults began to close. By age 22, the percentage of heavy drinkers subsided for both groups, although full-time college students still engaged in this behavior more often than other young adults.

There is, however, some evidence to suggest that the key variable may

46

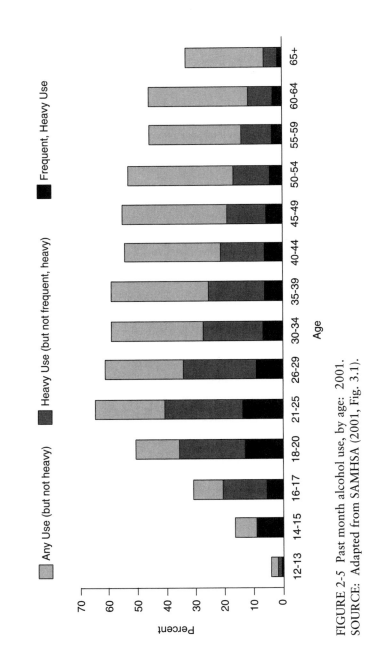

FIGURE 2-5 Past month alcohol use, by age: 2001.
SOURCE: Adapted from SAMHSA (2001, Fig. 3.1).

TABLE 2-4 Drinking Frequency and Intensity for Youths and Adults (current drinkers only)

Frequency and Intensity	Age	
	12-20	21 and older
Mean number of drinking days per month	5.79 (6.03)	8.02 (8.32)
Mean number of "usual" drinks on a drinking day*	4.48 (2.75)	2.78 (2.07)

*If respondents indicated that their usual number of drinks per occasion was some number greater than 12, that response was recoded as "missing." Missing values were imputed, using means for the same sex and age group.

NOTE: Standard deviations in parentheses.

SOURCE: Data from the 2000 NHSDA.

TABLE 2-5 Drinking Patterns for Youth and Adults (current drinkers only)

Drinking Pattern	Age				
	12-14	15-17	18-20	21-25	26+
Mean number of drinking days per month	3.40 (4.12)	4.98 (5.45)	6.54 (6.39)	6.87 (6.59)	8.16 (8.50)
Mean number of "usual" drinks on a drinking day	4.65 (8.09)	6.30 (7.70)	6.47 (8.30)	5.34 (7.71)	3.25 (5.02)
Mean number of days drank heavily per month	1.35 (2.74)	2.69 (4.09)	3.59 (5.11)	3.00 (4.76)	1.68 (4.25)

NOTE: Standard deviations in parentheses.
SOURCE: Data from the 2000 NHSDA.

be type of housing rather than college enrollment. Using data from the National Longitudinal Survey of Youth, Cook and Moore (2001) found that being in school actually reduced drinking and heavy drinking. The group with the highest prevalence of heavy drinking, other things equal,

TABLE 2-6 Past Month Heavy Drinking Among 18- to 22-Year-Olds by College Enrollment Status (in percent)

Age	Full-Time College Students	Other Young Adults	Difference Between Students and Others
18	33.8	29.8	4.0
19	39.1	31.7	9.3
20	42.9	35.6	7.3
21	48.0	43.7	4.3
22	44.8	40.7	4.1
Average, 18-22	41.4	35.9	5.5

SOURCE: Data from SAMHSA (2002).

were those living in a dormitory or fraternity house. Bachman et al. (1997) have found a similar "dormitory effect."

Race and Ethnicity

In general, drinking among racial and ethnic minorities is lower than among whites, and there is a great deal of variability across racial and ethnic groups. Among youths aged 12 to 20, drinking of all types (recent, heavy, frequent heavy) is highest for non-Hispanic whites, followed closely by Native Americans. Asian Americans and African Americans have the lowest prevalence of any racial or ethnic group. Hispanics and youth of multiple races fall about midway between the highest and lowest rates (Flewelling et al., 2004). For the 12- to 20-year-old population as a whole, the prevalence of alcohol use and heavy alcohol use increases among various racial and ethnic groups as they approach the legal drinking age (see Figures 2-6 and 2-7). "Due to sample size limitations, finer breakdowns by age groups and gender within the underage [whites, Hispanics, African Americans] population was only possible for the three major racial/ethnic groups" (Flewelling et al., 2004). This pattern holds for all three age groups and racial and ethnic groups.

Ethnic minorities consistently have lower rates of alcohol use than non-Hispanic whites, although it is unclear whether reporting bias contributes to these differences. Trend analysis of data from the Alcohol Research Group's National Alcohol Surveys showed that while rates of heavy drinking among 18- to 29-year-olds dropped between 1984 and 1995, rates among African American males remained the same (Caetano and Clark, 1998). This suggests the need to further explore explanations for racial and ethnic differences in drinking rates.

Gender

Alcohol use varies by gender as well as ethnicity. In the past, boys have consumed alcohol at notably higher rates than girls (National Center on Addiction and Substance Abuse [CASA], 2003). Unfortunately, this particular gender gap, most notably for younger children, appears to be closing. As of 2000, the prevalence of alcohol use among boys and girls aged 12 to 14 and 15 to 17 were within a few percentage points of each other (see Figure 2-6). Girls aged 12 to 14 in all three racial and ethnic groups, but most notably Hispanic girls, are actually more likely than boys to have used alcohol in the past 30 days—9.8 percent of Hispanic females, 8.3 percent of non-Hispanic white females, and 4.8 percent of African American females (see Figure 2-7). These rates compare with 6.3 percent of Hispanic males, 7.5 percent of non-Hispanic white males, and 4.2 percent of African American males. Clearly, a greater number of girls are initiating alcohol use at a younger age than boys. African American girls aged 15 to 17 also tend to drink more than African American boys of the same age. Among 18- to 20-year-olds, boys drink more than girls across the three racial and ethnic groups. However, the gap between boys and girls in each group is relatively small (see Figures 2-6 and 2-7)—for non-Hispanic whites the difference in any alcohol use in the past 30 days for 18- to 20-year-olds is 5.9 percent, 9.5 percent for Hispanics, and 8.4 percent for African Americans (with the exception of 12- to 14-year-olds). Males do consistently report engaging in heavy drinking at a higher rate than females.

In general, the differences between girls and boys is greater for heavy drinking than for recent use: for example, non-Hispanic white males aged 18 to 20 have a 13 percent higher prevalence for heavy drinking than non-Hispanic white females, compared to a 5.9 difference for any recent use. Similar patterns are observed in Hispanics and African Americans—Hispanic males have a 14.9 percent higher prevalence and African American males have an 8.6 percent higher prevalence for heavy drinking compared to their female counterparts. Males also have a higher prevalence of frequent heavy drinking than females: for example, more than 20 percent of non-Hispanic white males aged 18 to 20 are frequent heavy drinkers, compared with about 10 percent of non-Hispanic white females in this age group (Flewelling et al., 2004).

When considering these differences, however, we should be mindful of the biological differences between women and men that result in women processing alcohol more slowly. From a physiological perspective, five drinks is substantially more alcohol for a young female than a young male (NIAAA, 1990). As a result, women may be drinking somewhat less, but given their size and body weight, still drinking heavily. Acknowledging differences in body composition and alcohol metabolism, recent measures

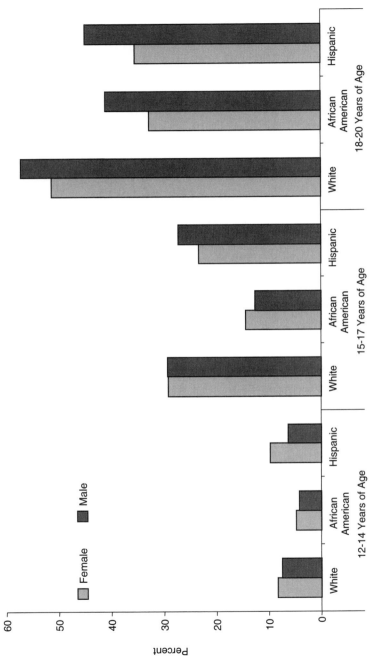

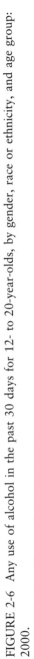

FIGURE 2-6 Any use of alcohol in the past 30 days for 12- to 20-year-olds, by gender, race or ethnicity, and age group: 2000.

SOURCE: Flewelling et al. (2004, Fig. 2).

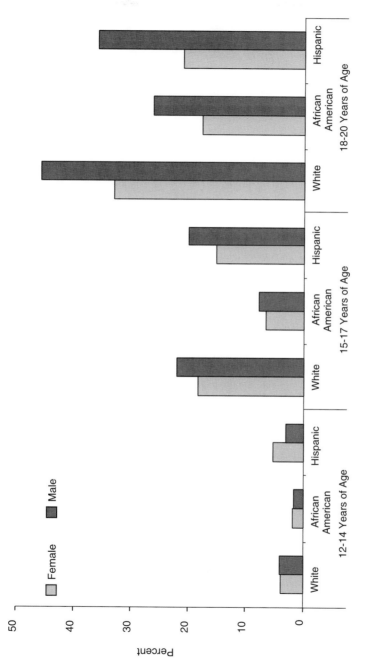

FIGURE 2-7 Heavy use of alcohol in the past 30 days for 12- to 20-year-olds, by gender, race or ethnicity, and age group: 2000.

SOURCE: Flewelling et al. (2004, Fig. 3).

of heavy drinking on college campuses modify the definition for women to four rather than five drinks in a row. Recent studies using this modified measure have reported increased rates of heavy drinking among women on college campuses; this may suggest that gender differences in heavy drinking are also beginning to erode (Wechsler et al., 2002).

Summary

Several generalizations about underage drinking emerge from these data. Substantial numbers of 12- to 14-year-olds are using alcohol, and more girls than boys are having their first drink at this age. When adolescents and young adults do drink, they generally do not drink often as adults, but they drink more heavily. Variation in prevalence and drinking patterns are found by ethnicity and gender: racial and ethnic minorities tend to have a lower prevalence than non-Hispanic whites, and although the gender gap appears to be eroding, older females (18 to 20 years) tend to have a lower prevalence than males.

While it is encouraging that racial and ethnic minority youth as a whole have lower rates of alcohol use than non-Hispanic white youth, it is notable to mention that alcohol abuse and alcohol-related problems affect these communities to varying degrees. While Asian American youth as a whole tend to have lower rates of alcohol use than other youth, specific subgroups (Koreans, 21.1 percent; Filipinos, 19.1 percent; and Asian Indians, 17.5 percent) report similar rates of past month use as some Latino subgroups (Central or South American, 22.3 percent; Cuban, 22.3 percent) and African American youth (18.5 percent) (NHSDA, 2001). Moreover, for youth aged 12 to 17, nearly one-third of all Filipinos (29.5 percent) and a quarter of all Koreans (24.9 percent) reported alcohol use within the past year (NHSDA, 2001). By ignoring the differences that occur both across and within youth subgroups, misperceptions about alcohol use among certain groups may lead to incorrect views of actual need.

It is also important to consider acculturation experiences as they affect drinking behavior. Research has shown that while newly arrived immigrants have lower rates of alcohol use, consumption and more liberal attitudes toward drinking increase as individuals become more acculturated (NIAAA, 1994; National Women's Health Information Center, 2002). This trend has serious implications for many minority communities as subsequent generations reside in the United States for longer periods of time.

OVERALL CONSUMPTION LEVELS

Efforts to estimate the proportion of alcohol consumed by underage drinkers have been bedeviled by the imprecision of quantity questions in drinking surveys and by concerns about the differing prevalence rates that result from the three major national surveys, with the NHSDA consistently reporting the lowest prevalence. The most recent and prominent effort, by Foster et al. (2003), used the NHSDA data to estimate the number of drinks consumed during the previous 30 days by current drinkers, based on multiplying together answers to questions on the number of drinking days during that period, and on how many drinks the respondent "usually" had on a drinking day.[3] But NHSDA data were *not* used to estimate the participation rates—the proportions of the youth and adult populations that were current drinkers. Instead, the authors chose to use the Youth Risk Behavior Survey (YRBS) of the Centers for Disease Control and Prevention to estimate the proportion of underage individuals (12 to 20) who were current drinkers, and the Behavioral Risk Factor Surveillance Survey to estimate the proportion of adults who were current drinkers. These estimated participation rates were then combined with the NHSDA data on average drinks per current drinker to estimate the total amounts of alcohol consumed by youths and adults. The authors (Foster et al., 2003) calculated that underage individuals consumed 19.7 percent of the total number of drinks consumed in the United States in 1999, amounting to more than 830.6 million drinks per month. It is easy to find fault with the procedure adopted by Foster et al. (2003), but it is nonetheless not clear a priori whether the estimate is high, low, or about right. Three problems may be especially important. First, the *average* number of drinks consumed on drinking occasions is not well captured by the NHSDA item, which asks about the *usual* number of drinks. For example, a respondent who drinks a beer with supper every night and an additional six-pack on Saturday nights will "usually" drink one drink per occasion, but will drink *an average* of two drinks per occasion (14 for the week, divided by 7 days). What is not known is how each respondent interpreted this question and whether he or she then answered one or two drinks or something else. Whether this problem is greater for underage or adult drinkers is not clear, so the possible bias in the Foster et al. estimate could be either positive or negative.

Second, the YBRS does not seem well suited for estimating the participation rate for all youth aged 12 to 20 because the YRBS sampling frame is limited to youth aged 12 to 18 who are in school. Unlike the NHSDA, dropouts and older youths are not included in the YRBS. If the omitted groups have a higher drinking participation rate, as seems reasonable, then

---

[3]Foster et al. (2003) excluded cases that reported 50 or more drinks as the usual number of drinks consumed on days they drank in the last 30 days because the response suggest a misunderstanding of the question. It is not clear to what extent inclusion of these responses in the analysis would have changed the outcomes.

the YRBS estimate will tend to underestimate the youth participation rate, and hence underestimate the bottom line.

Third, since the prevalence rates for NHSDA youth respondents are substantially lower than for YRBS respondents and since NHSDA conducts household-based interviews only when a parent is in the home, Foster et al. (2003, p. 990) assert, reasonably enough, that "the accuracy of the responses may be suspect." In contrast, YRBS is conducted in schools. But if, as also seems reasonable, current drinkers who deny drinking in the NHSDA interview also tend to drink less than average, then these youths will be excluded from the calculation (since they have denied drinking) of the average number of drinks per self-admitted drinker and the average may be too high. (There is no analogous problem with the adult estimates.) The effect would be an overestimate.

Unfortunately, the estimate of the underage share of alcohol consumption is very sensitive to the procedure used. The somewhat elaborate procedure preferred by Foster et al. (2003) produces an estimate of about 20 percent. The more straightforward procedure of using the NHSDA data for estimating not only average quantity of drinks per drinker, but also the participation rates, produces an estimate of 10.8 percent for 2000.[4] Based on their preferred quantity estimates, the researchers then estimate the expenditures made by underage drinkers for beer, spirits, and wine. They conclude that underage drinkers spent $22.5 billion, representing 19.4 percent of total consumer expenditures for alcohol (slightly lower than the proportion of consumption because youths are more likely to consume beer, a lower priced beverage).

The procedure used by Foster et al. (2003) does not account for the differences in the average prices paid by underage youths and adults. It seems likely that youths pay less because they are less likely than adults to buy their drinks at bars or restaurants and because they may drink lower quality beverages. Unfortunately, there are no systematic data on prices paid by age. Given these problems, there is a good deal of uncertainty about the shares of total quantity consumed and total expenditures accounted for by underage drinkers. Is the true share of quantity nearer the 20 percent estimate preferred by Foster et al. based on combining selected statistics from three different surveys, or the 11 percent estimate using only the NHSDA survey data? Is it reasonable to assume (as do Foster et al.) that

---

[4]This estimate is computed under the assumption that respondents who reported that their "usual" number of drinks per occasion was greater than 12 had misunderstood the question. Those and other missing values were recoded with imputed values based on the age and sex of the respondent. Other reasonable assumptions and imputation procedures produce only slight differences in the estimate.

underage drinkers pay the same amount for beer or other beverages as adult drinkers or that youths tend to drink more cheaply? Current data sources do not provide reliable answers to these questions, and there is a wide range of plausible possibilities. The committee concludes that one can only say that underage youths consume in the range of 10 to 20 percent of all drinks and account for a somewhat lower, albeit still substantial, percentage of total expenditures.

CONTEXTS OF UNDERAGE DRINKING

It is apparently not difficult for youth who want to drink to readily obtain alcohol. A majority of high school students, even eighth graders, report that alcohol is "fairly easy" or "very easy" to get, with the proportion increasing from eighth to tenth to twelfth grade. Although the proportion of eighth graders who report that alcohol is fairly easy or very easy to get has decreased over the past decade, it remains more than 60 percent. For twelfth graders, the percentage is more than 90 percent (Johnston et al., 2003).

The alcohol most favored by underage drinkers is beer. Based on 2000 MTF data, high school seniors, more than one-half of males and more than one-third of females drank beer in the past 30 days. Liquor (the term used in MTF) was a close second—41.7 and 30.7 percent of males and females, respectively—with far fewer drinking wine and wine coolers.[5] Among those who reported heavy drinking, a similar pattern is found (see Figure 2-8). However, there are differences by beverage types in the relative proportion of heavy drinkers. Most beer and liquor drinkers also tend to be heavy drinkers, particularly boys. This relationship is much weaker for wine and wine coolers (Flewelling et al., 2004). Although it is reasonable to assume that youth drink beer more often than adults, data comparable to the above are not available for adults.

Young people drink in a variety of locations and situations. Drinking at one's own home, friends' homes, outdoors, and in cars or other vehicles are the most commonly reported drinking contexts for young people. For example, survey data from high school seniors in Minnesota indicate that 38 percent of drinkers reported drinking in their own home, 83 percent drinking at another person's home, 22 percent in a bar or restaurant, 46 percent outdoors, 7 percent at work, and 41 percent in a moving car or vehicle (Lee et al., 1997). Similarly, for 15- to 20-year-old drinkers in a recent survey in

---

[5]It is unclear whether and how youth report drinking newer alcohol products such as "alcopops," which do not neatly translate into the current MTF categories of beer, liquor, wine, and wine coolers.

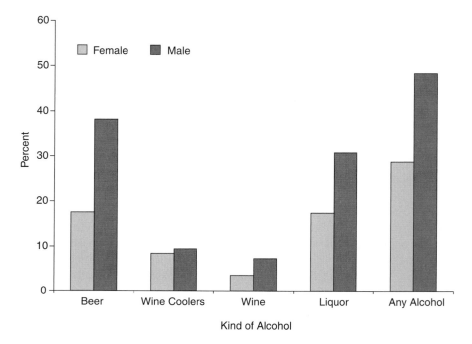

FIGURE 2-8   Kind of alcohol consumed by high school seniors who are heavy drinkers, by gender.
NOTE: Heavy drinkers consumed five or more drinks in a row during the past 2 weeks.
SOURCE: Flewelling et al. (2004, Fig. 5).

California (Table 2-7), parties and outdoor venues were the most frequently reported drinking locations during the past year followed by cars (Walker et al., 2001). In this same survey, drinking in bars and restaurants was rare among younger adolescents, but increased substantially with age. Some studies suggest that drinking in supervised settings (i.e., at home with parent present) decreases with age, while drinking in unsupervised settings (i.e., parties, cars, and outdoors) increases with age (Harford, 1984). For young people, drinking in friends' homes, bars, parties, cars, and parking lots and other outdoor locations is related to higher frequency of intoxication, drinking and driving, and riding with drinking drivers than drinking in the home (Jones-Webb et al., 1997; Lee et al., 1997; Snow and Landrum, 1986; Walker et al., 2001).

TABLE 2-7 Alcohol Consumption by Specific Locations, by Age, in California

Age Group	Location				
	Party	Bar	Restaurant	Outdoors	Car
≤ 15	75.8	9.7	19.4	56.5	38.7
16-17	80.8	17.2	20.2	54.5	32.8
18-20	85.7	45.3	30.1	53.0	31.0

SOURCE: Walker et al. (2001).

3

Consequences of Underage Drinking

U nderage drinking, especially heavy drinking and frequent, heavy drinking, is associated with numerous negative consequences. The consequences of alcohol use can be acute and immediate outcomes of a single episode of alcohol-impaired functioning, such as accidental death and injury, or they can be the accumulated and diverse effects of a chronic pattern of drinking, such as poor school performance and fractured relationships secondary to alcohol abuse and addiction. By ages 19 and 20, 70 percent of all drinkers engage in heavy drinking, suggesting that the majority of young people are at great risk of making poor decisions that have significant long-term consequences (Flewelling et al., 2004). But underage drinkers need not drink heavily to be at high risk of experiencing negative consequences. The crash risk associated with driving after drinking is higher for youths than for adults at all blood alcohol content (BAC) levels (Hingson and Kenkel, 2004). In other words, adolescents and young adults do not need to drink heavily to significantly increase their risk of negative consequences.

This chapter reviews some of the acute and chronic consequences of underage drinking. It covers such problems as drunk driving, as well as a range of other common consequences of acute impairment, such as violence. It also discusses long-term consequences of early drinking, including recent research on the possible effects of early onset of alcohol use on adolescent brain development.

Many adults may assume that the risks and potential consequences of underage drinking are more or less the same as they are for adults, but research suggests that the dangers of youth drinking are magnified. In 2000, 36.6 percent of youths (under age 21) traffic fatalities involved alcohol, a rate slightly lower than the rate for adults (41.7 percent). However, when the denominator is the number of licensed drivers, drinking drivers under age 21 are involved in fatal crashes at twice the rate of adult drivers (National Highway Traffic Safety Administration, 2002a). Moreover, alcohol use among youths is strongly correlated with violence, risky sexual behavior, poor school performance, suicide, and other harmful behaviors (Hingson and Kenkel, 2004). College students are also significantly and negatively affected by their peer's drinking (Wechsler, 1996; Wechsler et al., 2001a, 2001b, 2001c), including being assaulted, having one's property damaged or experiencing an unwanted sexual advance. Recent research also suggests that adolescent drinking can inflict permanent damage on the developing brain (Brown and Tapert, 2004). And as noted in Chapter 2, early onset of alcohol use greatly increases the probability of adult alcohol dependence. In addition to the negative consequences to individual youth who drink, the costs of underage drinking to society—in lost lives, lost productivity, and increased health care costs—are substantial.

CONSEQUENCES OF ACUTE IMPAIRMENT

Alcohol impairs one's decision-making capacity. As a result, young people who drink are more likely to engage in risk-taking behavior that can result in illness, injury, and death. Acute consequences of underage drinking include unintentional death and injury associated with driving or engaging in other risky tasks after drinking, homicide and violence, suicide attempts, sexual assault, risky sexual behavior, and vandalism and property damage. In addition, these consequences appear to be more severe for those who start drinking at a young age. Hingson and Kenkel (2004), report on a series of studies that controlled for history of alcohol dependency, frequency of heavy drinking, years of drinking, age, gender, race or ethnicity, history of cigarette smoking, and illicit drug use. These studies reveal that youth who started drinking before age 15, compared to those who waited until they were 21, were 12 times more likely to be unintentionally injured while under the influence of alcohol, 7 times more likely to be in a motor vehicle crash after drinking, and 10 times more likely to have been in a physical fight after drinking.

Drinking and Driving

The consequences of driving after drinking have received intense media attention and targeted policy responses. Laws have been passed to lower allowable blood alcohol content levels for underage drivers to near zero (typically 0.02, compared with the adult limit of 0.08 or 0.10). Although alcohol-related youth motor vehicle fatalities have decreased substantially over the past decade or so, youth are still overrepresented in alcohol-related fatal crashes compared with the older population. In 2000, 69 percent of youths who died in alcohol-related traffic fatalities involved young drinking drivers. It remains a very serious issue with extreme consequences, not only for the young driver but also for innocent victims. While only 7 percent of licensed drivers in 2000 were aged 15 to 20, they represented approximately 13 percent of drivers involved in fatal crashes who had been drinking (National Highway Traffic Safety Administration, 2002b). According to Grunbaum et al. (2002), 38.3 percent of Latinos, 30.3 percent of whites, and 27.6 percent of African Americans in this age group rode with a driver who had been drinking alcohol. And 14.7 percent of whites, 13.1 percent of Latinos, and 7.7 percent of African Americans aged 15 to 20 admitted to driving a car after drinking alcohol.

Alcohol-related traffic fatalities constituted almost 37 percent of all fatal youth traffic fatalities (National Highway Traffic Safety Administration, 2002b). Youths who drive after drinking are more likely to be in a crash than youths who have not had a drink, and the crashes underage drinkers are involved in tend to be more severe than those of adults, resulting in a greater number of deaths and more serious injury. Underage drinkers present greater risks than adults when driving, even at lower BAC levels. More 19-year-olds died in alcohol-related crashes with relatively low BAC levels than any other age (National Highway Traffic Safety Administration, 2002b).

When young people drink and get into a car, they also tend to make poor decisions that bear on their safety. For example, young people who have been drinking are less likely to wear a safety belt. They are more likely to get in a car with an intoxicated driver: 41 percent of frequent heavy drinkers reported riding with an intoxicated driver, compared with only 14 percent of those who never drank (Hingson and Kenkel, 2004). In alcohol-related traffic crashes, there were three times more deaths among young people who were not wearing their seat belts than among those who were wearing them. In sum, alcohol-related crashes involving underage drinkers are more likely to result in death and serious injury than those involving other drivers.

Homicide, Suicide, and Unintentional Injuries

Alcohol is implicated in a large proportion of unintentional deaths and injuries caused by other forms of dangerous behavior than driving. In 1999, nearly 40 percent of people under age 21 who were victims of drownings, burns, and falls tested positive for alcohol. Youth constituted 7 percent of nonfatal and 30 percent of fatal alcohol-related drownings and burns (Levy et al., 1999).

Drinking not only increases one's risk of being involved in a traffic accident or suffering another unintentional injury, it is also implicated in deaths and injuries associated with violence and suicidal behavior. Frequent heavy alcohol use is associated with increased feelings of hopelessness, suicide ideation, and suicide attempts. Alcohol has been reported to be involved in 36 percent of homicides, 12 percent of male suicides, and 8 percent of female suicides involving people under 21—a total of about 1,500 homicides and 300 suicides in 2000. Homicide is the second leading cause of death for 15- to 24-year-olds (Centers for Disease Control and Prevention, 2001). By racial and ethnic group, deaths due to homicide for ages 15 to 24 are the leading cause of death for African Americans, second for Latinos, and fourth for whites. In that age group, suicide is the second leading cause of death for whites, third for Latinos, and third for African Americans (Anderson, 2002). Caetano and Clark (1998) report that the incidence of social consequences from drinking among Latinas is almost three times higher than for white females, despite generally lower rates of drinking.

According to Levy et al. (1999), individuals under the age of 21 commit 45 percent of rapes, 44 percent of robberies, and 37 percent of other assaults, and it is estimated that 50 percent of violent crime is alcohol-related (Harwood et al., 1998).[1] A report by the National Center on Addiction and Substance Abuse (1994) found that on college campuses 95 percent of all violent crime and 90 percent of college rapes involve the use of alcohol by the assailant, victim, or both. Although it is difficult to disentangle alcohol use from other possible contributing factors, such as depression, emerging evidence demonstrates a causal link between alcohol and suicide (Light et al., 2003).

Sexual Activity

Sexual violence and unplanned and unprotected sexual activity constitute yet another set of alcohol-related problems. As reported in *A Call to Action: Changing the Culture of Drinking at U.S. Colleges* (National

---

[1]Underage drinkers are also more likely than their nondrinking peers to carry a weapon— 44 percent of frequent heavy drinkers had carried a weapon, and 22 percent had carried a gun in the past 30 days, compared with only 10 and 3 percent, respectively, of nondrinkers. Carrying a weapon increases the dangers associated with drinking; not surprisingly, injuries due to a physical fight were more common among frequent heavy drinkers (13 percent) than for nondrinking peers (only about 2 percent).

Institute on Alcohol Abuse and Alcoholism [NIAAA], 2002) more than 70,000 students aged 18 to 24 are victims of alcohol-related sexual assault or date rape. Studies of date rape and sexual assault on college campuses suggest that alcohol use factors into the behavior of both assailants and victims. For example, Harrington and Leitenberg (1994) found that date rape victims who reported being at least "somewhat drunk" at the time of the assault believed that their assailants were also under the influence of alcohol. A study of assailants showed that 44 percent of the men had been drinking when they committed a sexual assault (Abbey et al., 1996). Given that many sexual assaults—especially acquaintance rape—are believed to be unreported, it is possible that alcohol figures into many more assaults than these studies indicate.

In addition to being more vulnerable to experiencing (or committing) sexual assault, young people who are drinking are also more likely to engage in risky sexual behavior. According to research by the Kaiser Family Foundation, young people are more likely to engage in consensual sexual activity after drinking and report that they "do more" sexually while using alcohol than they had planned. According to Strunin and Hingson (1992), 44 percent of sexually active teenagers report that they are more likely to have intercourse if they have been drinking. Based on analysis of 2001 Youth Risk Behavior Surveillance data, Grunbaum and colleagues (2002) report that 23.4 percent of white youth, 24.1 percent of Latino youth, and 17.8 percent of African American youth reported using alcohol or other drugs at the time of their last sexual intercourse.

Young people are less likely to use a condom if they have been drinking, which puts them at risk for unplanned pregnancies and contracting sexually transmitted diseases and HIV (the virus that causes AIDS). More disturbing still is that young people seem to be aware that using alcohol influences their decisions about sexual behavior: 29 percent of 15- to 17-year-olds and 37 percent of 18- to 24-year-olds said that alcohol or drugs influenced their decision to do something sexual. In other words, young people choose to drink even though they realize that alcohol affects their decision making and may cause them to engage in sexual behaviors they would not do while sober.

Early onset of alcohol use has also been associated with unplanned and unprotected sex. A college survey conducted by the Boston University School of Public Health showed that among drinkers, those who had their first drink before the age of 13 were twice as likely to have unplanned sex and more than twice as likely to have unprotected sex (Hingson and Kenkel, 2004).

Vandalism and Property Damage

Vandalism and property damage represent yet another set of consequences influenced by alcohol. Intoxicated youth are more likely to commit these acts regardless of their age, but vandalism and property damage are a particular problem on college campuses. Wechsler et al. (2002) report that about 11 percent of college students admitted to having damaged property while drinking. The cost of these behaviors is picked up by the college or by the local communities if the vandalism happens off campus.

LONG-TERM CONSEQUENCES

A single episode of alcohol-impaired judgment can have immediate consequences (leading to death, injury, or arrest, for example) with long-term effects. In addition, heavy alcohol use at a young age has been implicated in long-term changes in the youths' life prospects. Individuals who begin drinking before age 15 appear to be at greater risk for serious lifelong problems (Hingson and Kenkel, 2004). For example, young people who begin drinking before age 15 are significantly more likely to develop alcohol dependence than those who begin drinking at older ages. Youth who begin drinking before the age of 15 have a 41 percent chance of future alcohol dependence, compared with a 10 percent chance for those who begin after the legal drinking age (Grant and Dawson, 1997). Some become dependent during adolescence.[2] Analyses of the 1999 Harvard School of Public Health National College Alcohol Survey of students age 19 or older, after controlling for a variety of factors, found that the earlier they had first drunk to intoxication, the more likely they were to experience alcohol dependence and frequent heavy drinking in college (Gruber et al., 1996).

Frequent heavy use is associated with low self-esteem, depression (which is probably related to greater suicide attempts among underage drinkers), conduct disorders, antisocial behavior, dependency on other drugs and tobacco, and anxiety (Brown and Tapert, in press). Adolescents and college-age students who use alcohol have higher rates of academic problems and poor performance than nondrinkers. *A Call to Action* (NIAAA, 2002) noted that about 25 percent of college students report that using alcohol resulted in problematic consequences, such as missing classes, falling behind in school work, performing badly on papers and exams, and receiving lower grades overall.

---

[2]Data from the NHSDA show that in 2000, between 4 and 12 percent of young people aged 12 to 20 met alcohol abuse or dependence diagnostic criteria.

Chronic health problems resulting from heavy alcohol use are generally not observed in adolescents because such effects take longer to accumulate. However, heavy drinking during adolescence, especially if this behavior is continued in adulthood, places a person at risk of such health problems as pancreatitis, hepatitis, liver cirrhosis, hypertension, and anemia. Chronic liver disease and cirrhosis among Latinos and American Indian and Alaskan natives are the sixth leading cause of death among these groups (Anderson, 2002). Recent research suggests that drinking during puberty may have deleterious effects on bone density development: for young women, failing to develop maximal bone density during adolescence puts them at risk later in life for osteoporosis.

Effects on the Adolescent Brain

New research on adolescent brain development suggests that early heavy alcohol use may also have negative effects on the actual physical development of brain structure (Brown and Tapert, 2004). Contrary to earlier beliefs, the brain continues to change physiologically well beyond childhood. Brain growth among infants and children is focused essentially on volume—creating as many brain cells with as many connections to other brain cells as possible. During adolescence, development shifts from producing a great number of neurons to creating efficient neural pathways, which occurs in two ways. First, the structure of neurons changes as they become encased by an insulating tissue (myelin) that helps to speed the movement of the electric impulses carried by brain cells. This change means that adults can relay information from one part of the brain to another more rapidly than can children. In adolescence, this myelination occurs predominantly in the frontal and prefrontal lobes, the part of the brain responsible for important functions such as planning, organization, and halting an impulse. The second change in brain development has to do with synaptic refinement, the process by which connections between brain cells are pruned and eliminated so that only the most efficient connections are used and maintained. Like myelination, synaptic refinement also contributes to increasing the speed and efficiency of transmitting information from one part of the brain to another, which in turn improves reaction time. Adolescent brain developments occur in areas of the brain critical for considering the consequences of actions and important for stress responses and managing drives (Spear, 2002).

Recent studies based on animal models suggest that alcohol use during adolescence may have deleterious effects on myelination and synaptic refinement. Rats that were given doses of alcohol in quantities and frequency that mimic the use of frequent heavy adolescent drinkers had problems with memory tasks (White et al., 2000). Another study showed that heavy alcohol use caused damage to the frontal regions of the brain (Crews et al., 2000).

New research using magnetic resonance imaging (MRI) technology to obtain a portrait of adolescent human brains support these animal studies, showing that the brain structure of youths with alcohol-use disorders is adversely affected. The hippocampus, which is responsible for forming new memories, was noticeably smaller in youth who abuse alcohol than in their nondrinking peers (De Bellis et al., 2000). Youth with alcohol-use disorders also performed worse on memory tests than nondrinkers, further suggesting that the structural difference in hippocampus size was affecting brain functioning. Neuropsychological studies also suggest that alcohol use during adolescence may have a direct effect on brain functioning: negative effects included decreased ability in planning and executive functioning, memory, spatial operations, and attention—all of which are important to academic performance and future functioning (Giancola and Mezzich, 2000; Brown et al., 2000; Tapert and Brown, 1999; Tapert et al., 2001).

THE CAUSATION QUESTION

Many consequences—both immediate and long-term—are correlated with youthful drinking. In the case of immediate consequences, drinking impairs one's perceptual and motor skills, and this impairment clearly increases the risk of a car crash if one drives after drinking—a risk that is demonstrably higher for young drivers. Similarly, the disinhibiting effect of alcohol use impairs judgment and increases the risk of violence and unprotected sexual intercourse. In this sense, the causal link between alcohol use and the outcomes and problem behaviors just reviewed is not in doubt. The empirical evidence also shows a clear correlation between early drinking and problematic adult drinking and other related longer term problems: that is, the earlier that young people start drinking, the more likely they are to have problems in their adult lives.

However, these outcomes and behaviors may not be entirely attributable to alcohol. For example, some youths who have alcohol-related crashes or engage in alcohol-related violence or other risk-taking behavior may have been otherwise strongly predisposed to engage in problem behaviors of all sorts due to genetics, family circumstances, or other factors. Similarly, the higher rates of alcohol dependence, disease, and dysfunction among adults who began heavy drinking as youths may not be attributable to the early drinking per se. Some of these long-term outcomes are also consistent with the possibility that some individuals have a particular vulnerability to developing bad drinking habits and that one of the characteristics of these individuals is that they start drinking early. (For example, children of alcoholics are more likely than children of nonalcoholics to start drinking during adolescence [NIAAA, 1997].)

Some of the strongest evidence of the causal role of alcohol in negative outcomes is derived from studies designed to assess the effects of policy interventions targeted on underage alcohol consumption. It is clear from these studies that reducing alcohol consumption among young people reduces such immediate outcomes as deaths, crime, and other consequences of impaired behavior. For example, research has shown that policies that affect alcohol availability, including excise tax rates and the minimum drinking age, have measurable effects on such outcomes as crime, highway fatalities, tobacco and drug use, and sexually transmitted diseases with greater availability associated with increases in these outcomes (Chaloupka, 2004; Chesson et al., 1997; Coate and Grossman, 1988; Cook, 1981; Cook and Moore, 1993a, 1993b; Cook and Tauchen, 1982, 1984; Kenkel, 2000; Ohsfeldt and Morrisey, 1997; Pacula, 1998; Ruhm, 1996; Saffer and Grossman, 1987; Wagenaar and Toomey, 2002). Given that the only plausible mechanisms by which such policies could affect these outcomes are through their effects on the volume and patterns of alcohol consumption, it is logical to conclude that alcohol consumption is indeed a causal agent for these outcomes.

In the case of long-term negative outcomes, the key question is whether reducing underage drinking would also reduce those outcomes. To the extent that individual vulnerability plays a large role, merely delaying the onset of drinking would not necessarily have much of an effect; the vulnerable people would eventually end up as problematic drinkers regardless of when they started. Moreover, many underage individuals who start heavy drinking in their late teens give it up as they reach their late 20s and 30s. The committee has carefully considered the evidence on this important issue—the extent to which early drinking causes later drinking problems, reduces them, or has no effect at all. Clearly predisposition and early alcohol use interact, and the effect of alcohol varies according to the degree of vulnerability of different individuals. However, notwithstanding the complexity of the inquiry, the committee concludes that the evidence establishes a prima facie case regarding the negative effects of early drinking on long-term welfare.

We think that prudent parents and a prudent society should assume, based on the current evidence, that underage drinking increases the risk of future drinking problems and contributes independently to the many deficits experienced by early drinkers over the course of their lives. However, additional research to further refine understanding of the interaction of the multiple interrelated factors on long-term outcomes is warranted.

SOCIAL COSTS

It has become standard practice in formal assessments of the social burden of an illness or harmful activity to translate the resulting disability and death into dollar figures. Underage drinking is no exception. For example, a recent report concluded that the cost of alcohol use by youth was $53 billion in 1996, including $19 billion from traffic crashes and $29 billion from violent crime (Pacific Institute for Research and Evaluation [PIRE]). If the costs of other consequences—such as low academic performance or medical costs other than those associated with traffic crashes—were quantified, it is possible that the cost would be even higher. Since numbers of this sort are potentially important in setting public priorities, it is worth understanding some of the controversies and practical difficulties in making such estimates (see Chapter 4; Cook and Ludwig, 2000; Cook, 1991).

Policy Relevance

It is natural to measure the burden of underage drinking in terms of the incidence of various consequences. As we have seen, those consequences include violent death, disability, disease, reduced academic and occupational achievement, and property damage, among many others. Estimating the causal role that underage drinking plays in each of these outcomes is the very big and difficult challenge for epidemiologists. But even with reliable estimates for the contribution of underage drinking for each consequence, one would be left with the question of how to sum them up. A summary statistic is useful in assigning relative priority to this particular problem in comparison with all the other problems requiring public attention. A summary statistic quoted in dollar terms is particularly useful because it lends itself to comparison with the budget costs of policies to remediate the problem.

What question is to be answered by the estimate of social cost? Ultimately the question is something like the following: *"How much would Americans' overall standard of living improve if underage drinking were somehow eliminated?"* In the PIRE study (1999) it is noted that the "cost" of underage drinking, based on the given assumptions, equaled $530 per year for every household in the United States; the suggestion is that eliminating underage drinking would be the equivalent of adding that amount to average household income.

Of course in practice there is no way to entirely eliminate underage drinking. But the total cost is nonetheless of some interest as a guide to how underage drinking can be compared with, say, cancer or illiteracy or terrorism in setting national priorities. The total is also useful to the extent that a partial reduction in underage drinking may confer benefit in proportion to the total. Thus, the study suggests that a 10 percent reduction would be worth about $53 per household, or 10 percent of the total cost per household. Of course, a complete analysis would require an assessment of the costs of achieving the reduction as well as the benefit; if the 10 percent reduction is achieved through a set of programs that cost $10 billion, then the net gain per household would be just $43.

An Accounting Framework

There are two problems in doing this sort of accounting exercise well. First is the epidemiologist's problem of discerning the actual consequences of eliminating (or reducing) underage drinking. What reduction would there be in highway crashes, crime, and school dropouts and in all the long-term effects of these events? All such consequences are the result of complex multicausal processes; knowing that there is alcohol involvement in some percentage of such cases leaves one far short of knowing the causal importance of drinking. A further complication is introduced by the realization that the actual effects of a reduction in underage drinking will depend not just on how much of a reduction is accomplished, but also on what sort of collateral consequences will occur. What effect will that intervention have on routine activities, such as weekend driving with friends, the use of other illicit drugs, or dating? The answers may be important in influencing the net consequences, which may well depend on the nature of an intervention to prevent or reduce underage drinking.

The second problem is to develop and implement a sound accounting system for translating outcomes into a measure of social burden. The choice of accounting rules in this context necessarily reflects decisions about deep issues in understanding the public good. Two specific issues are particularly thorny: whose preference should count in defining relevant consequences? Should the social cost computation include subjective losses or only production losses?

The presumption in our society is that the public good is the sum of individual preferences. A reasonable exception may be the preferences of teenagers, who tend to place too little emphasis on their long-term well-being and too much emphasis on pleasing their peers. That commonsense view of adolescent human nature, coupled with the fact that underage drinking is illegal, provides some justification for ignoring the pleasures of drinking as perceived by teens and accounting only for the harmful consequences.

Although few people think that the value of the life of someone killed or permanently disabled by a drunken teenager is limited to his or her lost earnings, that in fact has been the accounting rule used in the traditional "cost of illness" method of accounting. That method stipulates that the social cost of a harmful activity or illness is the sum of direct costs (property damage, medical costs, and so forth) and indirect costs (lost productivity). Lost productivity has little relationship to the value that individuals and those who care about them place on the value of health and continued life.

A comprehensive accounting framework, then, should take account of both tangible and intangible costs associated with the consequences of underage drinking. The PIRE analysis cited above does just that. Of the $53 billion in costs estimated for 1996, all but $4 billion is the result of lost quality and quantity of life.[3]

While this report is not the place to explain the methods used to arrive at this result, we note that it is based on the underlying principle that (adult) preferences should guide the valuation. Those preferences are observed in a generic sense in a variety of settings and choices, where people make risky decisions. For example, wages for risky jobs tend to be higher than safe jobs requiring comparable skill and effort: the "risk premium" reflects the amount that workers must be compensated to take on additional risk, and thereby form a useful basis for assessing the average "value of life." Note that what is being valued is not literally life itself, but rather a slight reduction in the probability of continued life. This valuation of small changes in safety is relevant for a forward-looking assessment. In assessing a proposed policy to reduce underage drinking, one does not know the identity of which lives will be saved; rather, the prospective accomplishment is a general reduction in risk for all, and that is what is to be valued.

The PIRE study is somewhat incomplete. For example, the study's estimate does not include medical costs other than those associated with traffic crashes (Hingson and Kenkel, 2004). Perhaps most important is that it neglects the possibility that drinking by teens may cause mild brain damage and lead to impaired academic performance and early termination of schooling. It also takes no account of the possibility that underage drinking engenders a greater likelihood of subsequent problems with alcohol dependence and abuse. In these respects the $53 billion appears to be an underestimate of the social costs of underage drinking.

In sum, the cost of underage drinking to society is substantial. Society is affected by loss of young lives, lost productivity and significant health care costs and stands to gain from reductions in underage drinking. The committee concludes that the PIRE estimate of $53 billion, while perhaps somewhat low, is a reasonable starting point for assessing social costs.

---

[3]The study reports separately the value of lost productivity ($11 billion) and of additional losses in quality and quantity of life ($38.5 billion). The reason for making this distinction is apparently a belief that some of the audience for the report expect to see the productivity measure as a separate statistic.

4

Understanding Youth Drinking

Adolescents in the United States grow up in a world filled with messages about alcohol (see Box 4-1 for select vignettes). Most of the messages present drinking in a positive light, and most of them show alcohol as a normal part of adult and teen social life. Warnings against underage drinking from parents or in health class may well be drowned out by the barrage of daily messages about alcohol in daily life.

Given this backdrop, it is not surprising that experimental or occasional use of alcohol is reported by the majority of adolescents in the United States, making it a normative behavior during the second decade of life. As noted in Chapter 2, about 50 percent of 20-year-olds report having recently drunk alcohol and the majority of twelfth graders (78 percent) report having drunk alcohol in their lifetimes. In this chapter we examine factors—primarily developmental and environmental factors—that are related to normative alcohol consumption. We do not discuss those involved in excessive or atypical use (e.g., youths with mental or addictive disorders). This is an important distinction because the factors that contribute to drinking patterns within the normative group of adolescents are different than those for youth who develop alcohol abuse patterns or dependency at a young age.

WHY DO ADOLESCENTS SAY THEY DRINK?

Adolescents say they drink for many of the same reasons as adults (Dunn and Goldman, 1996). Alcohol-related expectancies are well formed

---

BOX 4-1
Select Vignettes of Alcohol Messages to Youth

Twelve-year-old Jenna rides her bike to and from school most days. Her route takes her past a large billboard advertising a popular malt liquor.

Fourteen-year-old Joshua loves to watch basketball on television. During a typical game, he sees many beer commercials.

At 15, Sarah enjoys going to movies with friends. Many of the movies she has seen lately include scenes of adults drinking alcohol with dinner and at parties. A recent favorite showed teenagers getting into a nightclub using fake identification.

A favorite T-shirt for 16-year-old Sam says, "I'm trying to graduate with a 4.0 . . . blood alcohol level." His best friend's favorite sports shirt has an advertisement for a local bar on the back and "start drinking at 9 a.m. . . . it's gotta be happy hour somewhere" on the front.

Following the homecoming dance, 17-year-old Lynne attends an all-night party at a friend's home. The parents greet the guests as they arrive and take their car keys because they are serving beer. They prefer that their children and their friends drink at their home in a "safe environment" since they assume that their children will be drinking anyway.

After moving his belongings into his college dormitory and bidding his parents farewell, 19-year-old Jeremy attends an off-campus "welcome party" with a new acquaintance. He learns a lot on his first night on campus—how to play a drinking game, where to get a fake ID (identification), and which bars have happy hours on Thursdays.

---

by age 12, among drinkers as well as among those who have never consumed alcohol (Christiansen et al., 1982; Jones et al., 2001). Although it is always difficult to know if individuals can accurately report the reasons for their behavior, including drinking (see Nisbett and Wilson, 1977), both adolescents and adults indicate that alcohol is an important ingredient in social interactions, allowing them to lower their inhibitions and feel more relaxed in social situations (Jones et al., 2001; Wood et al., 1992). Other reasons given for drinking include reducing tension, fostering courage, reducing worry, increasing a sense of power, and causing cognitive and behavioral impairment (Prendergast, 1994). In addition, most individuals assign some costs to drinking, as well, which are discussed later in this chapter.

According to models such as the theory of planned behavior (Ajzen, 1991), social cognitive theory (e.g., Bandura, 1986), and alcohol expectancy theory (e.g., Goldman et al., 1991; Leigh, 1989), alcohol use can be largely explained by the alcohol-related expectancies for both positive and negative outcomes. Initiation and continuation of drinking, as well as the onset of problem drinking, are strongly and positively associated with expected benefits of drinking and negatively related to perceived negative expectancies (Christiansen et al., 1989; Christiansen et al., 1982; Chen et al., 1994; Grube et al., 1995; Jones et al., 2001; Smith et al., 1995; Wood et al., 1992; Goldberg et al., 2002).

Although children's and adult's alcohol expectancies are similar (Dunn and Goldman, 1996), younger children are more likely to report negative expectancies; perceptions of positive outcomes increase with age (Miller et al., 1990; Goldberg et al., 2002). Specific expectancies also differ by age: 12- to 14-year-olds rank reduced tension and impaired behavioral functioning highest; 15- to 16-year-olds cite enhanced social and physical pleasure and modified social and emotional behavior; and 17- to 19-year-olds cite enhanced sexual performance and increased power as top alcohol expectancies (Christiansen et al., 1982). There are also gender differences in alcohol expectations, with adolescent males perceiving more positive and fewer negative consequences of alcohol than do adolescent females. Although the relationship between quantity of alcohol use and social and physical outcomes was similar for adolescent males and females, the frequency of alcohol use may be associated with global positive effects, sexual enhancement, and pleasure for men, but reduced tension for women (Jones et al., 2001).

DEVELOPMENTAL FACTORS

During adolescence, individuals are going through rapid physical, social, and cognitive changes. These enormous changes to body, friendship, and thinking about the world are juxtaposed against changing expectations for behavior and increases in need and opportunities for autonomy. The desire to be *autonomous* and to be granted more decision making opportunities increases with age (Steinberg and Cauffman, 1996) and occurs in tandem with several other changes that serve to increase adolescents' desires for autonomy. First, the physical changes of puberty result in adolescents' seeing themselves as more deserving of adult-like privileges and opportunities to make decisions. In addition, as adolescents mature physically and develop secondary sex characteristics, they look older and are presumed to be able to take on more adult-like roles and responsibilities. Second, increased time spent with peers leads to more experiences and comparison of others' authority, power, and privileges. Third, cultural and societal beliefs suggest that adolescence is a time to practice adult roles. All of these factors serve to underscore the importance of autonomy from parents and push adolescents toward assuming more adult roles. In the United States, alcohol use is an important symbol of adult status.

The shift away from childhood and toward independence and adult roles is accompanied by a focus on peer acceptance and perceived norms in addition to parental standards. Adolescents need to develop their own sense of self or identity during this time, although expectations about the appropriate timing for increased autonomy during adolescence varies across cultures (e.g., Feldman and Rosenthal, 1990). Individuals adapt and modify their identities to enable them to function best in their particular social and cultural context (Baumeister and Muraven, 1996). Adolescents may "try on" various identities that will be defined, in part, by how time is spent and with whom it is spent. While constructing an identity, an adolescent's motivation may be to gain new experiences that will allow them to evaluate what fits and what does not with their newly developing identities. This process allows them to create adult selves that are realistic and comfortable (Curry et al., 1994). During this period, adolescents report having a "true self" (who they really are inside) and a "false self" (who they want other people to think they are, to impress or please them) (Harter et al., 1996). At this point, adolescents may knowingly make choices that they know they may later regret "just to see what it is like," to act more like an adult, or to impress others (e.g., Moffit, 1993). Some of these choices are likely to involve alcohol consumption.

In order to understand the shifts that adolescents are undergoing, it is important to consider both changes in cognition and in the social world in which adolescents find themselves during this period.

Cognitive Changes

Cognitive changes during adolescence include gradual improvements in social perspective, to about age 16 (Steinberg and Cauffman, 1996). These newfound perspective-taking skills allow an adolescent to recognize how the thoughts and actions of one person influence those of another and to imagine how others might perceive them. Although generally an indicator of greater maturity, a downside of this new ability is that adolescents are highly concerned with peer conformity, which may make them particularly susceptible to peer influence. The majority of studies indicate a positive relationship between susceptibility to peer pressure and risk-taking behavior (such as drinking). For reasons not yet known, there is variation in the extent to which adolescents succumb to social influence, including pressure to engage in behaviors that are undesirable (see Steinberg and Cauffman, 1996, for a review).

In general, thinking becomes more abstract and more future-oriented during adolescence, allowing adolescents to consider multiple aspects of any decision at one time, assess potential consequences of a decision, consider possible outcomes associated with various choices, and plan for the future. These cognitive changes enhance the adolescent's capacity for competent decision making (see, for example, Halpern-Felsher and Cauffman, 2001; Steinberg and Cauffman, 1996). However, these newly formed competencies are not always practiced when adolescents are confronted with real-world social situations. Many studies suggest that adolescents, as well as adults, may make less than optimal decisions when personal goals, beliefs, prior experience, values, social expectations, and emotions are added to the decision making equation (Jacobs and Klaczynski, 2002). This outcome is especially true for social decisions (like choosing whether to drink or how much to drink). This is so for a variety of reasons.

First, outcomes of decisions in social situations are probabilistic, meaning that negative consequences of bad decisions may not occur and may not even be highly likely, although they are devastating if they do occur. For example, while the probability of having a car crash after drinking is much higher than after not drinking, drinking and driving does not *always* end in a crash or a ticket. Because outcomes are probabilistic, adolescents may interpret the fact that they previously drank too much and drove home without a crash as evidence that they can drink and drive safely (Jacobs and Ganzel, 1994). In one study, older adolescents who had a lot of experience drinking and driving, but had not experienced a negative outcome, such as a traffic citation or crash, believed that they were in little danger of having an accident after drinking (Finken et al., 1998), this result suggests that engaging in risky behaviors without consequence may have caused them to lower their perceptions of the risks of drinking and driving. Other correlational studies have shown that greater involvement in risk-taking behaviors was related to lower perceptions of personal risk (e.g., Halpern-Felsher and Cauffman, 2001; Goldberg et al., 2002). Second, the norms for social decisions are not typically known. Instead, individuals are often forced to make judgments on the basis of their own estimates of the norms of social behaviors or attitudes. This general dilemma, faced by people of all ages, is even more difficult for adolescents because they must make decisions based on a limited amount of experience and little feedback from earlier decisions (Jacobs et al., 1995). Several studies indicate that most adolescents overestimate the number of others who drink alcohol (e.g., Basch et al., 1989; Jaccard and Turrisi, 1987). Not surprisingly, the overestimation is greatest for those individuals who drink. This same pattern has been found for other risk-taking and deviant behaviors (e.g., Benthin et al., 1993; Nucci et al., 1991), and it may be related to the fact that those who drink have friends who drink and so they begin to believe that everyone is drinking. In one longitudinal study, adolescents who spent time with peers who encouraged drinking later reported more positive views of drinkers (Blanton et al., 1997).

In addition, studies indicate that adolescents make more biased estimates when they are reasoning about populations with greater variability and when they are reasoning about unfamiliar others (Jacobs, 2004) Underage drinking and other forms of risk taking are likely to occur in social situations and when adolescents find themselves with large groups of unfamiliar peers. In these situations, they are left to estimate how others typically behave and what they think. The outcome may be overestimates of others' drinking and acceptance of such behavior, leading them to believe that the norm is to drink and that they should do it, too. However, providing adolescents with more realistic information about the extent to which people drink alcohol may not by itself reduce alcohol consumption. Instead, a focus on injunctive norms—views concerning what others think about one's drinking—might be more effective (Cialdini et al., 1990; Kallgren et al., 2000; Prentice and Miller, 1993).

Social Situations

The social situations in which adolescents find themselves also change during this period. Indeed, movement toward autonomy is accompanied by real and perceived changes in the social world as adolescents mature. Most move from environments in which they are protected, scheduled, and dominated by adults into environments that are primarily populated with other adolescents and in which they actually have much more autonomy. On average, middle-class adolescents spend about 20 percent of their time with parents and other relatives, 25 percent of their time alone, and the rest with friends and classmates (Csikszentmihalyi and Larson, 1984). Younger adolescents report that television and home- and family-centered activities fill much of their leisure time, but this shifts dramatically as they get older and report that peer-focused and solitary activities fill most of their time (Larson and Kleiber, 1990). Thus, as adolescents get older, they spend greater periods of their leisure time away from adult supervision, increasing the opportunities for becoming involved in such risk-taking behaviors as drinking alcohol.

In addition to the actual changes in supervision, teens are much more focused on real or imagined peer norms. They are most likely to attend to the standards set by their friends than by another same-age group. The often reported, "peer pressure" is, in reality, "friend pressure." As adolescents get older, they are more likely to choose friends who share their tastes and interests than when they were younger. Thus, they are likely to join crowds of teens who have similar values and life-styles. Crowd membership has been associated with alcohol consumption: some crowds or groups include drinking as part of how they spend their time, and an adolescent's choice to be involved in that crowd will include the knowledge that drinking is a typical activity for that group (Prinstein et al., 1996). For example, participation in competitive sports in high school has been related to higher rates of alcohol use (Eccles and Barber, 1999).

Unfortunately, information about a particular group's norms may not be available until after an adolescent has had one or more experiences with the group and has been faced with situations in which saying "no" to alcohol will be viewed unfavorably by peers. Younger adolescents report having more trouble moving between crowds than older adolescents, so it may be more difficult for them to go against the norms of a crowd if they feel uncomfortable (Brown et al., 1994).

INDIVIDUAL DIFFERENCES

Although we have concentrated on describing the normative changes that affect adolescents, there are clear individual differences in development as well, and some of these differences may be associated with higher alcohol consumption. These differences include personality, perceptions of risk, and self-efficacy, as well as gender and racial differences in adolescent alcohol consumption (noted in Chapter 2). Although numerous clinical studies indicate that individuals differ in their likelihood of experiencing alcohol dependency and related disorders (Kessler et al., 1997; Swendsen et al., 2002), our focus in this chapter remains on nonclinical populations.

Personality Differences

Is there a personality profile that is related to adolescent risk for alcohol abuse? Cloninger (1991) found that three traits, present as early as age 10, were associated with alcoholism at age 28: (1) being easily bored and needing constant stimulation; (2) being driven to avoid negative consequence for actions; and (3) craving immediate external rewards for efforts. In addition, antisocial personality disorder has been linked to alcohol misuse among adolescents (Clark et al., 1998). Similarly, a recent study of children aged 8 to 15 found that conduct disorder often predates and predicts later alcohol use (Clark et al., 1998).

In nonclinical populations, a major personality characteristic that has been related to adolescent risk taking is sensation seeking, defined by seeking novel, complex, or risky situations (Zuckerman, 1979). The appeal of drinking alcohol and other "forbidden" behaviors for adolescents may be the novel and intense sensations provided by the experiences (Arnett and Balle-Jensen, 1993); students who have higher needs for sensation seeking are more likely to report higher levels of drinking, as well as other delinquent behaviors. Others have also reported associations between sensation seeking or novelty seeking and alcohol use (e.g., Martin et al., 2002). Donohew and colleagues (1999) argued that sensation seeking influences alcohol use indirectly, through peer affiliations: teens who are sensation seekers tend to choose friends with similar sensation seeking desires, and such peer group affiliations increase alcohol use.

Beliefs About Risk

Although many adults believe that adolescents underestimate the risks of engaging in particular behaviors, most research indicates that adults and adolescents actually give similar estimates of various types of risk taking, including drinking alcohol (e.g., Beyth-Marom et al., 1993; Quadrel et al., 1993). Although sweeping age differences in risk estimates have not typically been found (Millstein and Halpern-Felsher, 2002), individuals' perceptions of risk vary, and their perceptions have been linked to their behaviors. In general, drinkers of all ages view consuming alcohol as less risky than nondrinkers (Goldberg et al., 2002), although the absolute accuracy of various risk perceptions has been the topic of debate (e.g., Slovic, 2000). Although adolescents generally overestimate their mortality risks for a variety of activities including alcohol (e.g., Fischhoff et al., 2000), recent studies suggest that adolescents who perceive a higher likelihood of negative consequences following alcohol consumption do not drink at all or drink more moderately than others (e.g., Goldberg et al., 2002; Halpern-Felsher and Cauffman, 2001; Small et al., 1993.)

Both adults and adolescents tend to overestimate how many other people are involved in activities in which they, themselves, are engaged (e.g., Kruglanski, 1989). Indeed, adolescents as well as adults who participate in high-risk activities generally believe that the rate of participation by others is higher than do nonparticipants (Benthin et al., 1993); thus, beliefs about normative practices may be related to older adolescents' decisions to engage in risky behaviors (Basch et al., 1989; Beck and Treiman, 1996; Olds and Thombs, 2001). In one recent study, adolescents who reported higher levels of alcohol consumption and other risk-taking behavior than their peers overestimated how much other adolescents in their school were participating in the same high-risk behaviors (Jacobs, 2000). Extreme overestimaters engaged in significantly more mild and severe deviant behaviors than either the moderate overestimaters or those whose estimates were correct, and they reported poorer self-esteem, lower grade point averages, and less rational decision-making skills. One of the most intriguing implications of the research focusing on individual differences is that some adolescents are more likely than others to perceive drinking as low risk, to overestimate the likelihood of others' drinking, and to look for sensation-seeking opportunities. This is the group that one would expect to drink the most and take the most risks when drinking.

Prior Experience

Although correlated with age, drinking experiences have a significant and independent effect on alcohol expectancies, which in turn play a role in alcohol use (Christiansen et al., 1989; Christiansen et al., 1982; Chen et al., 1994; Grube et al., 1995; Jones et al., 2001; Smith et al., 1995; Wood et al., 1992; Goldberg et al., 2002). More specific expectancies, such as enhanced sexual feelings, power, and reduced tension have been reported by those with greater drinking experiences, while youth with little or no alcohol experiences have more global expectancies of increased pleasure (Christiansen et al., 1982). As one gains more experience with alcohol, positive outcomes are reinforced and predict future drinking behaviors (Goldberg et al., 2002; Jones et al., 2001). Furthermore, positive drinking-related expectancies increase and negative expectations for risks decrease among adolescents with more drinking experiences (Halpern-Felsher et al., 2000; Goldberg et al., 2002).

Self-Efficacy

Drinking refusal self-efficacy, borrowed from Bandura's (1986, 1997) concept of general self-efficacy, refers to one's belief in her or his ability to resist urges or social pressures to drink, to drink in particular situations, or to consume large amounts of alcohol at one time. Adolescents with more positive self-efficacy are less likely to drink or drink excessively (Oei et al., 1998; Webb and Baer, 1995), and those with fewer refusal skills are more likely to drink (Hays and Ellickson, 1996). Refusal skills may be a better predictor of problem drinking than alcohol expectancies, especially for heavy or frequent alcohol use (Connor et al., 2000; Oei et al., 1998). Given that adolescents are more susceptible to peer pressure, it stands to reason that they will have lower drinking refusal skills. However, there is evidence that adolescents can be taught drinking refusal self-efficacy skills and that such skills can then result in less substance use (Bell et al., 1993; Ellickson et al., 1993).

CONTEXTUAL FACTORS

As noted in the previous chapter, the highest rate of both heavy drinking and frequent heavy drinking is found in young adults between the ages of 18 and 25. In addition, if adolescents between the ages of 14 and 20 drink alcohol, they are more likely to report heavy drinking than other drinking patterns (National Household Survey on Drug Abuse, 2001). These findings suggest that there may be something about the context of youth drinking that results in this particular pattern of alcohol consumption. Indeed, macrolevel and microlevel contextual factors are likely to contribute to both the number of underage drinkers and their patterns of alcohol use.

Community

U.S. culture is replete with messages touting the attractions of alcohol use, and—notwithstanding the legal norm—suggesting that drinking is acceptable for people under 21. Recent content analyses indicate that alcohol use was depicted, typically in a positive light, in more than 70 percent of a sample of episodes in prime-time television programming in 1999 (Christensen et al., 2000), and in more than 90 percent of the two hundred most popular movie rentals for 1996-1997 (Roberts et al., 1999b). Roberts et al. (1999b) also found that 17 percent of the 1,000 of the most popular songs in 1996-1997 across five genres of music popular with youth contained alcohol references, including almost one-half of the rap music recordings. The alcohol industry spent $1.6 billion on advertising in 2001, and probably twice that much in other promotional activity. Young people are exposed to a steady stream of images and lyrics presenting alcohol use in an attractive light.

Within any country, the specific community environment may contribute to drinking to a greater or lesser extent. The drinking environment can be characterized as varying on a "wet-dry" continuum. A "wet" community environment is one in which drinking is prevalent and common, public opinion is generally tolerant or positive, and alcohol is readily available both commercially and at private social occasions and is advertised as available. A "dry" community would be one in which drinking at social occasions is not the norm and is generally frowned on, and alcohol outlets are relatively scarce. One commonly used statistical indicator for the "wetness" of the environment is the per capita consumption of alcohol (the average number of drinks per person) for the population age 14 and over per year. In the United States, for example, per capita consumption ranged from 1.3 gallons of ethanol per capita in Utah to 2.8 gallons in Wisconsin, in 1997; see Table 4-1.

TABLE 4-1 Alcohol Consumption, 1999

State or Area	Ethanol*	Per Capita
Alabama	6,656	1.88
Alaska	1,346	2.88
Arizona	9,971	2.68
Arkansas	3,725	1.82
California	57,195	2.20
Colorado	8,305	2.57
Connecticut	5,953	2.26
Delaware	1,812	2.96
District of Columbia	1,647	3.74
Florida	32,773	2.66
Georgia	14,019	2.27

continued

TABLE 4-1 Continued

State or Area	Ethanol*	Per Capita
Hawaii	2,212	2.31
Idaho	2,355	2.39
Illinois	22,337	2.32
Indiana	9,371	1.97
Iowa	4,601	1.98
Kansas	3,925	1.85
Kentucky	5,662	1.76
Louisiana	8,678	2.50
Maine	2,348	2.26
Maryland	8,740	2.11
Massachusetts	12,290	2.45
Michigan	16,625	2.11
Minnesota	9,189	2.41
Mississippi	4,801	2.19
Missouri	9,962	2.26
Montana	1,828	2.55
Nebraska	2,979	2.24
Nevada	5,765	4.06
New Hampshire	3,943	4.07
New Jersey	14,416	2.20
New Mexico	3,308	2.43
New York	28,187	1.92
North Carolina	12,241	2.00
North Dakota	1,264	2.45
Ohio	18,203	2.01
Oklahoma	4,624	1.72
Oregon	6,239	2.32
Pennsylvania	18,723	1.91
Rhode Island	1,936	2.41
South Carolina	7,590	2.41
South Dakota	1,354	2.32
Tennessee	8,468	1.91
Texas	35,677	2.29
Utah	2,105	1.33
Vermont	1,144	2.34
Virginia	11,107	1.99
Washington	9,962	2.16
West Virginia	2,492	1.66
Wisconsin	11,664	2.75
Wyoming	961	2.48
Northeast	88,941	2.12
Midwest	111,474	2.20
South	170,712	2.21
West	111,551	2.32
U.S. Total	482,678	2.21

*Ethanol is the alcohol consumption measure used.
SOURCE: Data from National Institute on Alcohol
Abuse and Alcoholism (2002).

To what extent do environmental factors influence individual drinking choices by youth? It is interesting in this regard to analyze trends in youth drinking over time. Based on their analysis of Monitoring the Future data for high school seniors, Cook and Moore (2001) report that the 30-day prevalence of drinking and also of heavy drinking[1] peaked in 1979, and then declined by approximately one-third (30.6 and 37.5 percent, respectively), reaching a low point in 1993 and increasing only slightly since then. This downward trend is unrelated to demographic changes in the composition of the population of high-school seniors and cannot be fully explained by trends in prices, minimum drinking age, or availability (Cook and Moore, 2001). However, this trend in drinking prevalence closely tracks the societal trend in drinking, as measured by national per capita consumption. Thus, whatever the reason for the decline in youth drinking during the 1980s, it seems to be related to, and perhaps in some sense is the result of, the overall decline in drinking in the society.

More persuasive evidence of the link between "wetness" and youth consumption comes from a study of individual drinking behavior. Cook and Moore (2001) analyzed data from the National Longitudinal Survey of Youth (NLSY) that included annual items on individual drinking for 1982-1985 and 1988-1989. The initial cohort of 12,000 respondents ranged in age from 17 to 24 at the beginning of this period in 1982, so that the NLSY data provide information on drinking trajectories for older teens and those in their twenties. They found that, even after controlling for family, religion, schooling, aspirations, employment, and cognitive ability, various aspects of the environment contributed significantly to patterns of drinking. Specifically, youth with similar backgrounds and individual characteristics were more likely to drink if they lived in a state with relatively high per capita consumption.

The minimum drinking age and the excise tax on beer are also related to youth drinking. Thus, an 18-year-old living in a state in which his drinking was legal in 1982 would have been more likely to drink (and to drink heavily) than an identical twin living in a state with a higher minimum drinking age. Increases in the beer tax (which has a direct effect on average price) generally tend to lower drinking, although it is harder to pin down with the NLSY data; however, other studies are quite consistent at documenting that taxes and prices influence youth drinking (Chaloupka and Wechsler, 1996). This research suggests that a "wetter" environment may provide adolescents with more social occasions to drink, more positive attitudes about drinking, more advertising and outlets, and more lenient regulations concerning the sale and consumption of alcohol. In short, such environments have an enabling effect on underage drinking.

---

[1]Defined as five or more drinks in a row in the last 2 weeks.

In addition to specific community norms for drinking, several other societal factors may affect the prevalence of heavy drinking in adolescence. First, U.S. society is largely segregated by age. As adolescents get older, they spend more and more time alone or with other peers in unsupervised settings, and both age-segregation and lack of adult supervision have been related to higher levels of substance abuse and deviance, including greater alcohol consumption. "Hanging out" with friends in unstructured, unsupervised contexts is generally related to negative outcomes, while spending time with others in adult-sanctioned, structured contexts is generally related to positive outcomes (e.g., Osgood, 1998; Osgood et al., 1996).

A particularly vulnerable time for youth is the after-school period, 3:00 to 6:00 p.m. This time is especially likely to be unsupervised as adolescents get older and parents believe that it is "safe" to leave them at home unattended. Youth who participate in after-school programs, such as sports, clubs, library-based activities, and youth-serving organizations are less likely to use alcohol than nonparticipants (Eccles and Barber, 1999). The same point about age segregation and lack of supervision applies to adolescents' attendance at unchaperoned parties and other activities. It is not uncommon for caring parents to decide to host an all-night party with alcohol for their teenage children, taking the car keys from the guests as they arrive, on the theory that it is safer to allow drinking at home rather than to forbid it and have teens drink and drive. Individuals or organizations that host and support such events are providing opportunities that enable adolescents to drink to excess. Not surprisingly, having parents who sanction alcohol use (even in "controlled" settings) is related to heavier drinking among adolescents (Barnes et al., 1995; Peterson et al., 1994).

By and large, adolescents are even segregated by age in the workplace. Adolescents who work for pay are often employed in fast-food and similar jobs in which most of their coworkers are other adolescents (Mortimer et al., 1992). It is not uncommon for a 17-year-old to be managing a fast-food establishment and supervising 15- and 16-year-olds. Given this situation, it may not be surprising that part-time work during adolescence is positively related to involvement in drugs, alcohol, and other deviant behaviors (e.g., Bachman and Schulenberg, 1993; Greenberger and Steinberg, 1986; Steinberg et al., 1993).

The place in which adolescents are most segregated is likely to be at residential colleges. Although less than one-quarter of college students are in such settings, student-segregated apartments or college residence halls provide the conditions under which binge drinking is likely to occur: cultural norms that support drinking, little supervision by any adults, and peers who are likely to be heavily involved in drinking. In a recent study, Cook and Moore (2001) found support that college students are more likely to engage in drinking, especially heavy drinking, if they live in a dormitory than if they live off campus, even after controlling for other factors (such as age) that might explain this difference.

Social Setting

While adolescents are experiencing community-level influences related to the place of alcohol in our society, each adolescent is also making decisions about drinking within a particular social setting. Of particular importance with regard to social influences are adolescents' peers and friendship networks and their changing relationships with their parents. The effect of parents' and peers' alcohol consumption on adolescents' drinking patterns is both direct, through observation and modeling (Bandura, 1986) and indirect, through its influence on alcohol-related expectancies and attitudes (see Kuther, 2002, for a review).

Peers

Adolescents in the United States spend approximately twice as much time with peers as they spend with parents or other adults. Accordingly, peers are a major source of socialization and development for adolescents. Research supports the notion that both selection and socialization factors contribute to observed similarities in behavior among friends. That is, adolescents are influenced by the normative behaviors of their peers <u>and</u> they choose peers who reinforce their own norms and values (Kandel, 1978). The influences of peers are both direct and indirect (Bauman et al., 1989; Biddle et al., 1980; Ennett and Bauman 1991; Pruitt et al., 1991; Kandel and Logen, 1984). That is, adolescents are influenced directly (e.g., by observing peers' behavior or by peer pressure) and indirectly (e.g., by their perceptions of the extent to which their friends are drinking alcohol). The combination of the normative aspect of alcohol use and peer influences on underage alcohol use is also important. Youth are well aware of the normative nature of alcohol use, and they usually want to go along with their peer group (Aas and Klepp, 1992; Barnes et al., 1995; Beck and Treiman, 1996; Olds and Thombs, 2001). Perceived use of alcohol by one's peers and friends independently predicts self-reported alcohol use (e.g., Olds and Thombs, 2001; Reifman et al., 1998), with peers having a greater influence on adolescent drinking than do parents (Kuther, 2002).

It should be noted, however, that interventions that attempt to prevent or reduce alcohol consumption by focusing on changing perceptions of social norms must proceed cautiously. Research conducted by Cialdini and colleagues (Cialdini et al., 1990; Kallgren et al., 2000) points to the need to distinguish between descriptive norms (perceptions of what most others are doing) and injunctive norms (perception of what other people think one should be doing or not doing). Cialdini argues that focusing on injunctive norms is more effective at changing behavior than targeting only descriptive norms.

Parents

Although peers are one important influence on adolescents' choices, parents remain important during the teen years. Many adolescents report that they turn to their parents for advice regarding educational and career decisions, although they turn to their friends for advice about clothes and music (Montemayor, 1982). Indeed, most theoretical perspectives today suggest that close connections to both parents and peers are related to easier transitions to independence (e.g., Allen and Hauser, 1996). Yet peer influences also depend in part on the quality of parent-child relationships (Parke and Ladd, 1992). Adolescents who have positive relationships with their parents may be more likely to have friends who engage in socially valued activities than do adolescents with less positive parental interactions. Similarly, more involved parents may oversee and monitor their child's peer relationships more than do less involved parents, thereby reducing adolescents' engagement in undesired behaviors (see, for example, Fletcher et al., 1995). Parents also have a significant amount of influence on their children's choice of friends. Parents help shape prosocial and antisocial behavior, which leads children to gravitate toward particular crowds.

Parental monitoring and involvement are key components in reducing adolescent alcohol use. Monitoring of an adolescent's behavior involves the parent or guardian supervising the adolescent; knowing the adolescent's whereabouts; knowing the adolescent's friends and peers; setting expectations that are clear and optimally challenging; delivering consequences that are fair, affirming, and useful; and communicating with the adolescent (Connell et al., 1995; Connell and Halpern-Felsher, 1997; Halpern-Felsher et al., 1997; Lee and Halpern-Felsher, 2001). Similarly, parental involvement is the extent to which parents show interest in, are knowledgeable about, and put effort into their child's activities and development. Both parental monitoring and involvement serve to prevent or reduce adolescents' health-compromising behaviors through the setting of curfews, awareness of and participation in after-school and weekend activities, prevention of adolescents' association with risky peers, and the improvement of social skills (Beck and Lockhart, 1992; Cohen et al., 1994; Steinberg et al., 1994). Research on parental monitoring consistently shows protective effects on alcohol use (Barnes et al., 2000; Bogenschneider et al., 1998; Reifman et al., 1998; DiClemente et al., 2001).

Families also provide an arena in which fledgling decision makers try their new skills and in which more experienced decision makers model appropriate behavior or even provide instruction on how to make decisions (Jacobs and Ganzel, 1994). Learning to make decisions and live with their consequences and learn from them is an important developmental task that may be promoted or hindered by particular parenting practices. Although most parents give their adolescents increasing autonomy to make a wide range of decisions—in friendship, academics, extracurricular involvement, and consumer choices—many do so with little guidance or without letting adolescents experience the consequences of their actions. In addition, many parents provide an inconsistent pattern of restrictions and privileges (e.g., childlike restrictions about bedtime that don't match the adult privilege of driving the family car) that may lead adolescents to make choices that are aimed at rebelling against parental restrictions or that give them adult status (such as drinking alcohol).

Other aspects of parenting, such as parental norms and attitudes regarding adolescents' alcohol use and parents' own alcohol use, influence adolescent risk behavior. For example, Sieving and colleagues (2000) found that, in comparison with other variables, parent norms against underage drinking showed the strongest association with adolescents' abstention from alcohol use. In addition, parents, like other adults, may overestimate or underestimate drinking norms for adolescents, depending on their own experiences or their perceptions of societal norms. If parents believe that most adolescents drink, they may be more willing to "look the other way" when their children drink or to sponsor parties at which alcohol is served. Parents may benefit from knowing about other parents' practices and prohibitions concerning alcohol use by their children.

Parents' own alcohol use has also been linked to underage drinking (e.g., Pandina and Johnson, 1989), as well as to increased chance of experiencing alcohol-related negative consequences (Pandina and Johnson, 1990). However, family history of alcohol abuse and alcoholism alone may not be adequate to predict drinking patterns among children of parents with such drinking behaviors. It is possible that other factors, such as parental monitoring, personality, and stress coping strategies, mediate between family history of alcohol use and underage drinking (e.g., Johnson and Pandina, 1993; Reifman et al., 1998).

Two studies have demonstrated that sibling alcohol use is a risk factor. Of particular interest is the study by McGue and colleagues (1996) that examined the effect of both parental and sibling alcohol use on both adoptive and biological children raised in the same families: while parental alcohol use only had an effect for the biological children, sibling use had an effect on both adoptive and biological children. The effect was stronger if the sibling was similar in age, gender, and ethnicity.

CONFLUENCE OF FACTORS

In this chapter we have listed many social, cognitive, and contextual factors that are related to the reasons that adolescents drink. In a culture that promotes alcohol use, it is impossible to isolate one factor as the primary cause. Rather, understanding why adolescents drink is more likely to be found in the confluence of factors. Positive aspects of the normal developmental process (e.g., enhanced cognitive abilities and physical maturation) are directly related to the greater autonomy and freedom from supervision enjoyed by adolescents. However, increases in autonomy lead to more opportunities to obtain and use alcohol. Likewise, normal adolescent development includes focusing on peers and searching for one's own identity and friendship niche; however, these normal developmental processes lead to trying risky behaviors and conforming to peer norms that often include alcohol use. Thus, the trends that are typically associated with healthy adolescent development also set the stage for increased opportunities for alcohol use. In addition, adolescents are coming of age in the United States are doing so in a culture that promotes and enables underage drinking.

There is little that one can change about the timetable of cognitive and emotional development or personality characteristics, but one can consider interventions for some of the factors that have been related to adolescent alcohol consumption and can be changed. The most likely targets are adolescent, parent, and community attitudes about the acceptance of underage drinking. Media and educational campaigns with this goal, however, must keep in mind many of the factors that have been reviewed in this chapter. For example, messages to adolescents must consider factors such as developmental level; the need to act adult-like, try on new identities, and make decisions with little experience; and adolescents' peer norms and biased reasoning about these norms.

Communications aimed at parents and others must provide realistic information about the prevalence of underage drinking and the dangers associated with it. In addition, adults must be given clear messages about what they may be doing to enable underage drinking and concrete examples of what they can do to convey their expectations to their children, monitor their children, and provide a community environment that discourages rather than promotes underage drinking.

PART II

THE STRATEGY

5

Designing the Strategy

The committee was directed by Congress to "develop a cost-effective strategy to reduce underage drinking." This charge was admirably direct and simple. Still, to complete the task satisfactorily, the committee had to come to grips with some important issues raised by this mandate.

WHAT CONSTITUTES A "STRATEGY"?

The committee had first to consider what was meant by the idea of a strategy. To some, a strategy means a focused, sustained commitment to a single approach for accomplishing the desired result: for example, the adoption of a national media campaign designed to dissuade young people from drinking, or to restrict underage access to alcohol, or, a program to raise the price of alcohol through excise taxes. In this view, the important strategic decision would be to decide which of a variety of different policy tools or instruments is likely to produce the largest, most reliable effects at the least cost.

In the committee's view, a strategy is better understood not as a single approach, but rather as a portfolio of approaches or instruments—a multipronged effort to reduce underage drinking that can be refined and adjusted as knowledge and experience accumulate. There are several factors about underage drinking that lead to this view. The first is the heterogeneity of the problem. As shown in Part I, underage drinking encompasses several distinct phenomena that require different preventive approaches. For example, the actions needed to prevent and reduce frequent drinking by 12-year-olds are different from those that will be useful or necessary in dealing with the intermittent heavy drinking of a much larger group of 17- to 18-year-old young people in high schools: and this problem, in turn, is different from the challenge posed by underage drinking on college campuses or in neighborhood bars by groups of workers that include many underage drinkers in their midst.

The second factor is the interaction among policy instruments. The effectiveness of one instrument often depends on the extent to which other instruments are being used. For example, a new policy prescribing sanctions for underage drinkers and those who sell or give them alcohol might be expected to produce some effects. However, this same policy intervention might be expected to have a stronger effect if accompanied by a media campaign designed not only to inform individuals of the new sanctions, but also to mobilize other community organizations to intervene. Or, a high school could decide to "crack down" on drinking in and around school-sponsored events, but find that its efforts are undermined by parents who are not committed to enforcing the same policies on weekends in their homes. Even a "zero tolerance" policy toward underage drinking, which might be expected to maximize general deterrence, might do so only by injuring the future prospects of those young people who are severely punished. In fact, a policy of penalizing youthful drinkers might be most effective, overall, if it is combined with sustained, focused assistance for youth who have already developed serious drinking problems. To the extent that the effects of one policy can be enhanced by using another tool and to the extent that the negative effects of one policy can be mitigated by using a second instrument, it makes sense to have a strategy based on a portfolio approach.

The third factor is the problem of uncertainty. Even when research suggests that a particular approach is likely to be effective, one cannot be sure how effective it will be in particular situations. It is usually good investment advice to diversify the investment in the face of uncertainty—to avoiding putting "all the eggs in one basket"—and the same applies to public policy. Thus, uncertainty, and the desire to learn from experience, leads to a portfolio approach to the problem.

The fourth factor is the problem of diminishing returns. Even when one knows that a chosen intervention will succeed, the marginal benefits of investing an additional dollar in the intervention are likely to decline at some point. Thus, with, say $1 billion to invest in reducing underage drinking, one could decide to spend it all on a single intervention believed to be effective (e.g., reducing access to alcohol or a youth-oriented media campaign), but the greatest effect is likely to come from combined investments in both approaches.

The fifth factor is the lack of consensus. A portfolio approach gives many actors a chance to contribute. Different communities, institutions, and individuals have different resources and different ideas about which approaches will be useful and effective. In a world in which people disagree about which interventions are best and in which it will be valuable to engage many actors in the effort to deal with the problem, it would be a serious mistake to insist that only one approach be used.

To say that the committee decided to recommend a portfolio of approaches, however, is not to say that comparative judgments concerning the relative effectiveness of different instruments must be avoided or that individual components of the strategy cannot be implemented independently from the others However, we propose a comprehensive strategy that we believe will be cost-effective based on the notion that several instruments will be reinforced by the addition of other instruments as they help to reach a problem that is missed (or created) by a particular policy or as they provide hedges against uncertainty or opportunities to learn. Evidence from youth smoking prevention policy reinforces the notion that a comprehensive, multifaceted approach is likely to be more effective than any single approach (Lantz, 2004).

But the balance among these instruments has to reflect a clear conception of both the nature of the problem and the reasons for selecting the chosen strategy. We present our overall analysis of cost-effectiveness at the end of Chapter 12 after more fully discussing the individual components of the strategy.

WHAT DOES "COST-EFFECTIVE" IMPLY AND REQUIRE?

The committee also considered what Congress meant by a "cost-effective" strategy and what data and analysis are needed to assess cost-effectiveness. We note that such an assessment involves more than the usual question in program evaluation, which focuses simply on whether a particular policy "works" to produce the desired effect (or effects).

Assessing Effectiveness

What did Congress mean by effectiveness? Presumably, one key measure of effectiveness is simply reducing the numbers of youth who drink alcohol at all before they turn 21. To the extent that the law treats all drinking by people under 21 as illegal and to the extent that the goal of any law is to get to as close to complete compliance as possible, the ultimate test of effectiveness would be the degree to which underage drinking stopped altogether. However, given that alcohol use is regarded as entirely appropriate for adults and that this normative stance (and the policies it spawns) leads to ambivalent attitudes toward underage drinking and to easy opportunities for young people to drink, it is impossible as a practical matter to drive underage drinking to zero. Increasing the rate of abstention cannot be the *sole* measure of effectiveness.

Thus, it is necessary to develop different standards of effectiveness. In this light, it is important to recognize that some types of underage drinking are especially likely to be associated with harmful consequences, given the age of the drinkers, the characteristics of the drinking, and the contexts in which it occurs. Accordingly, effectiveness can be sensibly measured by reductions in these bad consequences, or in the intensity and dangerousness of underage drinking.

Relevant Outcomes

The committee has identified five goals that are pertinent to evaluating the effectiveness of a comprehensive strategy for preventing and reducing underage drinking.

- delaying onset (e.g., increasing the average age of first use or of first episode of heavy use);
- reducing the prevalence of (current) alcohol use;
- increasing the proportion of youths who are current abstainers and intend to continue to abstain until they meet the legal drinking age;
- reducing the intensity (frequency and quantity) of drinking (e.g., heavy drinking); and
- reducing the harmful consequences of alcohol use.

Delaying onset (meaning delaying the first episode of drinking, however measured) is an important outcome goal because of the documented relationship between early onset and adverse consequences, and because the average age of onset has been falling in recent years (see Chapter 2). Rates of prevalence (of use) and abstention are typically regarded as reciprocals of one another; however, in the present context, the committee believes that reducing prevalence and increasing abstention should be regarded as distinct objectives. In most surveys, prevalence of "current use" is operationalized as use within the last 30 days. As so measured, prevalence is not the reciprocal of abstention because individuals who are not abstaining and have no intention of doing so in the future may not have used alcohol within the last 30 days. This situation is particularly pertinent to underage drinking because many nonabstaining youths may not be current users (as measured by 30-day prevalence). As discussed in Chapter 2, young people who drink tend to drink heavily. One of the guiding assumptions of this report is that the most plausible goal for teenagers is to prevent or reduce drinking altogether, rather than focusing on reducing drinking intensity. Accordingly, rates of prevalence and abstention are particularly important outcomes for children and teens.[1]

Comparing Outcomes

Assessed independently, the effectiveness of specific policies depends on the aspect of the problem they are designed to address. Some policies aim to discourage initiation by young teens or preteens; others aim to reduce the prevalence of any drinking in a high school population; and others aim to reduce the number of occasions when high school students engage in heavy drinking or when they drive after drinking. For the most part, the current policy evaluation literature does not compare the effectiveness of different policies or interventions. Instead, a given intervention is evaluated in terms of one or more particular outcomes.

Ultimately, however, a sophisticated assessment of cost-effectiveness requires a common metric for comparing the outcomes of policies that address different components of the problem of underage drinking. For example, preventive interventions for disease or injury are often evaluated in terms of such outcomes as deaths prevented, years of potential life lost before age 65, or the quality-adjusted years "saved" by the intervention. Such consequence-based assessments of effectiveness are rarely possible for underage drinking. The dots cannot now be connected in any rigorous way between an incremental reduction in the prevalence, intensity, or age-of-onset of underage drinking and any "ultimate" outcome.

The committee considered what metric would be best for comparing the value of upward shifts in the age of onset, downward shifts in current use (prevalence) of drinking among 15-year-olds, reductions in levels of heavy drinking among high school students, or reductions in the prevalence of driving after drinking among underage drinkers. It seems clear that the most important factor in identifying and ranking outcomes is the harms or negative consequences associated with particular patterns of consumption. Just as different components of the problem might need separate targeting,

---

[1]Educational programs and media campaigns aimed at young adults (18 to 21) often must grapple with the reality of pervasive drinking, and they must decide whether and how to formulate a "harm reduction" message—i.e., one that says, in effect: "It's illegal to use alcohol, and you shouldn't do it at all, but if you do, do it responsibly..." Though such approaches might be useful for young adults, such a "harm reduction" or "responsible drinking" message is wholly inappropriate for children and young teens. Nonetheless, exploring such options was inconsistent with the committee's charge and the committee did not consider interventions with this objective.

so different components of the problem might have different long-term social consequences and therefore be more or less important as targets of public policy intervention.

In looking at harms, one needs to look at the adverse effects of particular underage drinking behavior on the well-being of the drinker and those around him or her—the drinker's immediate family, friends, neighbors, and strangers whom the drinker encounters. Ultimately, the effectiveness of a policy means having an important effect in reducing any or all of these negative consequences. When direct measures of these adverse consequences are available (such as truancy or fatal automobile crashes), they will be the preferred measures of policy effectiveness. However, because direct measures of these effects are rarely available, measures of prevalence, intensity, and circumstances are used as proxies for the negative consequences (both short-term and long-term). Because adverse effects are most closely correlated with early onset and with heavy drinking, these two indicators are likely to be particularly useful in comparing the effectiveness of different policies.

Assessing Costs

Even if a program is effective on some relevant outcome measure, it still might not be worth implementing if its cost is excessive in relation to the benefits achieved, or if the same benefits can be achieved by a less costly intervention. How, then, does one measure the cost of policies to reduce underage drinking? At first blush, this task may not seem too hard: all one has to do is to determine the costs of developing, implementing, and sustaining the program whose cost-effectiveness is being calculated. However, even leaving aside for a moment the practical difficulties of actually measuring the direct and indirect costs of a program, three important conceptual issues arise in measuring costs.

First, while it might be feasible to estimate the (resource) costs to the government of developing and implementing a particular government-sponsored program, it is far more problematic to assess the program's total resource costs to the society. After all, government often acts not only directly, but also indirectly by encouraging others to contribute. The encouragement can be through exhortation and the provision of financial incentives (which do not cover the full costs of the effort). Or the encouragement can be through regulation and enforcement efforts that require private organizations and individuals—companies, distributors, tavern owners, parents, or even the companions of underage drinkers—to restrain from activities that encourage underage drinking or to materially contribute their time, energy, and money to prevent or reduce it. Although government is generally applauded for these catalytic roles in leveraging the resources of others, it makes accounting for the full cost of the effort problematic.

Second, the costs of a policy have to include the negative (presumably unwanted) effects of a given policy, as well as the financial or material costs associated with implementing it. In judging the overall cost-effectiveness of a policy, it certainly makes sense to consider these unwanted, adverse effects of a policy as well as the desired, positive effects. And it certainly makes sense to enter these negative effects on the (negative) cost side of the ledger rather than the (positive) effectiveness side. But it is clear, we think, that the negative effects of a policy are costs in a much different sense than the resource costs necessary to carry out the program: they are often highly speculative and can rarely be quantified in monetary terms. Although they are no less important than costs that are easily quantified, they are much harder to account for in a cost-effectiveness analysis.

Third, it is important to recognize that one of the important costs of government policies is the burden that the use of government authority imposes on the freedom of private individuals. Government uses two different assets when it acts. It uses money raised through taxation—to mount media campaigns, provide incentives to states and localities to adopt certain programs that have proven effective in dealing with underage drinking, and so on. These costs can be captured relatively easily through financial cost accounting systems. The government also uses its authority to compel private individuals to take actions that are judged to be in the public's interest: for example, it penalizes package stores and bars for selling alcohol to underage drinkers, it creates very stiff penalties for those who drink and drive, and so on.

There is a measurable economic cost associated with these uses of state authority: one can estimate how much the state expends on its own efforts to enforce these laws and can try to estimate the economic consequences of these regulatory regimes for those affected by them. But what is missing from the calculation is that the state has reduced some individual liberty. All other things being equal, people in the United States usually prefer a policy that uses less coercive authority—that takes away less personal liberty—than a policy that achieves the same result with more coercive authority. As a result, when looking at alternative strategies for reducing underage drinking, it is important to try to account for the amount of coercive authority that is being used and treat its use as a cost in roughly the same way that the expenditure of public money is treated as a cost.

STANDARDS OF EVIDENCE

The committee has reviewed the pertinent evidence on the effectiveness of the various programs and interventions to prevent or reduce underage drinking, as well as those to prevent the use of tobacco and illegal drugs, and, when relevant, interventions that have been used to affect other health-related behavior. Occasionally, the available evidence is direct and clear—that an intervention does or does not affect alcohol use or other outcomes. Usually, however, the evidence is more equivocal—studies may be in conflict, the intervention may work for some groups but not others, the intervention lacks any direct evidence but is supported by a strong body of indirect evidence, and so on. It is necessary, under these circumstances, to assess the strength or weight of the evidence. In so doing, we draw on the concept of "standards of evidence," a phrase that generally refers to the methodological strength of and basis for a conclusion or recommendation.

Much of the research presented in this report describes empirical associations between the presence or absence of a prevention approach and alcohol use or other outcomes. These correlations do not provide conclusive evidence that the approach caused a reduction in alcohol use or other outcomes; they merely index the direction and magnitude of the association. Establishing that a particular intervention caused a given outcome (above and beyond the role of other factors) requires evidence from experimental and quasi-experimental research. As noted in Chapter 1 and further discussed in subsequent chapters, the effects of some policy interventions bearing on underage drinking (e.g., increasing the minimum drinking age to 21) have been assessed with research that presents clear evidence of causation.

Even in the absence of direct causal evidence, correlational evidence, together with other kinds of evidence, may be sufficiently compelling to suggest that an intervention represents a promising approach; we refer to this as suggestive evidence of effectiveness. In other cases, however, the causal connection is less plausible than other explanations for any association that exists, and so the evidence is too weak to support a conclusion or recommendation.

Empirical evidence, even of the associational kind, is not always available. However, this does not mean that a scientific judgment is not possible. In some cases, a conclusion or recommendation may be based on a formal, theoretically based, logical analysis of a phenomenon or empirical evidence in analogous domains. Finally, some conclusions or recommendations derive from the scientific judgment of the committee based on the members' experience and deliberation.

CONNECTING EVIDENCE AND STRATEGY

Reaching a judgment about whether or not a particular intervention is likely to be effective in relation to a particular outcome is only one step on the way to formulating a judgment about whether such an intervention is likely to be cost-effective and whether it should be a component of a strategy to prevent or reduce underage drinking. Inevitably, connecting the dots between evidence and policy requires a contextual judgment. How strong does the evidence bearing on effectiveness have to be to justify an intervention of this particular type in light of its likely range of costs? In making these judgments and designing the proposed strategy, the committee has been guided by several general considerations:

- In dealing with complex social phenomena, such as underage drinking, comprehensive, multipronged strategies usually work best. As we note above, one of the reasons to embrace a portfolio approach is to capture the synergistic effects of coordinated and reinforcing interventions. Moreover, although any one intervention may produce no effect at all or an effect too small to detect, it might make an important contribution to a multipronged strategy.

- It is necessary to distinguish between what is possible and what is likely. This distinction has two parts. One is between efficacy (what can be achieved in an experimental design?) and effectiveness (what can be achieved in the real world?) The second involves implementation. An intervention may be effective in a real-world context when it is carried out in faithful conformity with the recommended protocol, but not otherwise, or the effects may vary widely in relation to the quality of implementation. Whether a particular intervention should be included in a national strategy must depend on a judgment about implementation—how often would it be deployed effectively and with what cumulative effect—and whether that effect is worth the cost.

- One must carefully consider the risk that an intervention will produce a harmful effect. Some interventions may have a perverse effect—in the context of underage drinking, perhaps a media campaign or a school-based education program could have a boomerang effect that stimulates alcohol use rather than depressing it. This risk may be especially great if a program with proven effectiveness with a specific group is implemented for another group or is poorly implemented. Moreover, an intervention that is effective overall may have widely varying results for subpopulations, including harmful outcomes for some of them. This possibility raises an important ethical concern in balancing benefits and risks. The committee has been sensitive to any evidence that an intervention presents a risk of harm to any youth subgroup and suggests ways of reducing such risks when they might exist.

- Specific evidence of effectiveness for refinements of an intervention known to be effective and for which investments have already been made (e.g., limiting access) is not required. Because it is rarely possible, at this time, to quantify either the anticipated benefits or costs of proposed interventions, most of the committee's recommendations are based on qualitative judgments about likely cost-effectiveness.

UNDERAGE DRINKING AND LEGAL DRINKING

In designing the strategy, the committee also had to consider the extent to which the problem of underage drinking can be separated from the larger context of drinking in the general population. As noted in Chapter 4, the level and patterns of adult drinking importantly affect the level of underage drinking in the society. For example, the level of adult drinking determines how many liquor stores and bars exist in a particular area, how much alcohol is in home drinking cabinets, and, therefore, how conveniently available alcohol is to underage drinkers. The level of adult drinking also has a big effect on the level of advertising for alcohol products and, therefore, on the prevalence of mass media messages that expose young people to images and ideas about the virtues of drinking and also on the credibility of parents and others seeking to discourage it. The fact that the level and patterns of adult drinking shape the level and character of underage drinking in the society creates two important issues and concerns in relation to our charge.

First, given the potential influence of the adult drinking patterns on underage drinking, it is possible that the adult patterns sharply limit how much underage drinking can be reduced without also doing something to affect the adult drinking. The issue is the degree to which the problem of underage drinking can be disentangled or disaggregated from the overall pattern of drinking in the society. One possibility is that the level of underage drinking is nearly always more or less proportional to all drinking in the society: if adult drinking changes, underage drinking changes; if adult drinking does not change, underage drinking does not change very much, even with specific policies that try to discourage underage drinking while leaving adult drinking untouched. The implication of this analysis is that the only effective way to reduce underage drinking is to reduce the level of adult drinking; it would accordingly raise complex questions about the strength of the public commitment to reduce underage drinking. Another possibility is that the two phenomena are at least partly separable, that can have policies that focus explicitly on underage drinking that can be strong enough to produce a separate effect on underage drinking even when the aggregate patterns of adult drinking do not change.

Ultimately, the separability of underage drinking from general drinking patterns is an empirical question. The only way to answer the question definitively is by trying policies that are specific to underage drinking and measure their effects for prevention and reduction. However, as indicated in Chapter 4, the available evidence shows that the level of underage drinking does seem to be strongly linked to the level of adult drinking, and the level of adult drinking—at the very least—probably places clear upper bounds on the effectiveness of any given set of policies to control underage drinking. This evidence highlights the challenge, to which we referred in Chapter 1, of trying to suppress underage drinking in a culture in which drinking is normative behavior.

The relationship between underage drinking and adult drinking is relevant to our charge for a second reason. Since the level of adult drinking might be an important determinant of underage drinking, it is at least logically possible that the most "cost-effective strategy to reduce underage drinking" includes policies that produce their main effects not on underage drinking, but rather on the overall level of drinking in the population. The question to be faced, then, is whether to construe our mandate (to propose a cost-effective strategy to reduce and prevent underage drinking) as including: a review of *all* policy instruments that could produce an effect on underage drinking, including those that are not directed specifically at underage drinking, such as taxes and other general policies affecting price and availability, or a review only of policy instruments that are specific to underage drinking, such as the enforcement of laws prohibiting underage drinking, or the development of special media campaigns targeted only on underage drinking, or the strict regulation of venues in which underage drinking is most likely to occur.

The committee decided that it would focus on policies specifically aimed at underage drinking, but that it would not close its eyes, categorically, to policies that affect all drinking. Instead, we have carefully reviewed the evidence regarding the effects of *general* alcohol policies on underage drinking and have included in our proposed strategy one of these general components (raising excise taxes) because a substantial increase can be expected to have a robust impact on underage drinking and can also strengthen the nation's capacity to implement a strategy aiming to reduce underage drinking.

DO WE REALLY NEED A NEW STRATEGY?

Some people have argued that recent declines in underage drinking negate the need for significant new interventions. As noted in Chapter 2, the prevalence of alcohol use in the past 30 days among high school seniors has declined from a high of about 72 percent in 1979 to about 49 percent in 2002; similarly, the prevalence of heavy drinking within the past 2 weeks has declined from a high of 41 percent in 1981 to about 29 percent in 2002. The proportion of youth fatalities involving alcohol-involved underage drivers has also declined, from 55.8 percent in 1982 to 30.1 percent in 2000, although there has been little change in recent years (National Highway

Traffic Safety Administration, 2002). Nonetheless, most people acknowledge that these prevalence rates for underage alcohol use are still too high and that the adverse consequences of underage drinking are enormous, as discussed in Chapter 3. The 30-day prevalence rates have hovered at approximately 50 percent throughout the 1990s, and the patterns have been similar for rates of heavy use and daily drinking.

Thus, there has *not* been a steady decline in underage drinking over the past two decades. Instead, the decline in the prevalence of underage drinking was limited to the period from around 1981 to 1992, and the rates have been relatively stable since then. To explain this period, we can identify three things: a parallel decline in use of illegal drugs, a raise from 18 to 21 in the minimum drinking age across the country, and intensive campaigns to discourage drinking and driving and to encourage use of designated drivers. Peak use in the late 1970s and early 1980s may also be partly explained by the overall culture of youth experimentation in the United States in the 1960s and 1970s, and conversely, changes in the youth culture in the 1980s may have contributed to decreased use of alcohol, as well as illegal drugs. Economic conditions during the 1980s, with reduced resources available to youth, may also have contributed to the marked decrease in drinking.

Substantial evidence suggests that changes in the minimum drinking age laws also contributed to the decline in alcohol use during the 1980s. As noted in Chapter 1, between 1970 and 1976, 21 states reduced the minimum drinking age to 18, and another 8 states reduced it to 19 or 20; however, states began to raise the minimum age to 21 in the late 1970s. By 1984, when the Minimum Drinking Age Act was passed, 23 states had such laws in place. All states had minimum drinking age laws in place by 1988. This trend in implementation of minimum drinking age laws mirrors the national trend in declining alcohol prevalence among youth. Furthermore, research demonstrates a clear relationship between increases in the minimum drinking age and reduced rates of drinking (Wagenaar, 1981; Wagenaar and Maybee, 1986; O'Malley and Wagenaar, 1991; Klepp et al., 1996; Yu et al., 1997). Finally, O'Malley and Johnston (1999), while acknowledging the role of minimum drinking age laws, postulate that other initiatives, such as "zero tolerance" laws and national campaigns aimed at discouraging drunk driving, may also have contributed to the reduction. They observe that these campaigns peaked during a time of the decline in drinking.

In the committee's judgment, the salient lesson in these trend data is that the decline in underage drinking prevalence in the 1980s is largely attributable to specific interventions, including the increase in the minimum drinking age—perhaps supplemented by a secular decline in substance abuse and the grassroots campaign against drunk driving. We believe that decreases in prevalence did not continue into the 1990s because the immediate declarative effect of raising the drinking age had been exhausted by 1992 and media attention to drinking had abated.

There have been modest reductions in the 30-day and annual prevalence rates among high school seniors for the past 5 years. However, current rates are not significantly different than they were in 1993 and remain disturbingly high. Nearly half (48.6 percent) of high school seniors report drinking in the past 30 days—the same proportion as 1993, and significantly more than the proportion of youth that report either using marijuana (21.5 percent) or smoking (26.7 percent) in the past 30 days. The proportion of twelfth graders who report heavy drinking in the past 2 weeks declined slightly over the past several years, but was still higher (28.6 percent) in 2002 than it had been in 1993 (27.5 percent).

Thus, rates have remained essentially stable during the past decade despite a variety of efforts to address underage drinking. Many school districts have offered classroom interventions, the alcohol industry has included a "drink responsibly" message in many of its ads and implemented a variety of other programs, various state and national agencies and non-profit organizations have implemented interventions aimed at reducing use and have developed and disseminated a variety of informational materials, and grassroots community organizations have carried out diverse efforts. Absent some new intervention, there is no reason to expect any further substantial decline. The problem of underage drinking in the United States is endemic and, in the committee's judgment, is not likely to improve in the absence of a significant new intervention.

THE STRATEGY

In the following chapters, the committee details the major components of a cost-effective strategy to prevent and reduce underage drinking. The premises of the proposed strategy, its blueprint, and its key components are summarized here.

Premises

The committee's proposed strategy is based on three premises:

• Because alcohol use among *adults* is widespread, legally acceptable and deeply embedded in U.S. culture, youths receive mixed messages about the acceptability of underage drinking despite the fact that it is illegal. The proper message is that alcohol use by persons under 21 is both illegal and socially disapproved. A variety of institutions can play a role in establishing and sustaining a normative distinction that will reinforce the legal distinction between underage and adult drinking. Of special importance in this effort are parents, the alcohol industry, schools and other institutions that are responsible for adolescents, the media, and the entertainment industry.

• Although governments at all levels have an indispensable role to play in creating this boundary and in supporting actions to reduce underage drinking, voluntary initiatives taken by individuals and nongovernmental institutions are also of great importance.

• Although underage drinking is a national problem, and it must be addressed by the nation, much of the initiative must arise, and much of the work be accomplished, at the community level.

Blueprint

The preeminent goal of the recommended strategy is to animate and sustain a broad commitment to reduce underage drinking. Many actors can play important roles. Retail outlets and bars can reduce opportunities for young people to obtain and use alcohol. Parents and other adults can refrain from conduct that tends to encourage or facilitate underage drinking and use their authority and credibility to guide their children's choices about alcohol. Others who stand in the position of responsibility vis-à-vis young people—schools, landlords, employers with young employees, military commanders, and other community organization and business leaders—can contribute in a variety of ways to the community effort to prevent underage drinking and its associated harms.

Underage alcohol use, as we have said, is a pervasive problem. It follows, then, that numerous individuals and organizations are in a position to try to do something about it. Figure 5-1 depicts a schematic diagram depicting opportunities for intervention. Opportunities for effectuating a collective commitment can be sorted into three broad domains:

• Opportunities to reduce the *availability* of alcohol to underage drinkers (or to avoid practices that tend to increase availability).

• Opportunities to reduce the *occasions* and opportunities for underage drinking (or to avoid practices that tend to facilitate drinking opportunities).

• Opportunities to reduce the *demand* for alcohol among young people (or to avoid practices that tend to increase demand).

Availability

The major actors in any effort to reduce underage access to alcohol are the people and businesses engaged in the commercial production and distribution of alcohol: producers and importers of alcoholic beverages, whole-

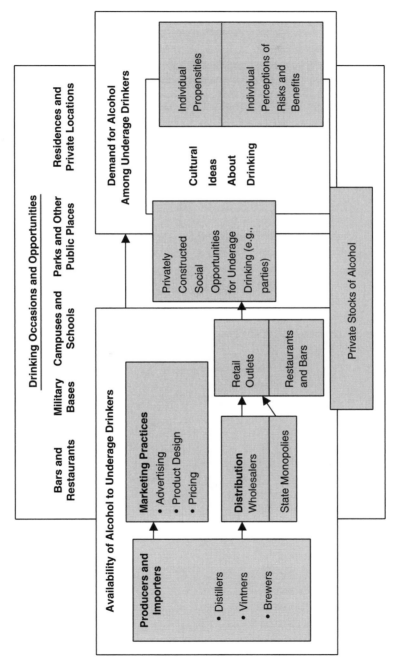

FIGURE 5-1 Opportunities for interventions in underage drinking: Occasions and opportunities; availability and demand.

salers, and retail distributors. In some states, some of these actors are government agencies. In principle, state control over distribution provides an opportunity for the state to achieve important social goals other than maximizing sale of alcoholic beverages, including keeping alcohol out of the hands of underage drinkers. It is also worth noting that an important source of supply to underage drinkers is not the commercial sector; instead, it is the diversion of alcohol from stocks kept in private homes to support adult drinking. Efforts to reduce underage access to alcohol are grounded in a legal prohibition, and the committee makes a variety of recommendations to strengthen this legal foundation and to increase the effectiveness of enforcement. However, given the diverse sources of supply to underage drinkers, it must be emphasized that the law cannot carry the weight of this obligation alone; it must be accompanied and reinforced by a genuine commitment to reduce underage drinking among these businesses and among parents.

Occasions

Responsibility for reducing drinking opportunities for young people, a distinctly practical task in everyday life, rests again with both commercial and noncommercial actors. Bars, taverns, public houses, restaurants, and other businesses that create opportunities for people to drink have an important responsibility to ensure that underage drinking does not occur. In addition, parents, schools, landlords, and everyone else with legal control over premises in which young people drink also have an obligation to take appropriate actions. Parents should not sponsor or facilitate underage drinking parties in the home on the assumption that "it will occur anyway" and that parental supervision can reduce the risks. Schools should work with community organizations to prevent drinking parties and to create alternatives. Local governments should develop strategies for preventing public parks and other public facilities from being used for underage drinking. Landlords who rent property to underage tenants should include lease provisions making drinking parties grounds for termination. Colleges and military installations have unique obligations in this context because such a large number of underage people in these settings are among slightly older peers.

Demand

Responsibility for reducing underage "demand" for alcohol and for teaching about acceptable drinking practices is generally thought to rest largely, if not exclusively, with parents and schools—perhaps supplemented by public service media messages funded by the government and private foundations. In the committee's view, however, responsibility for reducing underage demand for alcohol is much more widely dispersed. Alcohol producers and advertisers have a special responsibility to resist marketing initiatives whose effects may be to stimulate or reinforce youthful desires to drink. Many alcohol companies have accepted the responsibility to support prevention initiatives designed to counteract the strong commercial forces tending to encourage underage drinking, and the committee makes several recommendations to build on this foundation. Responsibility for reducing underage demand for alcohol also rests with the entertainment media who command so much of the time and attention of the nation's youth—these media exposures offer opportunities either to stimulate or reinforce youthful demand for alcohol or to reduce it. At a local level, schools, colleges and universities, healthcare providers, and other organizations are in a position to influence the drinking habits of young people; the good will and energies of individuals and community organizations need to be more effectively harnessed. Table 5-1 summarizes the collective responsibilities of the full array of individuals and organizations in a position to reduce underage drinking.

Key Components

Within this broad framework the committee has identified ten core components of the proposed strategy to reduce underage drinking:

- a national media campaign designed to animate and sustain a broad, deep, societal commitment to reduce underage drinking, to muster support for actions aiming to reduce underage drinking, and to encourage parents and other adults to refrain from conduct tending to encourage or facilitate underage drinking (see Chapter 6);
- a meaningful commitment by the alcohol industry to contribute to this effort by helping to establish and fund an independent, nonprofit organization to support programs to reduce underage drinking (see Chapter 7);
- self-restraint in marketing and strengthened self-regulation by the alcohol industry to reduce youth exposure to alcohol advertising (see Chapter 7);
- a meaningful commitment by the entertainment industry, especially the music recording industry, to avoid images and lyrics that tend to encourage drinking in products that are likely to be heard or viewed by predominately underage audiences (see Chapter 8);
- stronger restrictions on youth access to alcohol in both commercial and noncommercial settings, and intensified enforcement of these laws by state and local governments (see Chapter 9);

TABLE 5-1 Reducing Underage Drinking: A Collective Responsibility

Responsible Party	Reduce Availability	Reduce Demand	Reduce Drinking Occasions
Alcohol producers and importers	x	x	
Wholesalers	x	x	
Retail outlets	x		x
Restaurants and bars	x		x
Entertainment media		x	
Schools		x	x
Colleges/universities	x	x	x
Youth employers		x	
Military bases	x	x	x
Landlords			x
Community organizations	x	x	x
Parents and other adults	x	x	x
Peers and friends	x	x	x

• expansion of educational, counseling, and treatment programs of proven effectiveness in elementary and secondary schools, colleges and universities, and in other settings where natural opportunities arise to discourage underage drinking and assist young people with drinking problems (see Chapter 10);

• mobilization of communities to design and implement multipronged, comprehensive programs to prevent and reduce underage drinking (see Chapter 11);

• a commitment by the federal government to implement a national strategy to prevent and reduce underage drinking, to provide stable funding and technical assistance, and to mount the necessary surveys to monitor its effectiveness, and an analogous commitment by state governments to establish and fund the necessary infrastructure to implement state-based components of the strategy, such as enforcing access restrictions (see Chapter 12);

• increases in federal and state excise taxes on alcohol to help reduce underage consumption, reflect the social costs of drinking, and raise revenue for implementing the proposed strategy (see Chapter 12); and

• rigorous research and evaluation to assess the effectiveness of current interventions, to help design new ones, and to facilitate refinements of the strategy and its implementation (see Chapter 12).

The committee strongly endorses what it finds are compelling arguments for a multipronged strategy and believes the effectiveness of its proposed strategy for reducing underage drinking will be enhanced if the components are pursued simultaneously. However, we do not view the proposed strategy as an "all or none" proposition. In fact, implementation of the strategy requires the involvement of a range of decision makers from a variety of settings and levels of government, all of whom will be acting on different timetables with different constraints. Action on any one component should not be regarded as contingent on simultaneous action on any or all of the other components of our proposed strategy.

6

National Media Campaign

The committee was asked, particularly, to consider the role of a national media campaign in preventing and reducing underage drinking. As indicated in Chapter 1, we considered two mass media campaign approaches to affect youth alcohol consumption: a campaign directed primarily at youth, to affect their drinking decisions, and a campaign directed to parents and other adults who influence youth. On the basis of our review of the current evidence, we believe that an adult-oriented campaign holds more promise than a campaign directed at youth. Although there is limited direct evidence of effectiveness for either type of campaign, there is a clear and strong logical foundation for an adult campaign given the facilitative role of adult behavior in underage drinking and the potential preventive effect of parental monitoring. This logical argument is also strongly bolstered by the evidence of effectiveness of media campaigns in related public health areas. In the committee's judgment, this body of evidence provides reason for optimism regarding the potential effectiveness of an adult-oriented campaign on underage drinking and is sufficient to support a presumptive commitment to launch such a campaign after a carefully designed developmental phase. Our assessment of the possible effectiveness of a youth-focused campaign is presented in Chapter 10. In this chapter we address the adult-oriented campaign.

> Recommendation 6-1: The federal government should fund and actively support the development of a national media effort, as a major component of an adult-oriented campaign to reduce underage drinking.

The goals of the national media campaign would be to instill a broad societal commitment to reduce underage drinking, to increase specific actions by adults that are meant to discourage or inhibit underage drinking, and to decrease adult conduct that tends to facilitate underage drinking.

Such a campaign would be undertaken in the context of a comprehensive, society-wide effort to address underage drinking through the other mechanisms described in this volume. Those efforts could and should be undertaken while the media campaign is being developed. In this chapter we describe the underlying logic for the approach, what the campaign would look like, evidence concerning its promise, and its possible strengths and weaknesses. We conclude by outlining the developmental approach we propose. We believe that the development of an adult-oriented campaign warrants a substantial investment if its promise of effectiveness is borne out during the developmental period.

ADULT ATTITUDES AND KNOWLEDGE ABOUT UNDERAGE DRINKING

Attitudes

Many groups concerned with underage drinking claim that societal acceptance of, or at least ambivalence toward such drinking, reflected both in expressed attitudes and in the actions of many adults in facilitating underage drinking, is a substantial cause for such drinking (see National Center on Addiction and Substance Abuse [CASA], 2002). Yet, when asked, the great majority of adults express concern about underage drinking. For example 84 percent of respondents to the 2001 survey undertaken by CASA said that underage drinking was either "a big problem" or "somewhat of a problem" in their community, and 92 percent said they were personally "somewhat" or "very much concerned" with underage alcohol use. That survey also shows widespread support for many public policy actions, with 83 percent favoring regulation of location of alcohol outlets near school, and 78 percent, 71 percent, and 69 percent supporting undercover compliance checks, "cops in shops" checks, and "shoulder tap" checks, respectively, to reduce alcohol outlet sales to underage youth.

Despite the high level of expressed adult concern, most underage drinking requires involvement by some adults—in selling the alcohol to youth, in purchasing it on behalf of youth, or in permitting minors to have parties in their homes where alcohol is served. Obviously, many adults are not taking proper precautions to restrict underage drinking, and often facilitate it in violation of the law. And even if adults do not supply alcohol to minors directly, underage drinking is tacitly supported by many adults—such as parents who view youth drinking as an inevitable part of adolescence and do not respond to it, or who do not make sure that parties their children attend are alcohol free and properly supervised by adults. Even though adults tend to favor some strong measures to prevent underage drinking, the CASA study suggests that they are least enthusiastic about regulations that would affect them directly: only 60 percent favor restriction on the number of alcohol outlets, and 51 percent favor limitations on outlet days or hours. The reluctance of policy makers to enact alcohol restrictions that might reduce youth use but also affects adult use (such as controlling outlets) presumably reflects, in some part, perception of the lack of public support for such restrictions.

Adults themselves do not think that parents are doing all that they can do to prevent underage drinking. There is substantial recognition by adults that parents are the most important channel of influence on their children's underage drinking. When asked to choose what was most responsible for "preventing us from effectively reducing underage drinking" more than half of the adult respondents said "lack of or limited parental involvement in teens' lives" (see Table 6-1). This response indicates that there is another way that adult behavior may support underage drinking in addition to explicit or tacit support for alcohol use, which involves ineffective parenting more generally.

The parenting literature argues that effective parenting includes monitoring and supervising youth behavior. For younger adolescents, this parenting includes such things as: knowing who a child's friends are, making sure that children are always supervised by adults, knowing what a child's plans are for the coming day, knowing what children are doing

TABLE 6-1 Adults' Reports of Barriers to Reducing Underage Drinking (in percent)

Which of *(the following)* are most responsible for preventing us from effectively reducing underage drinking? (N = 900)

Barrier	Percent
Lack of limited parental involvement in teens' lives	52
Ineffective enforcement of current laws or regulations	19
Lack of effective prevention programs	7
The media	7
Insufficient laws or regulations	6
Alcohol advertisements	4
Lack of effective treatment programs	3
Other	3

SOURCE: Data from Roper Center at the University of Connecticut (2003a).

when away from home, and enforcing evening curfews. It also includes engagement with children's lives, including doing projects and activities with them, and the use of appropriate punishments for misbehavior and rewards for positive behavior. There is good evidence that such parenting is associated with a reduced risk of using all substances, including alcohol (see Chapter 4). A recent national longitudinal survey of parents and their 9- to 18-year-old children supports this claim. Children of parents who were relatively high on a supervision and monitoring scale were compared with children of parents who were low on the monitoring scale. Less monitored youth were more likely, subsequently, to progress to alcohol consumption in the next 12 to 18 months, and if they were already drinkers, were more likely to continue drinking.[1]

Knowledge

There is significant evidence that parents are unaware of the extent and riskiness of youth drinking. The national longitudinal survey mentioned above compared reports of alcohol use among youth aged 12 to 18 with their parents' perception of their alcohol use. Both parents and their children were asked about whether or not the child had used alcohol, more than a few sips, in the previous 12 months. Overall, parents moderately underestimated what their children reported as use: for 12- to 13-year-olds, the parents thought that 7 percent had used alcohol, but 11 percent of their children said they did; for 14- to 15-year-olds, the comparable numbers were 21 percent and 33 percent; and for 16- to 18-year-olds, the numbers were 44 percent and 56 percent.

An even more telling way to look at these data is to turn them around and ask how often parents knew when their own child was drinking. Including all of the children from 12 to 18 years old, 44 percent of all the youth who had had drinks in the past year were described by their parents as nondrinkers. Moreover, 31 percent of the youth who said they had been drunk in the past year were said by their parent to be nondrinkers, and 27 percent of those who said they had had five or more drinks in the past month were said by their parents to be nondrinkers. While a majority of parents may know whether or not their children drink, there is a substantial fraction who do not, even when their children admit to recent heavy drinking (see also Sieving, 1997; Beck et al., 1995).

A 1998 study by Bogenschneider and colleagues found that less than one-third of parents (29 percent of mothers and 31 percent of fathers) were

---

[1]Based on analysis by Robert Hornik of unpublished data collected by Westat for the National Institute on Drug Abuse for the evaluation of the Office of National Drug Control Policy's national youth antidrug media campaign.

TABLE 6-2 Parents' and Teenagers' Reports of Alcohol Use (in percent)

Alcohol Use	Parents	Teenagers
Has had more than a few sips in their life	17.0	65.2
Has been drinking in the past month	2.4	37.6
Has had five or more drinks in the past 2 weeks	1.0	20.4

NOTE: Two separate surveys were conducted; parents surveyed were not necessarily the parents of the teenagers surveyed.
SOURCE: Data from Strategic Marketing Services (2002).

aware of their adolescents' drinking even though all of the adolescents reported using alcohol at least once in the past month.[2] Parents were more likely to report use by their adolescents' close friends than by their own children. More than one-half of parents (56 percent of both mothers and fathers) reported that they were not sure or thought it was likely that their children's close friends use alcohol.

Bogenschneider and colleagues also found that adolescent children of aware parents were *more* likely to drink and drive than adolescent children of unaware parents. In response to these unanticipated results, the researchers postulated "episodes of drinking and driving serve to alert parents to the possibility that their offspring use alcohol" (1998:369). If this hypothesis is true, parents become aware of their children's drinking after they have engaged in a risky behavior.

Additional evidence that parents are not aware of teenage drinking comes from two surveys conducted by the state of Maine: one of parents of teenagers and the other of teenagers.[3] Although more than half of the parents surveyed (55.6 percent) reported that they are more concerned about teenage use of alcohol than tobacco, marijuana, other illegal drugs, or prescription drugs, these parents greatly underestimate the extent to which eighth to twelfth graders drink alcohol (Strategic Marketing Services, 2002). Table 6-2 presents the differences between the reports of the parents and the teenagers. The discrepancy between parent and youth reports is particularly notable for heavy drinking: although nearly all parents (99 percent) reported that they did not think their children had had five or more

---

[2]Awareness was defined as being unsure or believing that their adolescents' alcohol use was likely.

[3]The parents included in the parent survey were not necessarily the parents of the teens included in the teen survey.

drinks in the past 2 weeks, one in five youth (20 percent) reported having done so at least once.

While the majority of parents (56 percent) in the Maine Survey reported having serious talks about alcohol with their child several times a year, only slightly more than a third (34.2 percent) said that they had these discussions once a month or more. Not surprisingly, drinking and driving was the most common topic discussed, with 71 percent of parents reporting that they discussed this issue. Other primary topics, though less common, included the effects of alcohol on judgment or decision making (50.7 percent), peer pressure (48.9 percent), negative medical effects of alcohol (34.9 percent), and parental feelings about underage drinking (34.1 percent).

Clearly, many parents do not know when their children are drinking. However, even if the parents know their children are drinking, there is a question of whether they see underage alcohol consumption as risky. The evidence concerning whether or not parents perceive risks in underage drinking comes from the study by CASA (2002). In Table 6-3, we present the proportion of adult respondents who indicated that each of the named consequences of underage drinking was a concern.

There are two ways to read Table 6-3. One perspective notes that a majority of adults recognize every potential risk as a matter of concern. This is reinforced by the finding that, at most, only 14 percent of the respondents indicated that any of the potential consequences was not a concern at all. This view emphasizes that people recognize the risks. An alternative perspective notes the minimal discrimination among the various consequences. This lack of discrimination among consequences suggests

TABLE 6-3 Adult Reports of Concern for Potential Consequences of Underage Drinking (in percent) (N = 900)

Potential Consequence	Level of Concern		
	Very Much	Somewhat	Not at All
Delinquency or criminal behavior	64	30	6
Risk of sexual behavior	64	28	8
Risk of developing alcoholism or dependence	62	31	8
Gateway to illicit drug use	57	28	14
Physical health	55	36	9
Emotional or social consequences	54	37	9
Financial cost to society	53	39	8
Academic or work problems	53	38	10

SOURCE: Data from Roper Center at the University of Connecticut (2003b).

that the respondents have not thought about the consequences seriously and suggests that adults only recognize the risks in a rote fashion, when primed.

CAMPAIGN GOAL AND LOGIC

The primary role of a societal, adult-oriented media campaign would be to convince parents and other adults not merely that there is a general problem with underage drinking in their communities, an idea that they appear to accept already, but also that it is very likely a problem for their own children and their children's friends, that there are important negative consequences of such alcohol use besides those risks associated with drinking and driving, and that they have an obligation to their children and the community to do something about it. The campaign would argue that by taking specific personal actions to prevent underage alcohol use, by increasing recommended parenting behaviors, and by support of community-level policies, parents and other adults can affect underage drinking and reduce its bad consequences.

The campaign rests on five assumptions:

- Many parents do not recognize either the prevalence of or the many risks associated with underage drinking for their own children.
- Many parents effectively facilitate their underage children's drinking by giving youth access to alcohol, by not responding to known incidents of children's drinking, and by not adequately monitoring and supervising their children's lives, generally.
- If parents changed their beliefs about the nature of underage alcohol use and its consequences, they would increase monitoring and other actions to limit their children's use.
- Because many underage drinkers obtain their alcohol from adult acquaintances or even strangers, if adults' willingness to buy alcohol for young people or to facilitate their drinking decreases, it would be more difficult for underage youths to obtain or use alcohol.
- If parents and other adults increased monitoring and other actions aiming to limit use, there would be a reduction in underage drinking, particularly heavy drinking.

What are the arguments in favor of such an adult-oriented campaign? One argument is that campaigns that offer new information are more promising than campaigns that revisit information that already has been widely distributed. Youth have often heard anti-alcohol messages addressed to them, but they have shown little change in recent years in most drinking behavior, although they have been somewhat responsive to the drinking and driving message (see below). A new youth-focused campaign would be seen as old hat and redundant with what they are already hearing. In contrast, an adult-oriented campaign would present new messages. It would target parents and other adults, who are now facilitating youth alcohol use because they are not sufficiently aware of the problem for their children; not aware of the many harmful consequences of youth alcohol use; not aware that actions they take can affect the risks; and not aware that buying alcohol for underage persons or giving it to them, is socially irresponsible and usually illegal. For adults, in contrast with youth, there is the possibility of a communication program diffusing new information, which suggests greater effectiveness. In addition, it is possible that an adult-focused campaign may work to make what parents already believe more salient to them as they consider their actions to restrict their children's alcohol access. Effectively, a campaign can give them permission to act on the concerns they already have.

POTENTIAL EFFECTIVENESS

Disseminating Facts

An important question is what evidence is available that a large-scale communication campaign could affect awareness of extent and riskiness, and (assuming that such knowledge leads to motivation to act) teach effective actions (for review, see Atkin, 2004).

There have been a small number of campaigns that tried to affect adult awareness of the extent and perceived riskiness of underage drinking and parental actions to reduce underage drinking, but they do not provide a solid foundation for estimating the promise for this approach. For example, the Australian National Alcohol Campaign in 2000 and 2001 primarily addressed youth, with some magazine advertising and brochure distribution to parents. However, the parent component was probably too small to expect much effect, and the evaluation information for parents does not provide an adequate basis for determining its behavioral effect (Ball et al., 2002). We then turn to less direct evidence that such a campaign will influence parent knowledge and behavior, relying on a reasonable generalization of evidence from other programs. In some sense, it is possible to separate two aspects of such a campaign and ask about the availability of evidence for each.

Insofar as an adult-focused campaign is only presenting facts, not previously known by parents, there is good evidence that this can be accomplished readily. Diffusing facts is what communication programs do well.

There are many examples of diffusion of a new idea or set of facts through mass media. And there are some examples that suggest circumstances when simple diffusion of new facts was sufficient to produce behavior change. In one clear case, campaigns to encourage parents to put their infants to sleep on their backs to avoid sudden infant death syndrome have had fairly quick and widespread success (Willinger et al., 2000; Engelberts et al., 1991). This behavior required a small change by parents and the changed sleeping position promised to avoid a dreaded consequence. Of most relevance for this discussion, the value of the back sleeping position represented new information for most parents.

Closer to the alcohol area, the idea of the "designated driver" diffused rapidly in the United States. The first mention of the term in the Lexis-Nexis electronic news major papers database is the fall of 1982, which is presumably when it was introduced to public discussion. By 1987, 91 percent of the respondents to a Gallup Poll indicated they approved of the idea (Roper Center at the University of Connecticut, 1987). By 1988, the term could be used in questions without a parenthetical definition, suggesting that it was well known. The proportion of adults who reported using designated drivers also grew rapidly (Roper Center at the University of Connecticut, 1988; see also Winsten, 1994).

In terms of diffusing facts, the major issue is not whether it can be done, but whether a comprehensible and credible message can be transmitted with sufficient reach and frequency so that most people become aware of it and whether the particular facts encourage behavior change.[4]

Changing Behavior?

The more difficult claim to support is not whether a mass media campaign can diffuse facts but whether it can effectively teach and, most important, influence specific new behaviors by adults. We do not know of any studies of a specific intervention of this sort relating to alcohol. The closest published example comes from Project Northland (Perry et al., 2002), which used only community-level media, along with other community activities, to try and affect parenting norms and behaviors. That limited intervention showed little effect on parental attitudes or behavior (although, as we discuss in Chapter 10, the initiative overall provides evidence for positive effects on youth). However, like the Australian campaign described above, Project Northland is a much more limited program than we propose, which

---

[4]We recognize that any message encouraging parents to recognize that many children drink has the risk of containing an additional implied message: that all kids drink so maybe it is not a big concern. It will be important to test messages for parents to make sure they do not hear such a mixed message.

would involve a national focus, heavy use of mass media, and involvement of the alcohol industry and other important institutions.

There is evidence that mass media campaigns, usually combining publicity and law enforcement, have succeeded in influencing drinking and driving (Murray, 1991; Bierness et al., 2000; Voas et al., 1997; Nienstedt, 1990; Hurst and Wright, 1981; Cameron and Newstead, 1996; Tay, 2000). There is also evidence that campaigns have influenced the use of designated drivers (Winsten, 1994; Dejong and Hingson, 1998; Boots and Midford, 1999; Hingson et al., 1996).

Although there have been many campaigns to affect adult drinking behavior (other than driving), they have generally been understudied. For example, the National Institute on Alcohol Abuse and Alcoholism sponsored campaigns in 1971-1972, and in 1980-1982, and there is some published information about regular campaigns about drinking in Denmark from 1990 to 1996 (Strunge, 1998) and about single campaigns in other places. However the evaluations of those campaigns are weaker than those addressing drunk driving, and they often do not measure behavior or have credible comparison groups.[5] In any case, these results, even the favorable ones about drunk driving, are not the same as evidence that parenting behaviors concerning their children's alcohol use can be affected. We recognize that in contrast to these other campaigns, the recommended campaign does not focus on a single behavior, nor does it focus on specific changes in adults' own behavior with regard to alcohol use. It urges parents and other adults to accept and act on a broad social norm, and it therefore has a longer time horizon than many of these more focused campaigns.

Although the available evidence bearing on the effectiveness of an adult-oriented campaign is modest, the committee is reasonably optimistic about the potential value of such a campaign, for two reasons. First, there is associational evidence that periods of broad national campaigns incorporating a variety of channels and institutional change efforts have been matched by periods of reductions in risky behavior. Those examples include the National High Blood Pressure Campaign from 1972 to 1984 (Roccella, 2002), the anti-tobacco efforts of the late 1960s-early 1970s (Warner, 1981) and the late 1990s-early 2000s (Siegel, 2002), and the anti-drug campaigns of the middle 1980s (Institute of Medicine, 2002).

---

[5]The best evaluated of these, the winners campaign in California (Wallack and Barrows, 1982), showed some differences in levels of exposure between control and mass media communities and some hints about attitude difference, but none suggesting behavior change. However, the authors of the evaluation caution against generalizing too much from the results since they indicate how far the realized program departed from the proposed intervention.

Second, there is particularly strong evidence for the positive effects of media campaigns, which are able to link communication efforts with enforcement. The drinking and driving efforts described above were successful when they were able to link their messages to a specific expectation of enforcement. Similarly, seat belt use has climbed quickly when media publicity is linked to enforcement (Williams et al., 1996). Indeed one meta-analysis of the literature concludes that the largest effects evident in the mass media campaign literature come from campaigns which link media publicity with enforcement (Snyder and Hamilton, 2002).

Also pertinent to this aspect of the proposed campaign, both for parents and other adults, is the literature on compliance with the law. A central theme in the proposed campaign is that facilitating underage drinking is not only socially irresponsible but also illegal in most situations. Deterrence—through the threat of criminal prosecution or of civil liability for any injuries to third parties—can be part of the message, but the more powerful mechanism may be through the "expressive" or "declarative" function of the law, the mechanism through which the law registers social disapproval, teaches that the behavior is perhaps more dangerous than may have been appreciated, and thereby instills or reinforces the desired social norm. The mechanism here is not fear, but rather a powerful form of instruction drawing on the general desire to comply with legal rules (see Bonnie, 1985; Tyler, 1992; Tyler and Huo, 2002).

This discussion has focused on intervening with parents and other adults in ways that encourage their active prevention of underage drinking specifically. However, there is a second route of intervention with parents that might well be incorporated into the proposed campaign. Evidence shows that the extent of supervision and monitoring by parents of youth, in general, affects youth initiation of risky behaviors and that intensive individual or group parent counseling can affect parenting behavior and, in turn, youth risk behaviors, including alcohol consumption (Taylor and Biglan, 1998; Dishion and Andrews, 1995; Dishion et al., 2002). So a reasonable argument has been made that it would be worthwhile to attempt to communicate about new parenting behaviors, particularly through the use of advertising.

The Office of National Drug Control Policy (ONDCP) took this task on as a complement to its youth-focused campaign, described in Chapter 10. It dedicated nearly an equal amount of its ad campaign to parenting skills, particularly encouraging the close monitoring of children by parents. The expectation was that success in encouraging closer monitoring would in turn affect youth use of drug. Thus far the evaluation of this component of the anti-drug campaign suggests mixed results (Hornik et al., 2002). There is some evidence of an effect on the extent that parents talk with their children about drugs and for an effect on parental beliefs about the value of monitoring. The evidence for effects on actual monitoring and supervision is less strong, however. The ONDCP campaign is still ongoing, so definitive results are not yet available.

It may be possible that some actions to prevent youth drinking are easier to affect than general parent monitoring. For example, it may be easier to convince parents and other adults to stop facilitating drinking parties by their underage children than it is to encourage them to systematically monitor their children. Although this may be a sensible argument, there is not yet evidence to support it.

THE EVIDENCE FOR ACTION

In sum, there are several arguments in favor of a campaign aimed at parents and other adults: they often do not know about their children's drinking behavior; they probably do not have a well-developed understanding of the specific risks of drinking; communication campaigns are often quite good at diffusing new knowledge; such campaigns have been successful in promoting specific protective behaviors by parents and in changing attitudes and behaviors relating to drunk driving; and parental monitoring of their children is prospectively related to their likelihood of using alcohol. At the same time, the evidence is not clear as to whether such knowledge about their children's risk of alcohol use and abuse, and of the negative consequences of such use, affects parents' behavior with regard to alcohol. In addition, there is as yet no evidence of any campaign effects on relevant parental behavior, particularly on monitoring and supervision behaviors. Yet the campaign proposed here is sufficiently different than previous efforts that we ought not be constrained by the lack of clear prior success. It is different because it intends a more comprehensive approach, combining media attention with community efforts; it is different because it addresses both general parenting skills and specific adult behaviors that may facilitate underage drinking; and it is different because it is taking the long view, recognizing that there is a need for transformation in that community social norms underlie underage drinking.

A complex additional concern has to do with the indirectness of this approach. A campaign directed toward youth will be successful if it affects youth behavior, its immediate target. A campaign directed toward adults is only successful if it first affects adults' behaviors and if those behaviors then affect youths' behavior. Such a two-stage approach may appear to be less promising than a direct one if the goal is to reduce youth drinking. However, from a longer-term perspective, the goal is to change or strengthen the social norm against facilitation of underage drinking, and any effects on youth are secondary to this change in the normative climate. The goal is to convince parents and other adults to embrace the idea that they need to take their own obligation seriously and that they need to hold other parents and adults to a high standard as well. The success of this effort cannot be judged, in the short term, by whether it has an effect on underage drinking. A reasonable goal, in the very short term, would be to show an effect on adult knowledge and attitudes, and, in the intermediate term, to show an effect on adult behavior. If the campaign has these effects, the committee is reasonably confident that it would ultimately have an impact on youth drinking over the long term.

DESIGNING THE CAMPAIGN

It is premature for the committee to propose a particular structure or content for the media campaign before a program of formative research has been carried out.[6] However, to give Congress and other interested audiences a more concrete idea of what we envision, we briefly describe a possible structure for such a campaign.

An adult-focused campaign might have three major themes. At the start, much of the emphasis might on broad social norms. As detailed above, most parents consider youth alcohol use to be problematic, but do not accurately perceive the risk to their own children and fail to recognize their own role in influencing their children's alcohol use. The earliest phase of the campaign might work on these perceptions, readying parents and other adults for the need to change their own behavior insofar as it facilitates or condones underage alcohol use. If the legal messages are determined in the developmental phase to be significant with the target audience, this phase might also include information about the law governing underage drinking and the legal duties of parents and other adults.

The preparatory phase might serve as the foundation for the next phase a more action-oriented phase that might include two complementary approaches. One approach might focus on specific beliefs related to youth alcohol use that has been shown by preliminary research to motivate adult action—such as perception that youth drinking is harmful in specific ways other than drinking and driving or that parents expect other parents to take action to prevent youth drinking. The accompanying message might recommend specific actions to prevent youth alcohol use, such as not hosting

---

[6]During this period of formative research, consideration must be given to the growing diversity of the U.S. population. For example, the percentage of Hispanic children increased from 9 to 16 percent between 1980 and 2000 and is projected to increase to 22 percent by 2020. Cultural and linguistic factors will need to be taken in to account for specific racial or ethnic groups.

teenage parties that provide alcohol and not purchasing liquor on behalf of underage youth. The second, complementary approach might focus on parental monitoring—including supervision, engaging with children, and imposing consistent and appropriate discipline—on the grounds that those skills can have a major influence on underage drinking, as well as other risky behavior.

These themes might be delivered through a variety of channels. Paid media would probably have to play a substantial role in diffusing specific messages and would probably represent the most costly portion of the campaign. However, the messages conveyed through paid media would probably be insufficient to produce a change in parental norms and behavior unless messages supporting such changes were reinforced through other channels that reach parents and adults. Assuring that multiple sources of information and a wide variety of institutions are presenting reinforcing messages would be a crucial objective for the campaign.

Possible Models

One model for this approach can be found in one of the first and most successful national campaigns, the National High Blood Pressure Education Campaign. Although this campaign did some advertising of its messages, it relied heavily on actions by other institutions: campaign planners worked with physicians' organizations to encourage physicians to provide advice about high blood pressure consistent with national guidelines; they proposed stories to newspapers and television and radio that conveyed their priority messages; and they developed affiliations with, and provided materials to, grassroots organizations interested in hypertension (Roccella, 2002).

The California anti-tobacco campaign provides another possible model for this approach. That effort was able to mobilize statewide support for a dedicated tobacco tax: those revenues were then used to purchase media time for anti-tobacco advertising, to support school and community-level anti-tobacco programs, and to promote local policies limiting exposure to environmental tobacco smoke. The media campaign was expected to directly influence smokers or potential smokers, but it also served to energize the population around the state and to promote policy changes designed to further reduce opportunities for smoking. While the increased tax on tobacco surely had independent effects on consumption, there is evidence that the observed reductions in smoking in California reflected the interaction of higher cost, direct advertising, and complementary local activities (Pierce, 2002; Hu et al., 1995).

As we envision it, an adult-focused campaign to reduce underage drinking would work similarly to the California campaign and other successful campaigns. It would make use of a range of channels to reach its audience, continuously adjusting its message strategy, its mix of channels, and its links with grassroots organizations and national leadership groups and policy makers. It would both encourage policy changes and grassroots support for local and national policy changes and use policy changes as a basis for disseminating messages to individual parents and other adults and for encouraging specific behavioral actions.

A Developmental Approach

The committee believes that there is a sound, though limited, evidentiary and logical foundation for an adult-focused campaign. Given the limited knowledge, however, some people may be reluctant to support a national campaign and suggest, instead, pilot programs to test the strategy. The committee disagrees with this view because underage drinking is so well embedded in U.S. culture that small-scale prototype tests may miss the point or at least find it difficult to make much headway.

Because the acceptability of underage drinking is widespread, it will take more than an isolated campaign to affect it, no matter how well designed such a campaign might be. It will take a multipronged effort over a long period, making use of as many routes of influence as possible. We think the evidence is sufficient to support a presumptive commitment to the idea of launching such a campaign after a carefully designed, step-by-step developmental phase. Thus, while we do not favor a small-scale pilot test of the campaign as a whole, we do recommend pilot testing of specific features of the campaign during the developmental period, as discussed below.

The Challenge

The history of campaigns aimed at tobacco use and drunk driving are instructive in indicating why we think that the presumptive commitment is warranted. The anti-tobacco efforts have been successful because they changed the culture about smoking. That cultural change has permitted many other things about smoking to change (social and legal norms about where people can smoke, etc.). Drunk driving has been subject to a similar cultural shift. Grassroots lobbying from Mothers Against Drunk Driving and others, along with specific government-sponsored interventions and new regulations and enforcement policies, transformed a behavior that was once perceived as risky, but not strongly condemned, into conduct that is universally regarded as socially unacceptable.

If one assumes that the culture around underage drinking needs to change in the same way that the cultures around drunk driving and tobacco use have changed, then that history becomes the model. National campaigns are part of a broad effort to affect the culture. It is instructive that both of these exemplars reflect interactions between private and public entities. They are better described as social movements, in which the government's role is to respond to, support, and stimulate private action.

In this approach, a government-sponsored communication campaign has as its goal the support of changes in social norms that relate to adult behavior insofar as it enables and facilitates underage drinking. Such efforts are not to be evaluated by their short-term effects on youth drinking, but by their effects on broad social norms about that drinking, by the willingness of adults to take actions to reduce it, and by changes in public policies known to affect underage drinking rates.

An adult-focused mass communication campaign is also meant to support local efforts to reduce drinking. It is important not only because of what it does on its own, but also because its effects provide leverage for local efforts—and vice versa. It would link its activities to the broadest group of adult stakeholders—industry, colleges and universities, the military, and community organizations. Wherever possible, a national campaign would coordinate activities with local needs and provide for the tailoring of its messages for different communities. It cannot be tested as a prototype on a very local scale because its effectiveness depends on the involvement of a wide range of constituencies and, ideally, the engagement of the entire nation's attention.

Our Approach

In the end, the committee is faced with a conundrum in formulating its recommendation for developing and implementing an adult-focused media campaign. On one side, we find the idea to be highly promising, but lacking the kind of direct evidence needed for unequivocal endorsement of the high costs of such a campaign. On the other side, testing the campaign in a very limited way in order to gather more evidence is not a viable option because a small-scale effort (relying, for example, only on paid media messages delivered in one locality alone without any reinforcement by national or even regional media and other institutional partners) would almost certainly produce unimpressive results (see Institute of Medicine, 2002). In short, implementing an adult-oriented campaign in the absence of an opportunity to build the social movement around the idea would not be a fair test of the approach. Is there a middle course? We suggest a substantial effort to develop the program, with the aim of erecting circumscribed conditions of demonstrated efficacy that would have to be satisfied before the decision is made to implement a national campaign.

The proposed campaign would be developed over time on the basis of an intensive agenda of formative research designed to define the promising messages, the appropriate channels to reach target audiences, and the timing and weight given to various messages and channels over time. Campaign strategy would reflect initial research with target audiences and continual monitoring of how they respond to the campaign as it evolves. A central issue would be how best to link the campaign with local, state, and national policy changes about youth alcohol use, if they are adopted.

During the first phase, we suggest funding the basic formative work for the campaign, including intensive and multifaceted developmental research. This phase might involve controlled tests of whether high exposure to messages leads parents and other adults to be willing to change their behavior, particularly if this can be done in the context of actions by local organizations concerned about youth alcohol use or of local policy changes. While we would be reluctant to expect too much influence from such a highly localized campaign, given the lack of nonlocal sources of reinforcing information, a good deal might be learned about what is promising and what falls completely flat.

A second preliminary phase might build on that local effort and develop larger-scale efforts in one or two states where there was substantial interest among government or grassroots organizations. While the national media and national policy would not be engaged, there would still be opportunities for building a statewide social movement, with analogies to the state-level anti-tobacco campaigns in California, Florida, and Massachusetts. If these statewide efforts show enough promise to suggest that a nationwide effort would be worthwhile, then the decision to build the broad national effort would rest on a strong scientific foundation and would be fully justified.

If results were positive at each stage, a projected schedule might require 3 years for developmental and preliminary testing. This would be followed by 5 years of full operation. In subsequent years, booster efforts might be implemented, as monitoring evidence established a need.

7

Alcohol Industry

The alcoholic beverage industry—the brewers, vintners, and producers of distilled spirits—and the distributors and servers of these products—have been an important part of U.S. society from its colonial beginnings. Indeed, it was in the "public houses" where "potables" were served that much of the planning for the American Revolution was accomplished. Part of that tradition, however, has been a general understanding that while alcohol is woven into the fabric of the nation's collective life, it also has great potential for causing harm, and that producers, distributors, and servers of alcohol bear some of the responsibility for preventing that harm and for promoting safe and responsible drinking. That is at least part of what it meant to be a "publican"—a position of significant status and responsibility in colonial society. That idea survives today in the licensing requirements for drinking establishments, in the existence of a structure of server liability, and in the commitment of the alcohol producers to encourage responsible drinking.

It is clear, we think, that those who produce and distribute alcohol have the opportunity to act in ways that will either ameliorate or exacerbate the problem of underage drinking. We take at face value the industry's collective commitment to helping society manage and reduce underage drinking. Such a declaration of values and intentions is consistent with a common-sense understanding of the industry's social and legal responsibility with respect to underage drinking. Yet two important social realities are inescapable: first, that a significant amount of underage drinking occurs in violation of the law and against the stated intentions of the industry, and second, that the alcohol beverage industry gains financial returns (both revenues and profits) from underage drinking.

Some have taken these facts to suggest that the alcohol industry's commitment to reducing underage drinking may be equivocal. After all, today's underage drinkers are tomorrow's legitimate customers, and the industry has self-evident economic incentives to satisfy the underage demand. Suspicion that some new alcohol products and some alcohol advertising seem to be specifically targeted at the tastes and sensibilities of underage drinkers leads some industry critics to claim that at least some companies are not only being negligent with respect to underage drinking, but may (more culpably) be encouraging it (American Academy of Pediatrics, 1995; Center on Alcohol Marketing and Youth, 2002a; Community Anti-Drug Coalitions of America, n.d.).

In this report we take the industry's professed motives as its true motives and focus our attention on how the industry's collective efforts to reduce underage drinking could become both more effective and more credible. In the committee's judgment, a great deal can and should be done by the alcohol industry to help society prevent and ameliorate some of the harms associated with its otherwise legitimate efforts to produce and market a product valued by the adult population. Specifically, the industry's commendable investment in programs to reduce underage drinking or promote responsible adult drinking warrant more rigorous evaluation and improved coordination with other efforts. The committee makes several recommendations designed to increase and channel the industry's prevention efforts. In addition, the committee urges the industry to exercise greater collective self-restraint in its marketing practices in order to reduce underage exposure to alcohol advertising. Although the evidence regarding the causal effects of alcohol advertising on underage consumption is inconclusive, it has been amply documented that there is a large underage market for alcohol, that advertising reaches a substantial underage audience, and that many commercial alcohol messages are particularly appealing to youth. In the committee's judgment, this evidence warrants more aggressive self-regulatory efforts to reduce youth exposure to advertising. Specific recommendations, drawing on the industry's best practices, are presented later in the chapter.

THE UNDERAGE MARKET

Efforts to estimate the proportion of alcohol consumed by underage drinkers have been bedeviled by the imprecision of quantity questions in national surveys and by concerns about underreporting, particularly in the National Household Survey of Drug Abuse. The most recent effort, by Foster et al. (2003), estimated that underage drinkers consumed 830.6

million drinks per month, or 19.7 percent of the total alcohol consumed. As discussed in Chapter 2, the estimation procedure used in that study is subject to a number of criticisms, and the committee calculates that the proportion is likely somewhere between 10 and 20 percent.

Based on their quantity estimates, Foster et al. (2003) estimated the expenditures by underage drinkers for beer, spirits, and wine, and concluded that underage drinkers spent $22.5 billion, or 19.4 percent of total consumer expenditures for alcohol. (It is lower than the proportion of consumption because youths are more likely to consume beer, a lower-priced beverage.) As explained in Chapter 2, we think this revenue estimate is a bit high because underage drinkers probably spend less per drink than do adults for a variety of reasons: most important is the fact that most of the drinks consumed by underage youths are off premise, originally purchased in the form of bottles, kegs, or six-packs, rather than from restaurants and bars, and the average price for on-premise sales is probably three or four times as high as off-premise sales. Whatever the precise amount, however, it is highly likely that underage drinking accounts for a significant proportion of the alcohol market, especially for beer.

INDUSTRY PROGRAMS TO REDUCE AND PREVENT UNDERAGE DRINKING

In recognition of the high prevalence of underage and illegal drinking, the alcohol industry has declared its collective support of the 21-year-old minimum drinking age and has undertaken efforts to discourage alcohol use by underage youths. Various industry-sponsored initiatives and programs have been implemented with the stated objectives of reducing underage drinking and promoting responsible or moderate drinking among adults.[1] The Beer Institute, the national trade association for the nation's brewers, reported that the beer industry has "committed hundreds of millions of dollars to create effective anti-underage drinking programs."[2] For example, Anheuser-Busch and its wholesalers have "invested more than $375 million [time period not specified] to implement alcohol awareness programs to fight drunk driving, help retailers spot fake IDs, and encourage parents to talk with their kids about drinking."

---

[1]For brief descriptions of some of the industry-sponsored activities, see http://www. centurycouncil.org/under_age/prevention.cfm; http://www.centurycouncil.org/underage_age/ retail/cops.htm; http://www.discus.org/industry/underagedrinking.htm; http://www.discus.org/ ir/college_education.htm; http://www.beerinstitute.org/alcoholprograms.htm; and http://www. nbwa.org/advocates/respons.htm.

[2]Quotations included in this section are based on materials submitted to the committee by various industry organizations; they are available in the public access file for this committee at the National Academies.

Beer producers and wholesalers have produced numerous brochures, booklets, compact disks, videos, and public service announcements aimed at educating youth, parents, potential servers of alcohol to youth, and the general public. Programs for servers of alcohol (e.g., "We I.D.," "TIPS") are designed to promote enforcement of laws prohibiting sales to minors and to prevent serving underage and intoxicated persons. Other materials highlight the perils of drinking and driving, promote responsible drinking, or provide advice to parents on helping kids make responsible decisions. The industry also has sponsored activities specific to college campuses. They include the types of activities just noted, as well as support for the social norms approach (i.e., counteracting beliefs that the prevalence of drinking among peers is higher than it really is). Some companies in the beer industry also have sponsored public speakers and participated in community efforts to address underage drinking.

Representatives of the distilled spirits industry reported to the committee a similar commitment to reducing underage drinking. For example, the Distilled Spirits Council of the United States (DISCUS), a national trade association representing producers and marketers of distilled sprits and importers of wines sold in the United States, recently provided funding to a number of colleges to implement alcohol action plans. DISCUS also supports the programs funded by the Century Council,[3] a nonprofit entity established in 1991 that reports having invested "more than $120 million" over the last 10 years "in programs that fight against the misuse of their products." The Century Council defines its core activities as being aimed at four objectives, two of which focus on drunk driving and two of which focus specifically on underage drinking:

• educate middle-school through college students, their parents, teachers, and adult caregivers about the importance of making responsible decisions regarding beverage alcohol;
• inform the public about how gender, weight, and number and type of drink affect an individual's blood alcohol concentration (BAC) and increase awareness of state BAC driving laws;
• deter minors from buying beverage alcohol through joint programs with law enforcement, retailers, and wholesalers, using point-of-sale materials and public awareness campaigns; and
• reduce drunk driving through research and promising strategies, tougher state and federal legislation, treatment, and education.

---

[3]The Century Council is funded by Allied Domecq Spirits and Wine North America; Bacardi USA, Inc.; Brown-Forman; DIAGEO; Future Brands LLC; and Pernod Ricard USA.

In addition to activities similar to those described above, the Century Council (2001) has produced resource materials (e.g., *Promising Practices: Campus Alcohol Strategies*) aimed at helping colleges develop effective programs to reduce alcohol abuse. They also have developed and distributed Alcohol 101, a college-level interactive program on alcohol-related problems that is distributed to hundreds of campuses nationwide and Cops in Shops, a program aimed at deterring underage purchases.

Overall, the alcohol industry has apparently invested significant resources in a diverse range of efforts aimed at reducing underage drinking and its associated harms, including media messages, educational programs, and enforcement activities. Some industry members have also entered into partnerships with specific colleges and universities to reduce drinking problems on those campuses, often grounded in social norms marketing approaches (see Chapter 10).

The committee is aware of only one industry-sponsored education program that has been independently evaluated—Alcohol 101. The evaluation (Anderson and Cohen, 2001) used a naturalistic design with purposeful sampling, including attention to regional sampling, and included colleges and universities believed to have done a good job implementing the program. Anderson and Cohen reported that the program is viewed "with a high degree of positive regard" (2001, p. 22), with some campus personnel suggesting modest changes on their campuses, and others reporting positive student engagement. Anderson and Cohen reported, with the most robust implementations, measurable gains in relevant knowledge, willingness to act in emergencies, and intentions to modify drinking to reduce alcohol problems. Nonetheless, they suggested additional in-depth analysis of the campus-based findings involving additional institutions and types of settings and further statistical analyses of existing data.

A recent study by the Center on Alcohol Marketing and Youth (2003) studied "responsibility advertising" by the alcohol industry on television in 2001 and reported that industry spent $23.2 million to air 2,379 responsibility messages (discouraging underage drinking and drunk driving); they contrasted these with $811.2 million on 208,909 product advertisements. With regard to underage drinking in particular, they report that there were 179 product ads for every ad that referred to the legal drinking age. All of the legal-drinking age messages were broadcast by only two alcohol companies—Anheuser Busch ($12.2 million) and Coors ($3.6 million).

Many public health experts in the alcohol prevention field are highly skeptical about the value of the industry's underage drinking programs and other prevention activities and about the industry's collective motivation for sponsoring them. The criticism most frequently heard is that the main effect of these programs may be to promote brand identification, if not alcohol use itself. The committee is in no position to assess or ascertain the actual intentions underlying these programs. However, in the absence of documented evidence of effectiveness from independent evaluation, skepticism about the value of industry-sponsored programs is likely to continue. Based on our own review of the materials submitted by industry representatives, the alcohol prevention literature, and the other materials and testimony submitted to the committee, we believe that industry efforts to prevent and reduce underage drinking, however sincere, should be redirected and strengthened.

> **Recommendation 7-1: All segments of the alcohol industry that profit from underage drinking, inadvertently or otherwise, should join with other private and public partners to establish and fund an independent nonprofit foundation with the sole mission of reducing and preventing underage drinking.**

Other public health leaders have recently urged the alcohol industry to endow an independent foundation to curb excessive drinking by adults as well as underage drinking (National Center on Addiction and Substance Abuse, 2003). However, the committee believes that—at the outset, at least—the mission should be strictly limited to the prevention of underage drinking. If the mission is not limited to underage drinking, which is illegal, the committee is doubtful that agreement could be reached about the foundation's goals and the scope of its activities. While a very strong social consensus supports strong measures to reduce underage drinking, such a consensus does not yet exist about what it means to reduce "excessive" or otherwise "irresponsible" drinking or about the measures that should be taken to achieve this goal.

The committee believes that a foundation that is focused exclusively on preventing and reducing underage drinking—through activities, programs, and methods that can be carefully defined and specified in the founding charter—would provide an opportunity for the alcohol industry, interested business associations, advocacy organizations, and government to enter into a social contract grounded in, and manifesting, recognition of collective responsibility.[4] Primary funding for such a foundation would ideally be

---

[4]The agreement envisioned by the committee would differ substantially from the terms of the Master Settlement Agreement (MSA), executed by major tobacco manufacturers and the state attorneys general to settle the Medicaid lawsuits against the tobacco industry. The MSA established the American Legacy Foundation, charging it with specific functions relating to reducing youth smoking, and obligated the industry to fund the Foundation at least for a period of years. The Legacy Foundation grew out of a lawsuit and is currently in litigation over one tobacco company's claim that Legacy violated its obligation under the MSA to avoid "vilifying" the industry. The committee envisions a collaborative nonadversarial relationship among the parties to the agreement establishing a foundation to prevent underage drinking.

provided by alcohol producers and wholesalers as an offset to income they receive as a result of underage drinking. By contributing to the foundation, they would have an opportunity to acknowledge, without defensiveness, that marketing of alcohol to young adults contributes, however unintentionally, to the web of social influences promoting underage drinking. The foundation also would provide an opportunity for all member organizations to declare and implement a genuine and unequivocal commitment to try to curtail alcohol use by underage youths and to conduct impartial evaluation of the effectiveness of interventions undertaken.

As the committee envisions it, many, if not all, of the existing industry activities in the domain of underage drinking would be redirected to the new foundation. The committee is no position to write the charter for this entity, which will have to be negotiated among all the organizational participants. However, it is clear that the charter would have to ensure that the foundation's ability to operate is not hampered by the dominance of any single interest group or by the perception that it serves the commercial interests of its funders. A possible funding formula among all the participating industry partners could be developed along the following lines: Each alcohol producer, acting individually or through trade associations or other entities, would help to fund the activities of the foundation in a manner that is commensurate with the amount and proportion of industry revenues attributable to underage consumption. As indicated in Chapter 2, underage drinkers consumed between 10 and 20 percent of all alcohol consumed in 2000, representing about $11 to 22 billion, although the proportion differs substantially among beer, wine, and spirits. A reasonable target for the annual industry contribution to the foundation would be 0.5 percent of gross revenues (about $250-500 million) prorated according to the particular company's share of the underage market (estimated based on surveys about underage brand use, or, in the absence of such data, based on the particular company's share of the overall beer, wine, or spirits market).[5]

Until the proposed foundation has been established, the committee believes that the alcohol industry should take two immediate steps to redirect the resources and activities currently devoted to preventing underage drinking and to move toward the strategy recommended by the committee.

---

[5]A bill developed by the California Alcohol Policy Reform Initiative and pending before the California Assembly, would impose a "fee" on alcohol producers based on the producers' respective shares of the underage market. Under the bill, the California Department of Alcohol and Drug Programs would conduct an annual survey of youth drinking to determine brand preferences. Up to $100 million would be collected annually and distributed to the counties for youth prevention and treatment programs. The committee's proposal urges alcohol producers, advocacy groups, and other interested parties to reach agreement on such an approach in lieu of a governmental solution.

First, industry-sponsored media messages regarding underage drinking should be redirected away from youth audiences and focused instead on changing the attitudes and behavior of parents and other adults—to persuade them not to facilitate or enable underage drinking and to accept responsibility for preventing it. For example, industry-sponsored messages could be designed to alert adults to their legal responsibilities, including potential liability for injuries caused by underage drinkers to whom they give alcohol, or could show a shoulder-tap enforcement sting by undercover youths (see Chapter 9). Although the alcohol industry may not be the most credible source of messages aiming to reduce the demand for alcohol (by either adults or youths), messages aimed specifically at curbing behaviors that violate the restrictions on underage access can hardly be used as pretexts to stimulate demand. Indeed, they might be especially effective because the industry has both credibility and natural channels of communication with its adult customers. Second, industry-funded messages and programs should be delivered directly to young people only if they rest on a scientific foundation, as judged by qualified, independent organizations, or incorporate rigorous evaluation. Programs that have an exclusive focus on providing information have been demonstrated to be ineffective at reducing alcohol use and should be avoided (see Chapter 10).

ADVERTISING AND PROMOTION

In 2001, alcoholic beverage companies spent $1.6 billion on advertising in print media, broadcast media, billboards, and other venues—known as measured media purchases. At least twice that amount was spent on unmeasured promotion, which include sponsorships, product placement payment in entertainment media, point-of-sale advertising, discount promotion, apparel and other items with brand-name logos, and other activities (Federal Trade Commission, 1999, Appendix B; see Figure 7-1 for recent trends). Industry critics assert that some of these marketing activities are intentionally directed toward underage audiences (see, e.g., Center for Science in the Public Interest, 2002; Center on Alcohol Marketing and Youth, 2002a), but even if the companies are not targeting young people, abundant evidence shows that a large proportion of these commercial messages and promotional activities do, in fact, reach underage audiences. The current practice of some companies—advertising on television programs with an audience that is at least 50 percent adult—routinely allows placement of alcohol advertising on programs for which the percentage of underage viewers is higher than the percentage of underage children in the United States (Center for Alcohol Marketing and Youth, 2002b).

The effect on youth drinking of voluminous and pervasive alcohol advertising and promotional activity is one of the most highly contested

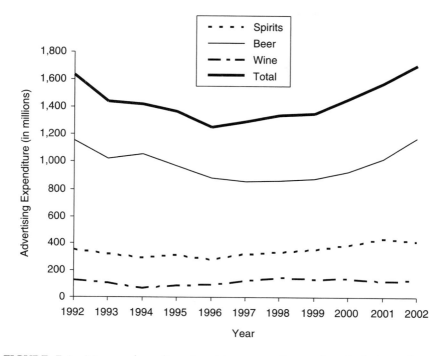

FIGURE 7-1 Measured media advertising expenditures for alcohol products, 1992-2002, in 2002 dollars (adjusted for inflation).
SOURCE: Data from LNA/Mediawatch multimedia service, competitive media reporting (expenditure) and McCann-Erikson world group (media cost-per-thousand composite index).

issues in the alcohol prevention field. The question is complex, both empirically and legally. Before turning to the controversial aspects, however, we present the undisputed points.

Alcohol advertising is designed to highlight the attractions of using alcohol, especially to enhance the enjoyment of social occasions, and to induce or persuade potential consumers to feel favorably toward the promoted product. Even though these messages may not be intentionally targeted at youths under 21, messages aimed at "young adults" (e.g., ages 21- to 25-year-olds) will inevitably reach older teens (e.g., ages 16- to 20-year-olds); moreover, many of those messages will also be attractive to children and teenagers (those under 16). A particularly troubling illustration of the youth-specific attractions of an alcohol marketing campaign concerns so-called "alcopops," sweet, flavored alcoholic malt beverages. Recent survey data suggest that these products are more popular with teenagers than with adults, in terms of both awareness and use. These concerns recently led

Congress to direct the Federal Trade Commission to study the impact of alcopop advertising on underage consumers (see Consolidated Appropriations Resolution, 2003). In sum, the widespread exposure of youth to alcohol marketing and the attractiveness of alcohol-related messages to them are well documented. The disputed issue, empirically, is whether alcohol advertising contributes, *in a causal sense*, to the prevalence and intensity of underage drinking. Although many people believe that it does (Community Anti-Drug Coalitions of America, n.d.) and there is some evidence of a correlation between exposure to alcohol advertising and drinking by young people (Atkin and Block, 1981; Atkin et al., 1984), a causal link between alcohol advertising and underage alcohol use has not been clearly established (e.g., Atkin, 1987, 1995; Smart, 1988; Lastovicka, 1995; Grube, 2004). A substantial body of research on the effects of advertising and promotion on alcohol consumption and its consequences, and specifically on underage alcohol consumption, has produced findings that are mixed and inconclusive (Grube, 2004). With some notable exceptions (e.g., Saffer, 1997), experimental and ecological studies have produced little evidence that alcohol advertising affects drinking beliefs, behaviors, or problems among young people.

Recent survey evidence (further described below) shows that young peoples' awareness of, and affect toward, certain types of commercial messages about alcohol are correlated with their drinking beliefs and behaviors (Austin and Nach-Ferguson, 1995; Grube, 1995; Slater et al., 1997), but because most of these studies are cross-sectional, the evidence is only suggestive. That is, it is possible that advertising affects young people's drinking beliefs and behaviors or, conversely, that preexisting predispositions to drink increase attention to alcohol advertising. Nonetheless, some research (Grube and Wallack, 1994) suggests that attention to alcohol advertising has a significant effect on drinking beliefs and intentions among school children, even when the reciprocal effects of these beliefs on attention are controlled. These effects, however, are modest and, overall, the evidence is best considered inconclusive.

It is sometimes assumed that, in the absence of compelling evidence of causation, there is no legitimate basis for limiting the exposure of young people to alcohol advertising. This assumption is wrong for three reasons. First, the absence of definitive proof may be caused by the methodological complexity of the inquiry rather than the absence of a contributing effect (e.g., see, Thorson, 1995; Calfee and Scheraga, 1994). Obviously, many social and cultural influences are propelling young people toward alcohol use, and it should come as little surprise that the available scientific tools cannot disentangle advertising from this web of influences. Second, there is a sound commonsense basis for believing, even in the absence of definitive proof, that making alcohol use attractive to young people increases the likelihood that they will become alcohol consumers as young people rather than waiting until they are adults. It is abundantly clear that young people attend to and are attracted to some alcohol advertisements. Moreover, young people who are drinkers or who are predisposed to drinking are more attracted to these advertisements than other young people (Martin et al., 2002; Casswell and Zhang, 1998; Wyllie et al., 1998a, 1998b; Grube and Wallack, 1994). Third, persistent exposure of young people to messages *encouraging* drinking by young people (even if they appear to be 21) contradicts and interferes with the implementation of the nation's goal of *discouraging* underage drinking. In this respect, the emphasis is less on causation than on contradiction and ambiguity.

The ongoing dispute about whether alcohol advertising causes underage drinking is tied to the legal controversy over whether government-imposed bans or restrictions on alcohol advertising would violate the First Amendment because the constitutionality of any significant limitations on advertising imposed by the government would probably turn on the strength of the evidence on causation. However, this emphasis on the constitutionality of government intervention, and the accompanying preoccupation with proof of causation, overlooks the paramount importance of self-regulation by the alcohol industry. The industry has the prerogative—indeed, the social obligation—to regulate its own practices and to refrain from marketing products or engaging in promotional activities that have a particular appeal to youngsters, irrespective of whether such practices can be *proven* to "cause" underage drinking.

In an important report on alcohol advertising, the Federal Trade Commission (FTC) (1999, p. 3) emphasized the virtues of self-regulation:

> Self-regulation often can be more prompt, flexible, and effective than the government regulation. It can permit application of the accumulated judgment and experience of an industry to issues that are sometimes difficult for the government to define with bright line rules. With respect to advertising practices, self-regulation is an appropriate mechanism because many forms of government intervention raise First Amendment concerns.

The FTC went on to fault the alcohol industry for the weakness of its current self-regulatory efforts, and that was the starting point for this committee's deliberations. The committee believes that greater self-restraint by the alcohol industry in its marketing practices is an essential component of a sound national strategy for reducing underage drinking.

In sum, the committee regards the empirical dispute about whether advertising causes underage drinking, and whether the existing evidence of causation is strong enough to justify government restriction under the First Amendment, to be an unnecessary distraction from the most important task at hand—strengthening industry self-regulation and promoting corporate responsibility. In the event that the industry fails to respond satisfactorily to this challenge, the case for some government action might become more compelling.[6]

> Recommendation 7-2: Alcohol companies, advertising companies, and commercial media should refrain from marketing practices (including product design, advertising, and promotional techniques) that have substantial underage appeal and should take reasonable precautions in the time, place, and manner of placement and promotion to reduce youthful exposure to other alcohol advertising and marketing activity.

Use of images or other content uniquely or unusually attractive to children provides highly persuasive evidence of an intention to target an illegal, underage audience. However, by far the more common situation involves advertisements that are not uniquely attractive to children and that have equivalent appeal to children or teenagers and adults. Should alcohol advertisers display or broadcast such messages knowing that they will appeal to young people? Obviously this is not a scientific question, and it highlights the challenge of defining socially responsible advertising behavior. This key issue is whether companies should voluntarily forgo potentially highly successful commercial messages (or display them only in adult-only venues) in order to avoid exposing them to young people who will find them attractive.

In the committee's opinion, alcohol companies should refrain from displaying commercial messages encouraging alcohol use to audiences known to include a significant number of children or teens when these messages are known to be highly attractive to young people. It is not enough for the company to say: "Because these messages also appeal to adults, who will predominate in the expected audience, we are within our legal rights."

---

[6]The committee emphasizes, in this connection, that government is not altogether powerless to regulate advertising, especially if effective industry self-regulation is not forthcoming. Even though banning or severely restricting the informational content of alcohol advertising as a means of preventing underage drinking may be impermissible in the absence of persuasive scientific evidence of causation, restrictions on the "time, place, and manner" of alcohol advertising to reduce its exposure to children and teenagers are probably permissible, on the basis of logic, experience, and common sense, as long as they do not substantially impede the industry's opportunity to communicate with its lawful consumers through equivalent channels. Few would doubt the authority of the government to preclude alcohol advertising in children's magazines, on television during daylight hours on weekdays, or on billboards immediately adjacent to an elementary or secondary school window. Furthermore, certain messages (e.g., "Hey kids, drinking is fun") would be precluded on the basis of the advertiser's illegal intention, and it can certainly be argued that use of cartoon characters or other images especially likely to attract children can also be restricted as long as informational content is unrestricted.

From the standpoint of industry self-regulation, there are two ways of responding to this situation. The most effective, and the easiest to administer, is to circumscribe the media locations (time and place) in which any alcohol messages can be placed. So, for example, there could be an industry guideline that no alcohol advertisement can be placed in a magazine or television show in which more than a designated percentage of the audience (say, 25 percent) is expected to be under 21. This approach is called a limit on the "placement" of advertising. The second approach focuses on the "content" of the advertising. Thus, the industry code might aim to preclude the use of certain types of images, sounds, or words that have particular appeal to youths. Obviously, formulating and applying a content-based standard is a difficult undertaking. The need to do so will depend in part on whether and to what extent the placement of advertisements is restricted. For example, there would ordinarily be less need for a content restriction if placements were precluded in any media for which more than 10 percent of the audience was expected to be underage than there would be if placements were precluded only if more than 50 percent of the audience was expected to be underage.

In 1998, Congress requested the FTC to assess the adequacy of self-regulatory efforts by the alcohol industry to prevent practices that encourage underage drinking. The FTC's report, issued in 1999, reviewed existing industry standards and practices, identified deficiencies and best practices, and recommended improvements in relation to advertising placement and content. Four years later, the 2003 appropriations bill directed the FTC to reexamine industry practice regarding liquor-branded "alcopop" advertising and expressed concern that the industry had not fully implemented the commission's 1999 recommendations. Although the committee believes the 1999 FTC recommendations are too weak in some respects, alcohol producers, wholesalers, and their trade associations should implement those recommendations forthwith, as an expression of good faith and as a signal of their willingness to become active partners in the nation's campaign to reduce underage drinking.

Recommendation 7-3: The alcohol industry trade associations, as well as individual companies, should strengthen their advertising codes to preclude placement of commercial messages in venues where a significant proportion of the expected audience is underage, to prohibit the use of commercial messages that have substantial underage appeal, and to establish independent external review boards to investigate complaints and enforce the codes.

Advertising Placement

Industry codes for beer and distilled spirits currently allow placement of alcohol advertising in media for which most of the audience is expected to be 21 or older. Because 70 percent of the population is 21 or over, this standard effectively allows placements almost anywhere except young children's television shows or magazines, and therefore allows alcohol messages to reach large numbers of children and teenagers on a regular basis. A good example is the pervasive beer advertising that accompanies sports broadcasts on weekday evenings and throughout the weekend. In 2001, for example, the alcohol industry spent $492 million dollars on advertising for sports television: Twenty percent of these ads (11,630 ads, with spending totaling more than $48 million) were on sports programs for which, based on expected proportions of the viewing audience, youth were more likely than adults to have seen the ads (Center on Alcohol Marketing and Youth, 2002b). In its 1999 report, the FTC recommended that the industry threshold be moved toward 25 percent, representing the industry's current best practices, and that companies be required by the codes to measure their compliance against the most reliable, up-to-date audience composition data available.

Since the 1999 FTC report, the wine industry and several individual beer and spirits companies have embraced a 30 percent threshold. These steps should be applauded, but the industry standard should continue to be reduced. In the committee's view, immediate implementation of an industry standard of 25 percent for television advertising, as suggested by the FTC, would signify meaningful self-restraint in alcohol marketing to reduce youth exposure. Based on data provided by the Center on Alcohol Marketing and Youth (CAMY) at Georgetown University, a 25 percent threshold would have a modest, but significant, effect on the volume of alcohol advertising on television and on the number of young people exposed to it. The current 50 percent voluntary standard for beer and spirits precludes advertising on only 6 percent of the television programs tracked by Nielsen if the denominator for the viewing population encompasses viewers as young as 2 and only 1 percent of the programs if the viewing population base excludes children under 12. A 25 percent threshold would preclude alcohol advertising on 16.4 percent of programs if the base includes children under 12 and 8.2 percent if it excludes children under 12.

Over time, the industry standard should move toward a 15 percent threshold for television advertising,[7] a standard currently being considered

---

[7]According to figures provided to the committee by the Center on Alcohol Marketing and Youth, a 15 percent threshold would preclude alcohol advertising on 34.0 percent of programs if the base includes children under 12 and 19.2 percent if it excludes children under 12.

by at least one industry member. Some advocacy groups have recommended that the audience proportion threshold be reduced to 10 percent and that it be coupled with a numerical maximum (e.g., 1 million youths) to take account of the size of the audience and the absolute number of young people likely to be exposed to the ads. However, the committee does not regard this as a practical suggestion, at least for the foreseeable future. Such a limit would preclude alcohol advertising on major "adult" viewing events, such as the Super Bowl, and the industry cannot reasonably be expected to embrace such a restrictive approach as a preferred practice.

Although most of the attention regarding alcohol advertising has focused on television, print advertising raises analogous concerns.[8] A recent study of alcohol advertising in magazines by Garfield et al. (2003) counted advertisements that appeared from 1997-2001 in 35 of 48 major U.S. magazines that tracked their adolescent readership. Variation was assessed in placement frequency for each alcohol product type according to size of adolescent readership and other variables. Garfield et al. (2003) found that the alcohol industry placed 9,148 advertisements, at a cost of $696 million, during this period, with adolescent readership of the magazines ranging from 1.0 to 7.1 million. Most (82 percent) of these advertisements were for liquor, with fewer placements for beer (13 percent) and wine (5 percent). The finding highlighted by the investigators was that, after adjustment for other magazine characteristics, the advertisement rate ratio for beer and liquor was 1.6 times higher for each additional million adolescent readers. However, the committee believes that the significance of this finding must be assessed in light of the accompanying finding that, for liquor advertising, the rate ratio is even higher (2.6) for every additional million young adult readers (defined as 20-24 because advertising industry data do not distinguish between 20- and 21-year-olds) than it is for increased adolescent readership.

This study calls attention to the basic policy problem in relation to alcohol advertising—increased exposure to the lawful young adult audience often involves increased exposure to older teens. In relation to liquor advertising, increasing young adult exposure was accompanied by increased youth

---

Assuming that alcohol advertising dollars would be redeployed to programs with audience compositions below the threshold, a 15 percent threshold (using a base of 12 and older) would reduce youth gross rating points (the industry standard measure of exposure) by 22 percent.

[8]In the context of billboards and other print media in local retail markets, allowing text-only advertising of price and key product characteristics, which may be less attractive to youth (Kelly et al., 2002), is a suitable alternative to a more sweeping restriction, whether self-imposed or enacted by local governments. The FDA's unsuccessful regulatory effort to restrict tobacco advertising to a text-only format, as recommended in *Growing Up Tobacco Free* (Institute of Medicine, 1994a), provides a useful model.

exposure, but at a lower rate. (By contrast, the advertisement rate ratio for beer advertising was only 1.0 for every additional million young adult readers, as compared with 1.6 for every additional million adolescent readers.) It is possible that a marketing strategy aiming for young adults could identify magazines with high young adult exposure but small youth readership. Indeed, although the numbers are small, Garfield et al. (2003) found that the wine advertisers were able to increase young adult exposure (advertisement rate ratio = 3.0) without increasing youth exposure (advertisement rate ratio = 0.72), and they also report that their findings regarding increased exposure of youth and young adults were statistically independent. In the overall policy context, however, the underlying problem remains—in order to avoid youth exposure, liquor advertisers might have to avoid placements in the magazines with the most promising young adult readership.

Setting a 25 percent threshold would be a useful improvement in the current industry practice, as a demonstration of good faith in the effort to find a formula that reasonably accommodates the industry's interest in communicating with its young adult consumers and the public's interest in minimizing underage exposure. According to CAMY, nearly 30 percent of alcohol advertising dollars spent in a sample of 98 magazines were spent in magazines with at least 25 percent adolescent readers. More than half of the money was spent in magazines whose adolescent and young adult (12-20) audience exceeded their proportion in the U.S. population (CAMY, 2002a). Based on these data, adoption of a 25 percent threshold, would reflect a meaningful commitment to alter otherwise lawful magazine advertising practices to reduce youth exposure to alcohol advertising.[9] As with television advertising, however, the industry should consider eventually moving toward a 15 percent threshold to further reduce the number of youth who are exposed to advertising intended for adults.

Advertising Content

As noted above, under some circumstances, the likelihood that a particular message will appeal to a youthful audience may be so great that the company will be said to have "intended" to target an underage audience

---

[9]The absolute size of the youth readership is obviously relevant for magazines, just as it is for television advertising. However, coupling a threshold for audience proportion with a ceiling on youth readership would selectively apply different rules to the largest circulation magazines with young adult audiences, and would have the effect of precluding alcohol advertising in these magazines altogether. Standing alone (rather than as part of a more complicated formula), a ceiling on youth readership does not appear to be a feasible solution.

with that advertisement, in violation of the existing codes and in violation of the federal and state laws prohibiting "unfair acts or practices" in advertising. The industry codes each ban the use of images or depictions, such as cartoons, uniquely attractive to youth.[10] However, the usual case is that the message is equally appealing to adults and young people. What should be done in these cases?

As suggested above, the answer depends in part on the nature and extent of any restrictions on placements. If placements of alcohol advertising are not permitted unless the expected audience is 85 percent or 90 percent adults, then the companies are presumably not targeting young people, and the message is being designed to be attractive to adults. Under these circumstances and in the absence of other evidence of youth targeting, it seems disingenuous to insist that a particular type of message be banned because it is also attractive to youths in an otherwise overwhelmingly adult audience. However, if the industry's current 50 percent threshold is maintained—or even if the threshold is reduced as suggested by the committee— the exposure of underage viewers will remain substantial. Under these circumstances, companies may properly be expected to avoid advertising content with strong appeal to young viewers.

Admittedly such a standard is not self-defining and self-executing. The committee joins the FTC in encouraging the companies and their trade associations to embrace and build on best practices to reduce the likelihood that alcohol advertising will have particular appeal to youths. Specifically, the kinds of practices to avoid would include any advertising content (a song, character, or idea) that would be effective in promoting a product that is explicitly meant to be used by children or young teens. Companies would also limit the "spillover" appeal to underage drinkers by targeting their alcohol messages to an audience that is no younger than 25.

---

[10]For example, the Wine Institute Code of Advertising Standards states that wine advertisements should not "use music, language, gestures, cartoon characters, or depictions, images, figures, or objects that are popular predominantly with children or otherwise specifically associated with or directed toward those below the legal drinking age, including the use of Santa Claus or the Easter Bunny." The Beer Institute Advertising and Marketing Code provides that "advertising and marketing materials should not employ any symbol, language, music, gesture, or cartoon character that is intended to appeal primarily to persons below the legal purchase age." To "appeal primarily" to youth means having "special attractiveness to such persons above and beyond the general attractiveness it has for persons above the legal purchase age, including young adults above the legal purchase age." The Code of Good Practice for Distilled Spirits Advertising and Marketing provides that distilled spirits advertising and marketing materials "should not depict a child or portray objects, images, or cartoon figures that are popular predominantly with children."

Internet Advertising

Many Internet sites sponsored by alcohol companies are easy for children to access. According to the FTC's 1999 report, there are more than 100 commercial alcohol websites, but only 43 percent of beer sites and 72 percent of spirit sites have some kind of age restriction (either a filter or a warning). Although these data are undoubtedly out of date, no recent review is available. While it appears that most sites now use "virtual bouncers" to check for age of viewers, the effectiveness of this approach is unknown. In keeping with their commitment to prevent underage drinking, alcohol companies should use their best efforts, based on evolving technology, to restrict underage access to their web sites and avoid using games and cartoons that are unusually attractive to children and teenagers.

Product Placement

As discussed in greater detail in the next chapter, the entertainment industry should acknowledge its own responsibility to avoid program content that glorifies, or presents in a favorable way, underage use of alcohol or that exposes young audiences to unsuitable messages relating to alcohol. The committee recognizes that the content of movies, television programs, web-based entertainment, and live theater lies at the heart of the First Amendment and that any governmental regulation is constitutionally precluded. However, these media have a social responsibility to try to avoid or reduce youth exposure to unsuitable alcohol messages.

Obviously, alcohol companies do not have complete control over artistic decisions to display or use their products in films or other entertainment media. However, an identifiable brand is not likely to be prominently displayed without the request or permission of the alcohol company. Moreover, it is a common practice within the industry to seek placements of alcohol products or logos in films, television programs, and music videos. In 1997-1998, eight companies responding to the FTC reported that they made product placements in 233 movies and one or more episodes of 181 different television series. The companies sometimes pay for these placements.

According to the FTC's 1999 report, alcohol companies avoid product placement in films, programs, or videos that actually show underage drinking, but otherwise do not seem to have a common practice regarding screening films and programs for alcohol-related content and for the likelihood of exposure to underage audiences. The FTC recommended that product placements be restricted to movies that are rated "R" (or NC-17), that they be avoided when an underage person is the primary character, and that the standards for placement of advertising (discussed above) also be applied to product placement. These recommendations seem sensible and the committee encourages the industry to implement them. At a minimum, product placements should be explicitly disclosed.

Code Enforcement

Among the most important recommendations in the FTC's 1999 report was its call for the industry to create independent external review boards with responsibility and authority to address complaints from the public or other industry members regarding alleged violations of the codes. In support of this recommendation, the FTC reported favorably on the experience of the National Advertising Division of the Council of Better Business Bureaus (CBBB), which receives and investigates complaints about the truthfulness of advertising, and the National Advertising Review Board, which receives advertiser appeals, and whose members are drawn from both inside and outside the advertising industry. Since the FTC's 1999 report, Coors is the only company to establish such a review mechanism. The company's "Advertising Complaint Evaluation" process opens company advertising and marketing materials to review by CBBB's Advertising Pledge program.

ACCOUNTABILITY

What should be done if the industry codes are not strengthened and the nation's young people continue to be exposed to such a large volume of messages portraying alcohol use in a favorable light? In the absence of external review mechanisms and in light of constitutional constraints on direct restrictions of advertising, the committee believes that the most fruitful governmental response would be to facilitate public awareness of industry advertising practices and thereby to promote industry accountability through the marketplace.

> **Recommendation 7-4: Congress should appropriate the necessary funding for the U.S. Department of Health and Human Services to monitor underage exposure to alcohol advertising on a continuing basis and to report periodically to Congress and the public. The report should include information on the underage percentage of the exposed audience and estimated number of underage viewers for print and broadcasting alcohol advertising in national markets and, for television and radio broadcasting, in a selection of large local or regional markets.**

In Chapter 12, the committee recommends that a market surveillance mechanism be established to monitor underage use of alcohol according to brand. Together with the advertising data collected and reported in accord with the recommendation set forth above, this information would enable the public to judge whether a company's marketing practices are attracting disproportionate numbers of underage consumers, whether wittingly or unwittingly. In such situations, the public will be in a position to bring market pressure to bear on the relevant company. And, of course, if the data suggest intentional targeting, or reckless disregard for the effects of the marketing on underage drinking, regulatory intervention might be undertaken.

THE SPECIAL CASE OF COLLEGES AND UNIVERSITIES

Colleges and universities should ban alcohol advertising and promotion on campus. Currently, 72 percent of colleges and universities prohibit on-campus alcohol advertising and 62 percent prohibit industry sponsorship of athletic events. The Congress (by "sense of the Congress resolution"), the Department of Health and Human Services, DISCUS, and the Wine Institute have urged all colleges and universities to adopt these policies. It should be emphasized, again, that this recommendation is not predicated on the argument that banning the advertising will, in itself, reduce the prevalence and intensity of drinking among underage college students. Instead, the objective is to declare and affirm colleges' genuine commitment to a policy of discouraging alcohol use among underage students.

8

Entertainment Industries

Since artistic expression inevitably reflects the culture in which it is embedded, it is hardly surprising that alcohol use and alcohol products are frequently displayed or mentioned in prime-time television, movies, and music recordings. Although the viewing or listening audiences for many of these media products are predominantly adult, some of them are disproportionately underage, and even the predominantly adult audiences typically include large numbers of young people.

The committee recognizes, of course, that the entertainment media and their adult audiences have a common interest in a robust free market in television programming as well as in movies, video games, and music recordings and that alcohol consumption is an inescapable element of modern U.S. culture. At the same time, it must also be recognized that images and lyrics depicting underage drinking in a favorable light or otherwise glamorizing alcohol consumption affect the perceptions and attitudes of children and teenagers toward alcohol consumption and that exposure to those images and lyrics is associated with youthful drinking.

Despite abundant correlational data from cross-sectional studies, however, there is no definitive evidence that youthful exposure to alcohol content in the entertainment media has a causal effect on underage drinking (Grube, 2004). Concern that such a relationship may exist is reinforced, however, by the findings of an important cohort study of adolescent initiation of smoking. Of more than 3,000 adolescents aged 10 to 14 who had never smoked, Dalton et al. (2003) report that 10 percent had initiated smoking 13 to 26 months later, and that 17 percent of those in the highest quartile of exposure to movie smoking had initiated smoking, in comparison with 3 percent of those in the lowest quartile of exposure. After controlling for baseline characteristics, the researchers concluded that adolescents in the highest quartile of exposure to movie smoking were 2.71 time more likely to initiate smoking than those in the lowest quartile, and that, in this cohort, 52 percent of smoking initiation was attributable to exposure to smoking in movies.

On the basis of this limited, but suggestive, evidence, the committee believes that there is a strong possibility that youthful exposure to alcohol content in entertainment media contributes to early initiation of alcohol use. In light of that possibility, the entertainment industries have a social responsibility to eschew displays or lyrics that portray underage drinking in a favorable light or that glamorize or promote alcohol consumption or irresponsible behavior in products that are targeted toward or likely to be heard or viewed by large underage audiences.

Recommendation 8-1: The entertainment industries should use rating systems and marketing codes to reduce the likelihood that underage audiences will be exposed to movies, recordings, or television programs with unsuitable alcohol content, even if adults are expected to predominate in the viewing or listening audiences.

By "unsuitable alcohol content," the committee means to include lyrics, images, depictions, or messages that portray underage drinking in a favorable light; that portray intoxication or otherwise excessive alcohol use by anyone in an attractive way; or that promote or glorify alcohol use in high-risk situations, such as while driving. Further specification of unsuitable alcohol content can be found in the advertising and marketing codes of the beer, wine, and distilled spirits industries. The committee urges the entertainment industries to review these codes to help develop specific standards for rating and marketing practices.

The challenge of promoting responsible industry practices regarding underage alcohol use is analogous to the challenge of reducing youth exposure to explicit sexual themes, violence, or illegal drug use. The committee accordingly reviewed industry practices in these areas—as well as the efforts of the Federal Trade Commission (FTC) to prod the industry into stronger self-regulation. In the context of violent programming, a recent series of FTC reports is highly instructive. In a 2000 report, the FTC found that members of all three major entertainment industries—motion pictures, music, and video games—had engaged in widespread marketing of violent movies, music, and electronic games to children under 17 by promoting their products on television, in magazines, and on Internet sites that have large underage audiences (FTC, 2000).

The FTC found that 80 percent of the 44 R-rated movies selected for study had been marketed to children under 17; as had 70 percent of the adult-rated video games and 100 percent of the explicit music recordings. In addition, the FTC found that advertisements for these products rarely contained rating information. The FTC also conducted undercover shopping operations to retailers and movie theaters with unaccompanied teens (aged 13-17); the young shoppers were able to buy M-rated electronic games and "parental advisory" labeled music recordings 85 percent of the time and to purchase tickets for R-rated movies 46 percent of the time.

Follow-up reports (FTC, 2001, 2002) noted progress by the movie and video game industries in disclosing rating information in advertising and in limiting advertising for R-rated movies and M-rated games in teen-oriented media. However, the report found little improvement in advertising by the music recording industry and only weak progress in strengthening self-regulation. The motion picture studios and video game manufacturers have developed an age-based rating system, designed to inform parents of the level of objectionable material suitable for children of different ages. In contrast, the music industry's "explicit content" warnings are not age specific and make no mention of the specific reasons for the warning (e.g., drug use, language, violence). However, one music industry member has begun including reasons for the warning on product packaging and advertising.

MOVIES

Extrapolating from recent national survey data, 11- to 13-year-olds spend an average of 6.2 hours per week, and 14- to 18-year-olds spend an average of 4.7 hours per week watching movies (Roberts et al., 1999a). In terms of alcohol content in films, recent content analyses indicate that alcohol was shown or consumed in 93 percent of the 200 most popular movie rentals for 1996 to 1997 (Roberts et al., 1999b). Although underage use of alcohol occurred in only about 9 percent of these films, alcohol and drinking were presented in an overwhelmingly positive light. Drinking was associated with wealth or luxury in 34 percent of films containing alcohol references and pro-use statements or overt advocacy of use occurred in 20 percent of the films. Anti-use statements appeared in 9 percent of films with alcohol references, 6 percent contained statements on limits as to when, where, and how much alcohol should be consumed, and 14 percent depicted refusals to drink.

Drinking in movies is often associated with such risky activities as crime or violence (38 percent), driving (14 percent), and sexual activity (19 percent). Portrayals of negative consequences of drinking are relatively rare. In all, 57 percent of films with alcohol references portrayed no consequences at all. Similar findings have emerged from other content analyses. Thus, at least one lead character drank in 79 percent of the top money-making U.S. films from 1985 to 1995 (Everett et al., 1998). Moreover, 96 percent of those films contained references supportive of alcohol use, while only 37 percent contained references discouraging alcohol use. Alcohol use even occurs in G-rated films. Among G-rated animated feature films released in U.S. theaters from 1937 to 2000 and available on videocassette, 47 percent showed alcohol use with, at best, ambivalent connotations (Thompson and Yokota, 2001). A review by Roberts, Henriksen, and Christensen (1999b) showed that alcohol use occurred in 76 percent of movies rated G or PG, 97 percent of movies rated PG-13, and 94 percent of movies rated R.

Ratings are assigned by a Rating Board appointed by the president of the Motion Picture Association of America (MPAA). According to the current MPAA Rating Board guidelines, the criteria taken into account by the board include theme violence, language, nudity, sensuality, and drug abuse. Films are rated as a whole. Under the rating system, films are rated G (all ages admitted), PG (parental guidance suggested because some material may be unsuitable for children), PG-13 (parents strongly cautioned because some material may be inappropriate for children under 13), R (restricted for children under 17 unless accompanied by parent), and NC-17 (no one under 17 admitted). Alcohol use is not explicitly mentioned as a rating criterion in the MPAA guidelines, and actual rating practice is not easily inferred. Although a film with illegal drug use cannot be assigned a G or PG rating, alcohol use (by adults) is widely depicted in films with these ratings.

> **Recommendation 8-2: The film rating board of the Motion Picture Association of America should consider alcohol content in rating films, avoiding G or PG ratings for films with unsuitable alcohol content, and assigning mature ratings for films that portray underage drinking in a favorable light.**

MUSIC RECORDINGS

Music is a popular form of entertainment for young people: 11- to 13-year-olds spend 11.2 hours per week and 14- to 18-year-olds spend 9.3 hours per week listening to music on radio, compact disks (CDs), or tape (Roberts et al., 1999a). Many parents and other adults are likely unaware of the extent of alcohol images in today's music and music videos, particularly rap music, which is especially appealing to young people. References to alcohol and drinking, including brand-name references and lyrics and images glamorizing alcohol use, are commonplace in today's music, particularly in hip hop songs and music videos. A recent content analysis (Roberts et al., 1999b) examined 1,000 of the most popular songs from

1996 to 1997 across five genres of music popular with youth. They found that 17 percent of all the lyrics contained references to alcohol: alcohol was mentioned much more frequently in rap music (47 percent) than in other genres, which included country-western (13 percent), top 40 (12 percent), alternative rock (10 percent), and heavy metal (4 percent). Overall, 22 percent of songs with alcohol mentions referred to beer or malt liquor, 34 percent to wine or champagne, 36 percent to hard liquor or mixed drinks, and 31 percent to generic terms such as "booze." A common theme was getting intoxicated or high (24 percent), although drinking was also associated with wealth and luxury (24 percent), sexual activity (34 percent), and crime or violence (13 percent). Consequences of drinking were mentioned in only 9 percent, and anti-use messages occurred in only 3 percent of the songs with alcohol references. Product placements or brand-name mentions occurred in 30 percent of them and were especially common in rap music (48 percent). An analysis of alcohol depictions in rap music (Herd, 1993) found the portrayal of alcohol use to convey elements of disinhibition, rebellion, identity, pleasure, sensuality, and personal power.

DuRant et al. (1997) analyzed 518 music videos from four television stations—MTV, BET, CMT and VH1—for portrayals of alcohol and tobacco use. In terms of music genre, rap music contained the highest percentage of depictions of alcohol use, and rhythm and blues videos showed the least alcohol use. Alcohol use was found in a higher proportion of music videos that had any sexual content than in videos that had no sexual content.

The music industry has been the slowest to implement rating and advertising restrictions in line with the FTC's recommendations in its reports on the marketing of recordings with violent content to young audiences. The deficiencies identified by the FTC in these reports are directly applicable to the marketing of recordings with alcohol content to young audiences. The recording industry has no independent review board for its decision to label recordings. There are also no stated standards for what sort of recording receives a label, and the current labeling system does not require recording companies to inform buyers of the reasons for the explicit-content label. The FTC's follow-up reports in 2001 and 2002 found that advertising for explicit-content labeled recordings continued to appear on television programs popular with teen audiences. Although there have been some recent improvements, these advertisements frequently failed to indicate that the advertised product had a parental warning label; even when this information was indicated, it was often too small to be read. Except for one recording company, the companies themselves provide little to no information as to the reasons for the parental warning label or where to find such information (FTC, 2002).

In the committee's judgment, more responsible self-regulation by the music recording industry is an essential component of a meaningful societal commitment to reduce underage drinking. At the present time, lyrics glamorizing alcohol use are proliferating in recordings that are marketed predominantly to teenagers, and the music recording industry has failed to take suitable steps to establish and enforce an appropriate rating system.

> **Recommendation 8-3: The music recording industry should not market recordings that promote or glamorize alcohol use to young people; should include alcohol content in a comprehensive rating system, similar to those used by the television, film, and video game industries; and should establish an independent body to assign ratings and oversee the industry code.**

Unlike the movie and video game industries, the music recording industry has not committed itself to meaningful self-regulation. It is time for the music recording industry to adopt such a code and to include in the code a specific ban against lyrics and images that depict underage drinking in a favorable light or otherwise glamorize or promote alcohol use in products that are marketed to underage audiences. These guidelines could be adapted from the FTC recommendations regarding alcohol advertising to youth (see FTC, 1999).

A music recording industry rating system of songs should provide consumers with brief descriptors of lyric and image content, including alcohol content, similar to rating systems adopted by the television, film, and video game industries. A rating system provides parents with information that can help them make informed decisions. While movies, television programs, and video games are rated on a gradient with specific guidelines for each of the ratings, the current system used by the music recording industry effectively classifies all products into two categories—with or without explicit content (on sex and violence). The packaging and marketing of music provides no other information as to the content of the product.

The system from the video gaming industry, established by the Entertainment Software Rating Board (ESRB), serves as the best model for a comprehensive rating system that can be adapted by the music recording industry. The system includes a rating that is displayed in a rating symbol on the front of the product's packaging and content descriptors that are located on the back of the product. The ESRB uses five ratings (early childhood, everyone, teen, mature, and adults only); fewer would probably be suitable for music recordings. The ESRB system has 26 content descriptors, including 2 for alcohol content—alcohol reference and use of alcohol—that can be used in any combination to describe the content found in the game; see Box 8-1.

The music recording industry should specify when the recording includes alcohol content, and when a rating system has been adopted, the

BOX 8-1
ESRB Rating System

Rating Symbols

EARLY CHILDHOOD: Content may be suitable for ages 3 and older; contains no material that parents would find inappropriate.
EVERYONE: Content may be suitable for persons aged 6 and older; may contain minimal violence and some comic mischief or crude language.
TEEN: Content may be suitable for persons aged 13 and older; may contain violent content, mild or strong language, or suggestive themes.
MATURE: Content may be suitable for persons aged 17 and older; may contain mature sexual themes or more intense violence or language.
ADULTS ONLY: Content is suitable only for adults; may include graphic depictions of sex or violence. Not intended for persons under the age of 18.
RATING PENDING: The product has been submitted to the ESRB and is awaiting final rating.

Examples of ESRB Content Descriptors

Alcohol reference: reference to images of alcoholic beverages.
Animated blood: cartoon or pixilated depictions of blood.
Blood and gore: depictions of blood or the mutilation of body parts.
Comic mischief: scenes depicting slapstick or gross vulgar humor.
Drug reference: reference to images of illegal drugs.
Gambling: betting like behavior.
Mature humor: vulgar or crude jokes and antics, including "bathroom" humor.
Mature sexual themes: provocative material, possibly including partial nudity.
Nudity: graphic or prolonged depictions of nudity.
Strong language: profanity and explicit references to sexuality, violence, alcohol, or drug use.
Strong sexual content: graphic depiction of sexual behavior, possibly including nudity.
Suggestive themes: mild provocative references or materials.
Tobacco reference: reference to images of tobacco products.
Use of drugs: the consumption or use of illegal drugs.
Use of alcohol: the consumption of alcoholic beverages.
Use of tobacco: the consumption of tobacco products.
Violence: scenes involving aggressive conflict.

SOURCE: Adapted from ESRB (2003).

rating board should classify any recording with unsuitable alcohol content, including name-brand reference of alcohol products, as appropriate only for "mature' audiences. Using this approach for name-brand references would be analogous to the FTC's recommendation that all films with paid alcohol placement receive an R or NC-17 rating (FTC, 1999). In conjunction with the alcohol industry, the music recording industry should work to bar alcohol placement in music videos aimed at underage audiences. Finally, the music recording industry should increase consumer and parental understanding of the improved rating system. In its December 2001 report on the marketing of violent entertainment to children, the FTC found that all of the 55 recordings in their study with explicit lyrical content (pertaining to violence) were targeted to children under the age of 17. With that type of marketing and pressure geared toward young people, parents must take an active role in regulating the images their children receive, and it is up to the industry to provide parents with the necessary information they need to make educated decisions regarding consumption. The recording industry should adopt a more comprehensive rating system, and it should provide literature on the reasons behind the ratings. This information should be made available either within the product packaging or in some other easily accessible area, such as through a telephone hotline or an Internet web site. The point is that parents be better able to access and understand information about the content of products they purchase for their children.

The MPAA has the Ratings Board and the Interactive Digital Software Association (IDSA) has the ESRB, but the Recording Industry Association of America (RIAA) has no separate governing body that rates the content of their industries products. MPAA's rating board and the IDSA's ESRB are both governing bodies established by their respective industry associations to provide nonbiased review and ratings of products for the purpose of educating parents. After viewing the content of a game (using video clips) or a movie (in its entirety), the boards make a rating decision on each game or film that is submitted to them; see Box 8-2.

The RIAA's Parental Advisory Program consists of a set of guidelines that regulate the placement of the parental advisory label on the packaging and marketing of music, but it establishes no authoritative board to review the content of products. Individual record companies and their artists determine whether each individual recording warrants a parental advisory label. Asking record companies to rate their own records is akin to asking studios to rate their own movies. Without an independent review board, any determination of explicit content is probably both unreliable and inconsistent. Furthermore, without a comprehensive ratings system (similar to the one used by the video game industry), the determination of explicit content in records is of little use to parents.

RETAIL ACCESS TO MOVIES AND RECORDINGS

FTC's recent reports on violence in the entertainment media, described above, recommended that all three industries (movie, music recording, and video game) improve the usefulness of their ratings and labels by establishing codes that prohibit marketing R/NC-rated/M-rated/explicit-labeled products in media or venues with a substantial under-17 audience. The reports also emphasized that restricting children's retail access to entertainment containing violent content is an essential complement to restricting the placement of advertising. Such restriction could be implemented by checking identification or requiring parental permission before selling tickets to R or NC movies and by not selling or renting products labeled "explicit" or rated R or M to children. In addition, the FTC suggested that each industry's trade associations monitor and encourage their members' compliance with these policies and impose meaningful sanctions for noncompliance.

We fully endorse the FTC's recommendation and suggestion. We believe that these would also be appropriate actions to reduce the exposure of underage audiences to unsuitable images relating to use of alcoholic beverages in the entertainment media.

TELEVISION

Adolescents are heavy users of television. Each week, 11- to 13-year-olds watch 27.7 hours, and 14- to 18-year-olds watch 20.2 hours of broadcast and taped television programming (Roberts et al., 1999). As a result, they are immersed in drinking portrayals and alcohol product placements. A recent content analysis of prime-time television from the 1998-1999 season, for example, showed that 71 percent of episodes sampled from prime-time programs depicted alcohol use, typically in a positive light, and that 77 percent contained some reference to alcohol (Christensen et al., 2000).

Among those programs most popular with teenagers, 53 percent portrayed alcohol use: 84 percent of TV-14 rated programming, 77 percent of TV-PG programming, and 38 percent of TV-G programming depicted alcohol use. More episodes portrayed drinking as an overall positive experience (40 percent) than a negative one (10 percent), although negative consequences were mentioned or portrayed in 23 percent of episodes. Underage drinking was relatively rare. Only 2 percent of regular characters under the age of 18 were depicted drinking alcohol. In another recent content analysis, however, characters between the ages of 13 and 18 accounted for 7 percent of all alcohol incidents portrayed (Mathios et al., 1998). When it occurs, youthful drinking or expressed desire to drink is often presented as means of appearing to be adult and grown-up (Grube, 1995).

The television networks have adopted a mandatory rating policy. Shows are rated for age-appropriate content under seven grades:

BOX 8-2
Ratings of the MPAA

G: "General Audiences—All Ages Admitted"

This is a film which contains nothing in theme, language, nudity and sex, violence, etc. which would, in the view of the Rating Board, be offensive to parents whose younger children view the film. The G rating is not a "certificate of approval," nor does it signify a children's film.

Some snippets of language may go beyond polite conversation but they are common everyday expressions. No stronger words are present in G-rated films. The violence is at a minimum. Nudity and sex scenes are not present; nor is there any drug use content.

PG: "Parental Guidance Suggested. Some Material May Not Be Suitable For Children"

This is a film which clearly needs to be examined or inquired into by parents before they let their children attend. The label PG plainly states that parents may consider some material unsuitable for their children, but the parent must make the decision.

Parents are warned against sending their children, unseen and without inquiry, to PG-rated movies.

The theme of a PG-rated film may itself call for parental guidance. There may be some profanity in these films. There may be some violence or brief nudity. But these elements are not deemed so intense as to require that parents be strongly cautioned beyond the suggestion of parental guidance. There is no drug use content in a PG-rated film.

The PG rating, suggesting parental guidance, is thus an alert for examination of a film by parents before deciding on its viewing by their children.

Obviously such a line is difficult to draw. In our pluralistic society it is not easy to make judgments without incurring some disagreement. So long as parents know they must exercise parental responsibility, the rating serves as a meaningful guide and as a warning.

PG-13: "Parents Strongly Cautioned. Some Material May Be Inappropriate For Children Under 13"

PG-13 is thus a sterner warning to parents to determine for themselves the attendance in particular of their younger children as they might consider some material not suited for them. Parents, by the rating, are alerted to be very careful about the attendance of their under-teenage children.

A PG-13 film is one which, in the view of the Rating Board, leaps beyond the boundaries of the PG rating in theme, violence, nudity, sensuality, language, or

---

- TV-Y—appropriate for all ages
- TV-Y7—appropriate for ages 7 and above
- TV-Y7-FV—suitable for ages 7 and up but containing some elements of fantasy violence
- TV-G—appropriate for most children

other contents, but does not quite fit within the restricted R category. Any drug use content will initially require at least a PG-13 rating. In effect, the PG-13 cautions parents with more stringency than usual to give special attention to this film before they allow their 12-year olds and younger to attend.

If nudity is sexually oriented, the film will generally not be found in the PG-13 category. If violence is too rough or persistent, the film goes into the R (restricted) rating. A film's single use of one of the harsher sexually-derived words, though only as an expletive, shall initially require the Rating Board to issue that film at least a PG-13 rating. More than one such expletive must lead the Rating Board to issue a film an R rating, as must even one of these words used in a sexual context. These films can be rated less severely, however, if by a special vote, the Rating Board feels that a lesser rating would more responsibly reflect the opinion of American parents.

PG-13 places larger responsibilities on parents for their children's movie going. The voluntary rating system is not a surrogate parent, nor should it be. It cannot, and should not, insert itself in family decisions that only parents can, and should, make. Its purpose is to give prescreening advance informational warnings, so that parents can form their own judgments. PG-13 is designed to make these parental decisions easier for films between PG and R.

R: "Restricted, Under 17 Requires Accompanying Parent Or Adult Guardian"
In the opinion of the Rating Board, this film definitely contains some adult material. Parents are strongly urged to find out more about this film before they allow their children to accompany them.

An R-rated film may include hard language, or tough violence, or nudity within sensual scenes, or drug abuse or other elements, or a combination of some of the above, so that parents are counseled, in advance, to take this advisory rating very seriously. Parents must find out more about an R-rated movie before they allow their teenagers to view it.

NC-17: "No One 17 And Under Admitted"
This rating declares that the Rating Board believes that this is a film that most parents will consider patently too adult for their youngsters under 17. No children will be admitted. NC-17 does not necessarily mean "obscene or pornographic" in the oft-accepted or legal meaning of those words. The Board does not and cannot mark films with those words. These are legal terms and for courts to decide. The reasons for the application of an NC-17 rating can be violence or sex or aberrational behavior or drug abuse or any other elements which, when present, most parents would consider too strong and therefore off-limits for viewing by their children.

SOURCE: MPAA (2003, pp. 4-5).

- TV-PG—containing some elements that may be inappropriate for young children
- TV-14—containing material that may be unsuitable for children under 14
- TV-MA—programming appropriate for people over 17

However, the ratings are typically assigned by the producers of the programming, and there is no independent board responsible for standardizing or enforcing these ratings. Moreover, although the networks rate programs, only conscientious use of the "v-chip" by parents serves to block programming.

The main criteria governing ratings under the prescribed categories are sexual content, violence, coarse language, and suggestive dialogue; if these elements are present, a notice is displayed on the screen at the beginning of the program, as well as in most television programming guides. While depictions of underage alcohol use or abuse may be rated as TV-14 or TV-MA, no specific criterion governs this type of content under existing standards, and, as a result, alcohol content is not one of the special criteria communicated to parents in advance (see www.tvguidlines.org).[1]

> Recommendation 8-4: Television broadcasters and producers should take appropriate precautions to ensure that programs do not portray underage drinking in a favorable light and that unsuitable alcohol content is included in the category of mature content for purposes of parental warnings.

ACCOUNTABILITY

The committee believes that standards to minimize underage exposure to lyrics, images and depictions with unsuitable alcohol content should be implemented on a voluntary basis by the pertinent industry trade associations and individual companies. However, as with the alcohol industry, some independent oversight of these standards is warranted. In both contexts, the committee believes that the most promising strategy is to promote industry accountability by facilitating public awareness of industry practices. Accordingly, the committee recommends that the U.S. Department of Health and Human Services be authorized and funded to monitor these media practices and report to Congress and the public.

> Recommendation 8-5: Congress should appropriate the necessary funds to enable the U.S. Department of Health and Human Services to conduct a periodic review of a representative sample of movies, television programs, and music recordings and videos that are offered at times or

---

[1]Direct regulation of content by the FCC is exercised only for obscene and indecent material, which has been interpreted almost exclusively to cover sexual depictions (http://www.fcc.gov/eb/broadcast/obscind.html, accessed November 15, 2002).

in venues likely to have a significant youth audience (e.g., 15 percent) to ascertain the nature and frequency of lyrics or images pertaining to alcohol. The results of these reviews should be reported to Congress and the public.

The Secretary of Health and Human Services should include this information in the Annual Report on Underage Drinking recommended in Chapter 12.

9

Access

This chapter addresses components of the strategy to reduce access to alcohol by youths under 21. Most developed societies that permit alcohol consumption by adults prescribe a minimum legal drinking age. Laws ban distribution of alcohol to underage persons and usually also proscribe underage purchase and possession of alcohol. As discussed in Chapter 1, these laws rest primarily on an instrumental rationale rather than a moral one—that is, they aim less to condemn immoral behavior than to protect young people from the potentially serious negative consequences of engaging in a behavior for which they may not be developmentally prepared. Their moral force lies mainly in the efforts to hold adults accountable for the harms caused by underage drinkers to whom they give or sell alcohol.

The prescribed minimum age differs substantially among countries; see Table 9-1. Whatever the prescribed minimum age, countries must decide what measures will be used to curtail access by minors through the otherwise lawful channels of distribution. Naturally, this is a daunting challenge, especially in countries like the United States, in which alcohol is widely available to adults through a multitude of outlets.

There is ample evidence that raising the minimum drinking age in the United States reduced drinking and its associated harms among youth. In all likelihood, these effects on underage consumption were mediated in part through the reduced accessibility of alcohol to youths. It is also clear that significant rates of noncompliance impede the effectiveness of the laws that restrict the provision of alcohol to underage youths. The question is what

TABLE 9-1 Minimum Legal Drinking or
Purchase Age Across 64 Countries

Minimum Age	Number of Countries
None	5
< 16	4
16	6
17	1
18	38
19	1
20	2
21	7

NOTE: Some countries have different minimum legal ages for the purchase and consumption of alcoholic beverages or for different beverage types (e.g., beer and wine versus spirits), and in some cases there are regional variations within countries. The numbers in this table reflect the lowest minimum age for purchase or consumption of any alcoholic beverage in any state, province, or region within a country.
SOURCE: International Center for Alcohol Policies (2002).

can be done to increase compliance and, thereby, alcohol's availability to underage youths. In order to promote compliance with any laws, they must be communicated to, and understood by, the intended audiences (in this case, primarily adults), and there must be a credible threat of enforcement to deter violations by those who have strong incentives to offend—in this case, by selling or giving alcohol to underage drinkers. Maximizing the incentives for voluntary compliance will minimize the need for enforcement.

The effectiveness of laws to restrict access to alcohol by youths can be increased by closing gaps in coverage, promoting compliance, and strengthening enforcement. Although particular methods for increasing effectiveness along these lines have been tried in various jurisdictions, and some data are available regarding their success, others have not been evaluated. The strength of the evidence in support of any particular intervention varies, and in some cases the available evidence is contradictory. However, the committee believes that the preponderance of the available evidence, including recent evidence from studies on the prevention of youth smoking, supports an emphasis on efforts designed to increase the effectiveness of restrictions on youth access to alcohol.

Given that youth usually obtain alcohol—directly or indirectly—from adults, the committee also believes that the focus of these efforts should be on adults. A key component of the committee's strategy is the proposed media campaign to help strengthen public commitment to the goal of reducing underage drinking and to promote adult compliance with youth access restrictions (see Chapter 6).

This chapter begins with a discussion of minimum drinking age laws and specific recommendations about the scope of the laws. It then moves to a discussion of how youths obtain alcohol. Given that youths obtain alcohol from a variety of venues, the committee believes that a range of approaches targeting different venues is necessary. The remainder of the chapter reviews various approaches to improving the effectiveness of access restrictions and summarizes the available evidence in four domains: (1) reducing access through commercial sources; (2) reducing access through noncommercial sources; (3) focused efforts to reduce drinking and driving by underage drinkers; and (4) prescribing and enforcing penalties directly against underage consumers.

Given that it is unreasonable to expect a measurable effect on consumption for any one isolated change in the fabric of access restrictions, most evaluations rely on measuring changes in enforcement behavior or in compliance on the assumption that, over time, increased enforcement will result in increased compliance, and that increased compliance (whether or not attributable to increased enforcement) will lead to reduced access, and in turn to reduced consumption. The level of evidence for specific recommendations varies, as discussed through this chapter. The committee has used its judgment in assessing the plausibility of these connections. In some cases, the committee's general recommendations include specific details that are based on the informed judgment of the committee. As with all aspects of the proposed strategy, particular interventions should be subjected to ongoing research to enable continued refinement of the strategy based on new empirical evidence.

The committee has assessed the potential value of each intervention not in isolation, but rather as part of a comprehensive set of steps that can be taken to curtail alcohol access to minors—mainly by promoting voluntary compliance, in both commercial and noncommercial contexts, but also by establishing and sustaining a credible threat of enforcement. Although there is robust evidence concerning the effects on consumption of increasing the legal minimum drinking age (and the accompanying, but unspecified, efforts to implement it), there is less evidence on the effects on youth consumption of comprehensive multipronged efforts to strengthen implementation of the underage drinking laws on the kind envisioned in this chapter.[1]

---

[1]An evaluation of the effects of the Enforcing the Underage Drinking Laws program on law enforcement and youth drinking behavior in the jurisdictions funded by the program is in the very early stages. The funded jurisdictions have wide latitude in the type of activities they can

IMPLEMENTING LAWS ON THE MINIMUM DRINKING AGE

Effectiveness

Strategies aimed at reducing youth access to alcohol focus on the nature and scope of the access restrictions and the policies and practices used to implement and enforce them (Holder, 2004; Grube and Nygaard, 2001; Toomey and Wagenaar, 1999). Overall, the purpose of these policies and practices is to raise the "full price" of alcohol by increasing the effort and resources necessary to obtain it or by increasing the threatened consequences for its use. Importantly, such policies and procedures can also communicate community norms—to young people regarding the unacceptability of their drinking and to adults about the unacceptability of providing alcohol to minors (Bonnie, 1986). These aims are analogous to those sought by laws curtailing youth access to tobacco (see Institute of Medicine, 1994a) and restricting nonmedical access to marijuana, cocaine, and other illegal drugs (see National Research Council, 2001).

Limiting youth access to alcohol has been shown to be effective in reducing and preventing underage drinking and drinking-related problems. Studies routinely show that increasing the minimum drinking age significantly decreased the number of fatal traffic crashes, the number of arrests for "driving under the influence" (DUI), and self-reported drinking by young people (Klepp et al., 1996; O'Malley and Wagenaar, 1991; Saffer and Grossman, 1987a, 1987b; Wagenaar, 1981, 1986; Wagenaar and Maybee, 1986; Voas et al., 1999; Yu et al., 1997). Similarly, implementation of zero tolerance laws—which ban underage youths from driving with a blood alcohol content (BAC) above measurable levels (usually 0.01-0.02)—has been shown to significantly reduce underage drinking and driving (Hingson et al., 1994; Voas et al., 1999; Wagenaar et al., 2001; Zwerling and Jones, 1999). Community interventions also provide evidence for the effectiveness of comprehensive approaches to reduce drinking and drinking

---

implement, and there is significant variation in the type and intensity of interventions implemented across communities; moreover, the evaluation was not designed to consider the effectiveness of a particular intervention or set of interventions within individual communities. The outcomes evaluation reported to date was also based on a single year of intervention (future evaluation reports will include 2 years of data), which is highly unlikely to affect alcohol use outcomes. Not surprisingly, the evaluation documents increases in enforcement activities, but no significant decreases in youth alcohol use (Wolfson et al., 2003). For the current fiscal year, the Office of Juvenile Justice and Delinquency Prevention (OJJDP) has shifted toward a more prescriptive approach that will require local communities participating in the discretionary grant component to implement identified best and most promising practices (OJJDP, 2003). If continued, this would better enable the evaluation to assess the effectiveness of particular interventions and further refine the program.

problems, including reducing underage access to alcohol (Holder et al., 1997a, 1997b, 2000; Wagenaar et al., 1999, 2000a; Wagenaar and Perry, 1994).

To some extent, merely declaring that alcohol should not be sold or given to underage youths will curtail access because many adults support the prohibition and are in the habit of complying with the law (Tyler, 1992; Tyler and Huo, 2002). However, these "declarative" effects of the law (Bonnie, 1982) can easily be eroded if youthful drinking is regarded as an unimportant or expected deviance and if no meaningful efforts are taken to enforce the prohibition. For example, bans against selling tobacco to minors became trivialized over decades of inattention until the public, and the government, began to take them seriously in the 1990s (Institute of Medicine, 1994a). Although youth access restrictions to alcohol have never fallen into such complete disregard, they are easily evaded because alcohol is so widely available through so many channels and because the adult world is ambivalent about how forcefully they should be enforced. In this context, the declarative effects of the law cannot be expected to do all the work; deterrence through threatened sanctions, both legal and social, is needed. In this sense, enforcement, and public awareness of enforcement, are essential if restrictions on youth access to alcohol are to be effectively implemented.

It is clear from the available research that the effectiveness of youth access restrictions and other alcohol control policies depends heavily on the intensity of implementation and enforcement and on the degree to which the intended targets are aware of both the policy and its enforcement (Grube and Nygaard, 2001; Hingson et al., 1988a, 1988b; Voas et al., 1998). Another potentially important element in increasing the effectiveness of youth access restrictions or other alcohol control policies is public support. Implementing effective polices will be very difficult if law enforcement officers and community leaders believe that there is little community support for such activities (Wagenaar and Wolfson, 1994, 1995). The strategic use of media can help overcome such resistance and elicit public support for limiting access (Holder and Treno, 1997).

Scope

Alcohol control is primarily a state responsibility under the 21st Amendment to the Constitution. In some states, counties and municipalities are permitted to take steps to control drinking that may be stricter than those required by state law. However, the National Minimum Drinking Age Act, enacted by the Congress in 1984, requires states to adopt a minimum drinking age of 21 for "purchase or public possession" of alcohol as a condition for receiving federal highway funds. As a result, all 50 states and the District of Columbia now set the minimum drinking or purchase age at 21.

A preliminary question concerns designation of the minimum age. Some experts in the field have suggested that the United States would be better off by lowering it (Hanson, 1990). A key argument made in favor of lowering the minimum age is that although the legal purchase age is 21, a majority of young people under this age consume alcohol anyway. Thus, the current age is seen as forcing young people to flout the law, thus undermining its legal authority and credibility. Furthermore, according to this perspective, the current age might actually encourage abusive drinking by young people by making alcohol use a rite of passage to adulthood or a symbol of rebellion and by forcing it to occur in uncontrolled and risky environments.

European countries are frequently held up as examples of societies in which young people can drink at an early age and thus learn to consume alcohol responsibly within a controlled and safe environment (e.g., the family). The facts, however, do not support this argument. Research clearly shows that most European countries not only have higher levels of consumption (an expected consequence of the lower drinking age), but also higher levels of problematic drinking (e.g., intoxication) among youth (Grube, 2001). Analyses of data from a 1999 survey of 15-year-old European school children (Hibell et al., 2000) and the 1999 Monitoring the Future U.S. survey of tenth graders (Johnston et al., 2002) show that U.S. students are less likely than young people from most European countries to report alcohol use in the past 30 days; see Figure 9-1. Similarly, U.S. adolescents are less likely than those from a majority of European countries to report becoming intoxicated in the past year; see Figure 9-2. In several countries—the United Kingdom, Ireland, Poland, and Denmark—the proportion of teenagers reporting drinking heavily on at least three occasions in the last month is substantially greater than the proportion of U.S. teenagers who report drinking that much on at least one occasion during the past two weeks (Room, 2004). In short, there is no evidence that the lower drinking ages in Europe are protective. Finally, and most importantly as noted above, raising the minimum drinking age in the United States significantly decreased self-reported drinking, fatal traffic crashes, alcohol-related crashes, and arrests for DUI among young people (Klepp et al., 1996; O'Malley and Wagenaar, 1991; Saffer and Grossman, 1987; Wagenaar, 1981, 1986; Wagenaar and Maybee, 1986; Yu et al., 1997).[2] The 21-year-old minimum drinking age may also moderate drinking beyond adolescence (O'Malley and Wagenaar, 1991).

Although every state now sets the legal age at 21, state laws vary greatly in the scope of the restrictions relating to underage purchase, pos-

---

[2]Research showing these effects led Congress in 1984 to use the leverage of highway funds to induce all the states to raise the drinking age to 21.

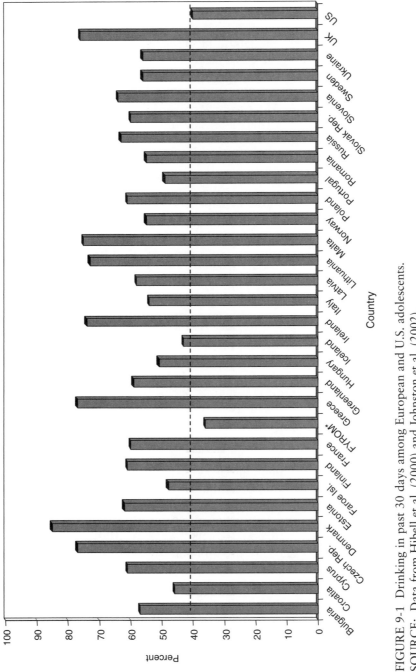

FIGURE 9-1 Drinking in past 30 days among European and U.S. adolescents.

SOURCE: Data from Hibell et al. (2000) and Johnston et al. (2002).

*FYROM is the accepted abbreviation for The Former Yugoslav Republic of Macedonia.

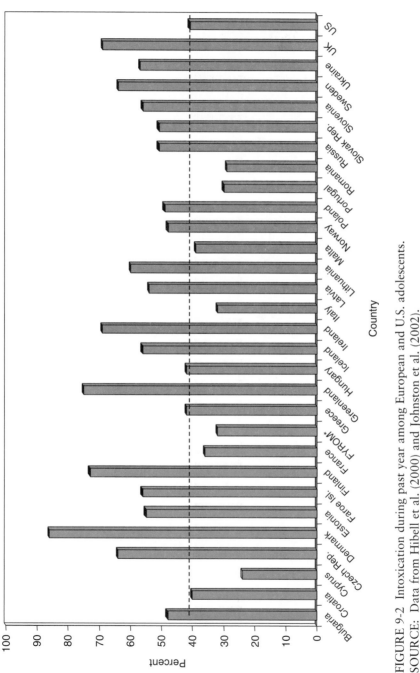

FIGURE 9-2 Intoxication during past year among European and U.S. adolescents.
SOURCE: Data from Hibell et al. (2000) and Johnston et al. (2002).
*FYROM is the accepted abbreviation for The Former Yugoslav Republic of Macedonia.

session, or consumption of alcohol and for the use of false identification to purchase alcohol. In 1993, the President's Commission on Model State Drug Laws (1993) recommended that states prohibit all of these activities. Moreover, although it is generally illegal to provide alcohol to minors, some states allow parents or guardians to give alcohol to minors or for underage drinking to take place in a private residence or private club. These weaknesses can compromise the effectiveness of minimum age laws.

Recommendation 9-1: The minimum drinking age laws of each state should prohibit

- **purchase or attempted purchase, possession, and consumption of alcoholic beverages by persons under 21;**
- **possession of and use of falsified or fraudulent identification to purchase or attempt to purchase alcoholic beverages;**
- **provision of any alcohol to minors by adults, except to their own children in their own residences; and**
- **underage drinking in private clubs and establishments.**

HOW YOUNG PEOPLE OBTAIN ALCOHOL

Young people obtain alcohol from a variety of sources; see Tables 9-2 and 9-3. Parties, friends, and adult purchasers are the most frequent sources of alcohol among college students and older adolescents (Harrison et al., 2000; Preusser et al., 1995; Schwartz et al., 1998; Wagenaar et al., 1996), and younger adolescents also often obtain alcohol from family members. Use of friends under 21 and adult strangers as sources for alcohol appears to increase with age while reports of parents or other family members as sources decrease with age. Thus, in a study in Minnesota (Harrison et al., 2000), 39 percent of drinkers in the sixth grade, 69 percent of drinkers in the ninth grade, and 72 percent of drinkers in the twelfth grade reported getting alcohol from friends within the past 30 days. The comparable figures for family members as sources for alcohol were 49 percent, 29 percent, and 18 percent, respectively. Purchase of alcohol was relatively low in this sample, with only 8 percent, 8 percent, and 9 percent of drinkers at the three grade levels, respectively, reporting buying alcohol from stores. Similarly, another Minnesota survey (Wagenaar et al., 1996) found that 46 percent of ninth graders, 60 percent of twelfth graders, and 68 percent of 18- to 20-year-olds obtained alcohol on their last drinking occasion from a friend over 21, 29 percent, 29 percent, and 10 percent of these age groups, respectively, obtained alcohol from a friend under 21. Only 3 percent, 9 percent, and 14 percent of respondents in each age group, respectively, reported purchasing alcohol; 27 percent, 6 percent, and 11 percent, respectively, obtained alcohol from home.

TABLE 9-2 Sources of Alcohol Used by Underage Drinkers in Minnesota During Past 30 Days (in percent)

Source	Grade 6	Grade 9	Grade 12
Friends	39.3	69.3	72.3
Family	48.7	28.8	18.2
Parties	32.1	55.6	59.8
Took from home	33.1	33.2	11.8
Took from friend's home	15.9	17.7	5.0
Got someone to buy it for me	14.0	35.3	52.6
Bought at store	8.3	7.6	8.5
Bought at bar or restaurant	8.1	4.6	7.5
Took from store	10.0	6.5	2.5

SOURCE: Data from Harrison et al. (2000).

TABLE 9-3 Sources of Alcohol for Underage Drinkers (in percent)

Study and Measure	Sample Population	Purchased	Source Person		
			Person Under 21	21 or Older	Parent
Preusser et al.	New York College	75	69	73	31
(1995);	Pennsylvania College	59	64	76	22
ever used	New York High School	43	67	44	23
	Pennsylvania High School	30	55	50	14
Schwartz et al.	Virginia Pediatrician's Office	30	—	—	—
(1998);	Virginia College	44	—	—	—
ever used	New York High School	35	—	—	—
	Southeast Substance Abuse Program	52	—	—	—
Wagenaar et al.	9th Graders	3	29	46	27
(1996);	12th Graders	9	29	60	6
used past 30 days	18- to 20-year-olds	14	10	68	11

Use of commercial sources appears to be much higher among college students, in urban settings, and where possession and purchase laws are relatively weak or unenforced. Thus, for example, in one survey, 75 percent of college students from New York—where the purchase and possession of alcohol by minors were not illegal at the time of the study and where the use of false identification was punishable by a relatively small fine—reported ever having tried to purchase alcohol, in comparison with 59 percent of college students in Pennsylvania where the laws regarding purchase, possession, and the use of false identification of alcohol were much stricter (Preusser et al., 1995). Similarly, 43 percent of New York high school students and 30 percent of Pennsylvania high school students reported ever having tried to purchase alcohol.

Ultimately, adults are responsible for young people obtaining alcohol by selling, providing, or otherwise making it available to them. Given the fact that young people use multiple sources for alcohol, efforts to target underage access should not focus exclusively on commercial access to alcohol, but should also address social availability through parents, friends, and strangers (Holder, 1994).

ACCESS TO ALCOHOL THROUGH COMMERCIAL SOURCES

Commercial access to alcohol takes place primarily through on-license and off-license establishments. On-license establishments are permitted to sell alcohol for consumption at the location where the sale is made; they include bars, restaurants, roadhouses, theaters, and similar places of business. Off-license establishments are permitted to sell alcohol for consumption at other locations; they include liquor stores, markets, convenience stores, and similar venues. In addition to on- and off-license establishments, some states allow home delivery and Internet sales of alcohol.

States differ considerably in their regulatory practices, ranging from those with complete state-run retail or wholesale monopolies and distribution systems to those where retail and wholesale alcohol sales and distribution are completely private. To some extent, retail alcohol sales can also be regulated at the local or municipal level through the use of local ordinances, conditional use permits, and zoning. Some states also allow for a "local option" through which municipalities or counties can prohibit or limit alcohol sales. Local ordinances can send a very strong message about what a community considers to be acceptable norms concerning underage drinking.

As noted above, young people under 21 can and do purchase alcohol in commercial settings, notwithstanding the fact that such sales are illegal everywhere. Purchase surveys in the United States show that anywhere from 40 percent to 90 percent of outlets sell to underage buyers, depending on location (e.g., Forster et al., 1994, 1995; Preusser and Williams, 1992; Grube, 1997). In part, these high sales rates result from low and inconsistent levels of enforcement against adults who sell or provide alcohol to minors and from perceptions on the part of law enforcement officers that there is little community support for such prevention efforts (Wagenaar and Wolfson, 1994, 1995).

Compliance Checks

Increasing enforcement against retailers who sell to minors can have a substantial effect on sales of alcohol to young people. Even moderate increases in enforcement can reduce sales of alcohol to minors by as much as 35 percent to 40 percent, especially when combined with media and other community activities (Grube, 1997; Wagenaar et al., 2000a). Effective compliance checks are conducted on an on-going basis, with regular enforcement actions (e.g., two or more times per year) against all outlets, rather than sporadic actions against "problem" outlets (Willingham, n.d.).

Further support for the importance of reducing retail access to alcohol can be obtained from the literature on tobacco control and youth smoking. Most notably, recent research suggests that increasing compliance with age identification for the purchase of tobacco not only reduced tobacco sales to minors and youth smoking, but also reduced underage drinking (Biglan et al., 2000). In a variation of compliance checks, the primary intervention in this research comprised repeated visits to tobacco outlets in which underage youth attempted to purchase tobacco. These young people gave a reminder of the law to clerks who agreed to sell. Clerks who refused to sell received a gift certificate worth $5 to $10, and local media publicized their refusal. This intervention was implemented within the context of a community-wide proclamation against selling to youth, visits to each merchant with information about the proclamation and the law, community-wide publicity about outlet refusals, and feedback to outlets about their rate of sales to young people. Across all communities, the average percent of outlets willing to sell decreased from 57 percent to 22 percent, a 61 percent relative decline. Although the community-based interventions focused on limiting youth access to tobacco products, a 60 percent relative reduction in weekly alcohol use among ninth graders also was achieved (Biglan et al., 2000). Whereas prevalence of weekly alcohol use increased from about 10 percent to 18 percent in the control communities, it remained virtually unchanged in the intervention communities, increasing from about 13 percent to 14 percent. The significant effect on ninth grade alcohol consumption may have been due to the intervention sensitizing clerks not to sell either tobacco or alcohol to minors.

Recommendation 9-2: States should strengthen their compliance check programs in retail outlets, using media campaigns and license revocation to increase deterrence.

- **Communities and states should undertake regular and comprehensive compliance check programs, including notification of retailers concerning the program and follow-up communication to them about the outcome (sale/no sale) for their outlet.**

- Enforcement agencies should issue citations for violations of underage sales laws, with substantial fines and temporary suspension of
  license for first offenses and increasingly stronger penalties thereafter, leading to permanent revocation of license after three offenses.
- Communities and states should implement media campaigns in conjunction with compliance check programs detailing the program, its
  purpose, and outcomes.

States may need to consider the adequacy of funding for their alcohol
control agencies including how efficiently resources are utilized, to enable
the agencies to undertake the committee's recommended enforcement efforts. Communities might also consider programs that reward retailers for
compliance and remind them of the law, as a complement to law enforcement compliance checks (Biglan et al., 2000).

A model for enforcing compliance with underage alcohol sales laws at
the national level can be found in the Synar Amendment, which applies to
tobacco. The Synar Amendment, enacted in 1992, requires states to enact
and enforce effective laws prohibiting the sale of tobacco products to children under 18 years of age. States failing to comply lose a portion of their
block grant funds for substance abuse prevention.

Recommendation 9-3: The federal government should require states to
achieve designated rates of retailer compliance with youth access prohibitions as a condition of receiving relevant block grant funding, similar
to the Synar Amendment's requirements for youth tobacco sales.

Specifically, under this requirement, all states, as a prerequisite for
receiving funds under one or more block grants (e.g., substance abuse
prevention and treatment, enforcing the underage drinking laws), would be
expected to:

- enforce effective laws prohibiting sales of alcohol to persons under
21 years of age in a manner that can reasonably be expected to reduce the
availability of alcohol products to individuals under the age of 21;
- conduct annual random, unannounced inspections of both on- and
off-license outlets to ensure compliance with the law;
- conduct these inspections in such a way as to provide a valid sample
of outlets accessible to youth;
- develop a strategy and a time frame for achieving an inspection
failure rate of less than 20 percent of outlets; and
- submit an annual report detailing (a) the state's activities to enforce
their law, (b) the overall success the state has achieved during the previous
year in reducing alcohol availability to youth, (c) how inspections were

conducted and the methods used to identify outlets, and (d) plans for enforcing the law in the coming fiscal year.

Responsible Beverage Service and Sales

Responsible beverage service and sales programs implement a combination of outlet policies (e.g., requiring clerks or servers to check identification for all customers appearing to be under the age of 30; requiring all servers to be over 21), manager training (e.g., policy development and enforcement), and server training (e.g., teaching clerks and servers to recognize altered or false identification). Such programs can be implemented at both on-license and off-license establishments and have been shown to be effective in some circumstances. They have been found to reduce the number of intoxicated patrons leaving a bar (e.g., Dresser and Gliksman, 1998; Gliksman et al., 1993; Saltz, 1987, 1989) and to reduce the number of car crashes (e.g., Holder and Wagenaar, 1994).

Few studies have evaluated the effects of responsible beverage service and sales programs on underage drinking. In one study of an off-license program, voluntary clerk and manager training were found to have a negligible effect on sales to minors above and beyond the effects of increased enforcement (Grube, 1997). Similarly, a study in Australia found that, even after training, age identification was rarely checked in bars, although decreases in the number of intoxicated patrons were observed (Lang et al., 1996, 1998). In at least one study, however, training was associated with an increase in self-reported checking of identification by servers (Buka and Birdthistle, 1999), and the apparent changes in behavior persisted among trained servers for as long as 4 years. Another study reported an 11.5 percent decrease in sales to minors and a 46.0 percent decrease in sales to intoxicated patrons following individual manager training and policy development (Toomey et al., 2001). Voluntary programs appear to be less effective than mandatory programs or programs using incentives such as reduced liability (Dresser and Gliksman, 1998).

How responsible beverage service and sales programs are implemented and what elements are included in a particular program may be important determinants of their effectiveness. Policy development and implementation within outlets may be as important, if not more so, than server training (Saltz, 1997). Research indicates, for example, that establishments with firm and clear policies (e.g., checking ID for all patrons who appear under the age of 30) and a system for monitoring staff compliance are less likely to sell alcohol to minors (Wolfson et al., 1996a, 1996b). There are six key elements of successful outlet policies: (1) minimum age of 21 for all servers and sellers; (2) staff awareness of legal responsibility; (3) staff awareness of outlet policies and consequences for violating those policies; (4) identification required for all patrons who appear to be under 30;[3] (5) guidelines and training as to what constitutes acceptable and valid identification; and (6) retailer-initiated compliance checks and enforcement of consequences for violation of policies.

Recommendation 9-4: States should require all sellers and servers of alcohol to complete state-approved training as a condition of employment.

State alcohol agencies should prescribe responsible beverage service and sales training, including all of the elements described above as a condition of licensing for retail outlets, and could consider using server licensing fees to offset the cost of this training. Aside from state alcoholic beverage control (ABC) regulatory requirements, all managers or owners of retail outlets have a social responsibility to develop and implement alcohol service policies to prevent sales to minors, to train their staff on these policies, and to enforce them. As discussed below, implementation of such a program might also serve as a defense against civil liability.

Dram Shop Liability

Dram shop liability laws allow individuals injured by a minor who is under the influence of alcohol to recover damages from the alcohol retailer who served or sold the alcohol to the minor who caused the injury (Mosher, 1979; Mosher et al., 2002; Sloan et al., 2000). In some states, the retailer can also be liable for the damages the minor causes to himself or herself. Owners and licensees can be held liable for their employees' actions under most or all dram shop liability laws (Mosher et al., 2002). Many state courts have recognized dram shop liability as a common law cause of action—that is, the courts themselves establish the plaintiff's right to sue under ordinary principles of common law negligence. The plaintiff must show that the retailer knew or should have known that the person being served was a minor, that the minor in fact consumed the alcohol, and that the consumption was a contributing cause of the harm.

Many courts recognized common law dram shop claims during the 1980s and early 1990s, overruling the traditional rule that the drinker was solely liable for any damage that he or she caused as a result of drinking. State legislatures have become increasingly active in this policy area, estab-

---

[3]Electronic scanning of driver's licenses is a promising method of assuring that IDs are valid. However, not all states currently issue scannable licenses, and the cost and inconvenience of scanning devices may reduce the willingness of some retailers to use them (National Highway Traffic Safety Administration, 2001).

lishing statutory-based claims that typically supersede and extinguish a plaintiff's right to sue under common law negligence principles. The general legislative trend has been to limit the scope of liability (Mosher, 2002; Holder et al., 1993). California, for example requires that the plaintiff show that the minor was obviously intoxicated at the time of sale (California Business and Professions Code § 25602.1). Other state legislatures have required proof of reckless, rather than negligent, conduct on the part of the retailer or have imposed caps on the amount of damages that can be collected (Mosher et al., 2002). Some states do not recognize dram shop liability at all, either because a court has ruled that common law negligence principles do not impose liability in this situation or because the legislature has overridden a judicial ruling finding retailers liable. Currently, 44 states permit dram shop liability suits (Mothers Against Drunk Driving [MADD], 2002b). However, a simple count does not adequately describe the wide variation in state approaches. Many state laws are so restrictive that they effectively preclude or severely limit plaintiffs' right to sue (see Mosher et al., 2002).

Dram shop liability laws and common law rights of action are a potentially powerful tool for changing the environment in which alcohol is sold (Mosher, 1979; Holder et al., 1993). Research suggests that the threat of liability may lead to a significant increase in checking age identification and to greater care in service practices (e.g., Sloan et al., 2000). The available studies also suggest that dram shop liability laws can significantly reduce single vehicle nighttime crash deaths, alcohol-related traffic crash deaths, and total traffic crash deaths among minors (Chaloupka et al., 1993; Sloan et al., 1994, 2000). Other research indicates that such laws also reduce alcohol-related traffic crashes, total traffic crashes, homicides, and other unintentional injuries in the general population (Chaloupka et al., 1993; Sloan et al., 1994, 2000). Overall, dram shop liability has been estimated to reduce alcohol-related traffic fatalities among underage drivers by 3 to 4 percent (Chaloupka et al., 1993). The perceived likelihood of being successfully sued under dram shop liability statutes may be important. Thus, two highly publicized successful dram shop liability lawsuits in Texas were found to be related to decreases of 6.5 percent and 5.3 percent, respectively, in single vehicle nighttime crashes, which is a surrogate measure for drinking and driving (Wagenaar and Holder, 1991). These presumably occurred because owners, managers, and servers changed serving practices as a result of the suits and accompanying publicity.

Three states—Maine, New Hampshire, and Rhode Island—have passed key elements of the Model Alcoholic Beverage Retail Licensee Liability Act of 1985 (reprinted in Mosher et al., 2002), developed under a grant from the National Institute on Alcohol Abuse and Alcoholism. The model act includes a "responsible business practices" defense. This provision allows retailers to avoid liability if they can establish that they took reasonable steps to avoid serving minors and obviously intoxicated adults. Key to the defense is evidence that the retailer trained his or her staff, including both servers and managers, established management policies designed to deter such sales and service, and that the training procedures and policies were fully implemented at the time of the illegal sale or service.[4] The model act seeks to establish a positive incentive for retailers to implement prevention policies and enhance the positive public health benefits of dram shop liability policies.

> **Recommendation 9-5:** States should enact or strengthen dram shop liability statutes to authorize negligence-based civil actions against commercial providers of alcohol for serving or selling alcohol to a minor who subsequently causes injury to others, while allowing a defense for sellers who have demonstrated compliance with responsible business practices. States should include in their dram shop statutes key portions of the Model Alcoholic Beverage Retail Licensee Liability Act of 1985, including the responsible business practices defense.

Internet Sales and Home Delivery

Surveys of underage purchase of alcohol over the Internet or through home delivery show that small percentages (10 percent) of young people report obtaining alcohol in this manner (Fletcher et al., 2000); however, increasing use of the Internet may increase the percentage. Although an argument can certainly be made for banning Internet and home delivery sales altogether in light of the likelihood that these methods will be used by underage purchasers, the committee recognizes that some states may not be willing to curtail legitimate access to alcohol through these means and so recommends, instead, tightening access.

> **Recommendation 9-6:** States that allow Internet sales and home delivery of alcohol should regulate these activities to reduce the likelihood of sales to underage purchasers. States should
>
> • require all packages for delivery containing alcohol to be clearly labeled as such;

---

[4]States allowing retailers to recover their fines and other costs by suing underage drinkers who use false identification should also condition the retailers' recovery on proof of compliance with responsible business practices, including electronic scanning of driver's licenses if the state issues scannable licenses.

- require persons who deliver alcohol to record the recipient's age identification information from a valid government-issued document (such as a driver's license or ID card); and
- require recipients of home delivery of alcohol to sign a statement verifying receipt of alcohol and attesting that they are of legal age to purchase alcohol.

ACCESS THROUGH NONCOMMERCIAL SOURCES

As noted above, young drinkers most often obtain alcohol from social sources, through friends, acquaintances, family members, and other adults who buy or provide alcohol to them. It is thus important for any effective strategy to reduce social access to alcohol for minors. In this regard, it is essential to communicate strong norms about the unacceptability of adults providing alcohol to minors or facilitating alcohol use by minors. Media campaigns highlighting the responsibility of adults in preventing young people from obtaining alcohol are one means of communicating such norms that should be implemented. Similarly, using media to increase awareness of laws prohibiting adults from providing alcohol to minors and drawing attention to enforcement efforts can further increase the effectiveness of legal approaches to preventing social provision of alcohol to minors and may help establish or reinforce community norms against this behavior. Such media activities are thus an important part of any enforcement activities to reduce provision of alcohol to minors (see Chapter 6).

Third-Party Transactions

Third-party transactions occur when young people ask adults to purchase alcohol for them. Third-party transactions are a common means through which underage drinkers, especially older teens, obtain alcohol (see Tables 9-2 and 9-3 above), partly because young people may believe it is less risky than trying to purchase alcohol themselves. Often, young people wait outside outlets and approach strangers whom they ask to buy alcohol.

"Shoulder tap" interventions are a strategy to directly reduce third-party transactions of alcohol by enforcing laws prohibiting provision of alcohol to minors. Underage decoys who are working with the police wait outside outlets and ask randomly selected passing strangers to buy alcohol (usually beer) for them. A plainclothes police observer is stationed nearby to witness the transaction. If a stranger agrees to make a purchase, he or she is given money to do so by the decoy. The buyer is cited or warned for providing alcohol to a minor when he or she completes the transaction and gives the alcohol to the decoy. Although rigorous evidence for effectiveness is lacking, case studies suggest that such programs can generate a relatively large number of citations and thus may have a deterrent value (Powell and Willingham, n.d.). Such programs, when accompanied by sufficient media coverage, may also help instill or reinforce community norms against buying alcohol for minors or otherwise providing it to them. Retailers should be involved in shoulder tap operations. In many states, retailers might be held responsible for allowing minors to solicit adults to purchase alcohol within the immediate vicinity of their outlet. In such cases, the retailer has legal responsibility to curb such activities.

> Recommendation 9-7: States and localities should implement enforcement programs to deter adults from purchasing alcohol for minors. States and communities should
>
> - routinely undertake shoulder tap or other prevention programs targeting adults who purchase alcohol for minors, using warnings, rather than citations, for the first offense;
> - enact and enforce laws to hold retailers responsible, as a condition of licensing, for allowing minors to loiter and solicit adults to purchase alcohol for them on outlet property; and
> - use nuisance and loitering ordinances as a means of discouraging youth from congregating outside of alcohol outlets in order to solicit adults to purchase alcohol.

Keg Registration

Keg registration laws require the purchaser of a keg of beer to complete a form that links his or her name to a number on the keg. It is seen primarily as a tool for prosecuting adults who supply alcohol to young people at parties. Keg registration laws have become increasingly popular in local communities in the United States. The committee found only one published study on the effectiveness of these laws in reducing underage drinking problems. In that study of 97 U.S. communities, it was found that requiring keg registration was significantly and negatively correlated with traffic fatality rates (Cohen et al., 2001). Although the effectiveness of keg registration has not yet been convincingly established, the committee believes that the evidence is sufficient to endorse it as a potentially valuable tool for strengthening the enforcement of underage drinking laws at relatively little additional cost.

> Recommendation 9-8: States and communities should establish and implement a system requiring registration of beer kegs that records information on the identity of purchasers.

Social Host Liability

Some courts have expanded the dram shop liability principles so that they apply to noncommercial servers, including social hosts, employers, fraternities, and other alcohol providers that are not licensed to sell or serve by the state. Under social host liability laws, adults who provide alcohol to a minor or serve an intoxicated adult can be sued through civil actions for injury caused by that minor or intoxicated adult. Social host liability laws may deter adults from hosting underage parties and purchasing alcohol for or providing alcohol to minors. Currently, 30 states have some form of social host liability law (MADD, 2002b). Many state legislatures have placed strict limits on social host liability and courts have historically been reluctant to impose it absent clear statutory authority. There is some evidence that this trend is changing. State legislatures are more willing to consider at least some form of social host liability for service to minors, and courts in recent years have been more willing to construe statutory limitations narrowly and impose social host liability, relying on common law negligence principles (Mosher et al., 2002).

There is very little research on the effectiveness of social host liability laws and what evidence exists is conflicting. In one study across all 50 states for 1984-1995, the presence of social host liability laws was associated with lower rates of alcohol-related traffic death among adults, but not with such deaths among minors (Whetten-Goldstein et al., 2000), and it was not related to single vehicle nighttime crashes for either group. Surprisingly, the presence of social host liability laws was related to *increases* in total motor vehicle fatalities among minors in this study. In a second study, however, using self-reported drinking data spanning the 1980s to 1995, social host liability laws were associated with decreases in self-reported heavy drinking and in self-reported drinking and driving by lighter drinkers, but not in self-reported drinking and driving by heavier drinkers (Stout et al., 2000). Separate data were not presented for minors.

The conflicting findings on social host liability laws may reflect the lack of a comprehensive program that ensures that social hosts are aware of their potential liability exposure. The prospect of liability for social hosts could send a powerful normative message to adults that providing alcohol to underage youth is unacceptable. However, that message must be effectively disseminated before it can have a preventive effect, either as a deterrent or as a moral injunction (see Holder and Treno, 1997). Media campaigns to educate the public would have to be an integral part of implementing social host liability laws. As a practical matter, imposing a criminal sanction, especially a jail sentence, on a parent who hosts a drinking party for minors may be more likely to attract media attention than a civil award of damages. For this reason, direct enforcement of the prohibition may be a more effective way of reinforcing the social norm than the rare and often invisible imposition of social host liability. Nonetheless, states may want to consider enacting or strengthening civil social host liability statutes that allow negligence-based civil actions against non-commercial providers of alcohol for serving or providing alcohol to a minor who subsequently causes injury to others.

Restricting Drinking in Public Places

Allowing the service of alcohol at child- and family-oriented public events may promote underage drinking. One way to control alcohol at public events, in parks, beaches, sports arenas, public recreation facilities, parking lots, and other publicly accessible locations is through the use of conditional use permits. Conditional use permits, used by a city or county, allow local communities to set standards for how and when alcohol will be sold and served. These local ordinances can reduce sales to minors by such means as requiring the use of responsible beverage sales and service practices at public events, limiting advertising, and restricting hours of sale. Conditional use permits allow communities to enforce laws and exact penalties locally. Case studies suggest that they can be used effectively to reduce sales to minors and excessive drinking at public events (Streiker, 2000; Reynolds, n.d.). Little or no rigorous research has been conducted on the effectiveness of conditional use permits. However, cities and counties may want to use conditional use permits to set standards for how and when alcohol will be sold and served at public events.

YOUNG DRINKERS AND DRIVING

Zero Tolerance

Zero tolerance laws specify a lower BAC for underage drivers. Usually this limit is set at the minimum that can be reliably detected by breath testing equipment (i.e., 0.01 to 0.02). Zero tolerance laws commonly invoke administrative penalties, such as automatic confiscation of a driver's license for driving after consuming even small amounts of alcohol.

Zero tolerance laws have now been enacted in all 50 states. There is strong evidence that zero tolerance laws can reduce underage drinking and driving and crash fatalities. Differences in effectiveness are thought to be related to differences in enforcement and in awareness among young people (Balmforth, 1999; Ferguson et al., 2000; Hingson et al, 1994). Impediments to the enforcement of these laws include requirements that zero tolerance citations be supported by evidential BAC testing, undue costs to police (e.g., paperwork, court appearances), and lack of behavioral cues for stopping young drivers at very low BACs. The most effective zero tolerance laws are those that allow passive breath testing, are implemented in combination with sobriety checkpoints, involve streamlined administrative procedures, and invoke administrative penalties (e.g., immediate loss of driver's license). Education and media can significantly increase the effectiveness of zero tolerance laws by increasing awareness of them on the part of young people.

Recommendation 9-9:   States should facilitate enforcement of zero tolerance laws in order to increase their deterrent effect. States should:

- **modify existing laws to allow passive breath testing, streamlined administrative procedures, and administrative penalties and**
- **implement media campaigns to increase young peoples' awareness of reduced BAC limits and of enforcement efforts.**

Graduated Driver Licensing

Graduated driver licensing places limits on the driving circumstances of new or young drivers, such as restrictions on nighttime driving or driving with young passengers. Graduated driver licensing policies also often include zero tolerance provisions. There is strong evidence that graduated licensing programs are associated with reductions in car crashes (Boase and Tasca, 1998; Langley et al., 1996; Smith, 1986; Ulmer et al., 2000), self-reported drinking and driving (Mann et al., 1997), and alcohol-related crashes (Boase and Tasca, 1998) among young people. Recent evidence, however, suggests that they may have limited effects on alcohol use and alcohol-related crashes, above and beyond that of zero tolerance laws (Shope et al., 2001). Nonetheless, graduated driver licensing may be an important adjunct to zero tolerance laws, for example, by providing cause for stopping young drivers who may be drinking.

Recommendation 9-10:   States should enact and enforce graduated driver licensing laws.

Sobriety Check Points and Random Breath Testing

Research strongly suggests that intensive use of sobriety checkpoints or mobile random breath testing can substantially reduce drinking and driving. In the United States, these policies can be implemented only under prescribed circumstances as determined by state laws, often involving prenotification about when and where they will be instituted. Breath tests at checkpoints can usually be given only if there is probable cause to suspect that a driver has been drinking. Even under these restricted circumstances, there is evidence that sobriety checkpoints can reduce alcohol-related crashes, injuries, and fatalities (Lacey et al., 1999; Stuster and Blowers, 1995). However, the committee did not find any studies addressing the effects of these programs on drinking or drinking and driving among adolescents. Sobriety checkpoints may be a particularly important component of zero tolerance laws, given the difficultly of detecting young drinking drivers with very low BAC levels. Public awareness and publicity appear to be important factors in the success of sobriety checkpoints.

Recommendation 9-11: States and localities should routinely implement sobriety checkpoints.

POSSESSION AND PURCHASE

Underage Drinking Parties

One major way that underage drinkers gain access to alcohol is at parties. In one study, for example, 32 percent of sixth graders, 56 percent of ninth graders, and 60 percent of twelfth graders reported obtaining alcohol at parties (Harrison et al., 2000). Underage drinking parties frequently involve large groups and are commonly held in a home, an outdoor area, or a hotel room. Law enforcement can respond to noise complaints to investigate such gatherings. Even when it is not possible to cite underage drinkers or the person who supplied the alcohol, awareness of increased police activity in this regard can act as a deterrent and can express community norms to adults regarding the unacceptability of providing alcohol to minors.

Recommendation 9-12: Local police, working with community leaders, should adopt and announce policies for detecting and terminating underage drinking parties, including:

- routinely responding to complaints from the public about noisy teenage parties and entering the premises when there is probable cause to suspect underage drinking is taking place;
- routinely checking, as a part of regular weekend patrols, open areas where teenage drinking parties are known to occur; and
- routinely citing underage drinkers and, if possible, the person who supplied the alcohol when underage drinking is observed at parties.

Cops in Shops

"Cops in Shops" is a voluntary program developed by the Century Council, a prevention organization sponsored by the alcohol industry. In this program, police or ABC agents pose as employees or customers in retail outlets in order to apprehend underage persons who attempt to buy alcoholic beverages or adults who attempt to purchase alcohol for minors. The program often includes prominent signs that warn that the establishment is participating in the Cops in Shops program. The participating officers can also use the program to review a retailer's policies and procedures and identify risky practices. Case studies indicate that Cops in Shops programs can generate a large number of citations, both against minors attempting purchase or using false identification and against adults who are purchasing for minors. The effects of the programs on underage drinking are unknown. Media coverage to increase public awareness again seems to be important for the success of these programs. In light of the greater importance of assuring retailer compliance, enforcement programs that focus on purchasers, including "Cops in Shops" programs, should be used only to supplement compliance check enforcement against retailers, not to displace it.

False Identification

The use of false identification for alcohol purchases is significant although there is a great deal of variability from study to study; see Table 9-4. In one survey, for example, only 7 percent of New York state high school students and 14 percent of Virginia college students indicated that they had

TABLE 9-4 Use of False Identification (ID) to Obtain Alcohol by Young People

Study and Measure	Sample Population	Age	Used False ID (percent)
Durkin et al. (1996); ever used	Virginia College	18-20	46
Preusser et al. (1995); ever used	Pennsylvania High School	16-18*	14
	New York High School	16-18*	28
	Pennsylvania College	18-20	37
	New York College	18-20	59
Schwartz et al. (1998); used in past 2 years	Virginia Pediatrician's Office	Mean, 17.2	13
	Virginia College	Mean, 8.5	14
	New York High School	Mean, 17.2	7
	Southeast Substance Abuse Programs	Mean, 16.9	9

*Complete age data not available: age ranges provided for 95 percent of high school students from Pennsylvania and New York combined and 92 percent of college students from the two states combined.

used false identification to purchase alcohol at least once in the previous 2 years (Schwartz et al., 1998). In another study, however, 28 percent of New York and 14 percent of Pennsylvania high school students and 59 percent and 37 percent of college students from those states, respectively, reported ever using false identification to purchase alcohol (Preusser et al., 1995). In a third study, nearly one-half (46 percent) of Virginia college students reported that they had ever used a false ID to purchase alcohol.

The reported use of false identification appears to be greater in urban areas and in states where enforcement is lax or penalties for purchasing alcohol, possessing alcohol, or using false identification are absent or minimal (Preusser et al., 1995). In Pennsylvania, where fines for using false identification were substantial ($500 fine and driver license suspension) and where purchase, attempted purchase, possession, and transportation of alcohol were prohibited at the time of the study, use of false identification was relatively infrequent. In contrast, in New York, where it was not illegal for a minor to possess or purchase alcohol and where the penalties for using false identification for purchase of alcohol were substantially less ($100 fine), use of false identification for alcohol purchase was more frequent.

Other factors also seem to be related to use of false identification for purchase of alcohol. In a survey of Virginia college students (Durkin et al., 1996), those who were members of fraternities or sororities were more likely to report use of false identification to purchase alcohol than other students (70 and 39 percent, respectively) and African American students were less likely to report use of false identification than students of other ethnicities (10 and 48 percent, respectively). False identification can be easily obtained in the United States through magazine advertisements and mail order or from acquaintances or friends who manufacture it (Schwartz et al., 1998). Use of false identification may increase as it becomes more easily available through the Internet. A recent search on the key words "novelty id," for example, turned up 21 web sites offering falsified identification or templates for producing false identification. Electronic scanning is potentially an effective tool for verifying the validity of driver's license IDs. Although it is premature to require universal use of this technology, due in part to resistance among some retailers because of the cost and perceived inconvenience (see National Highway Traffic Safety Administration, 2001), states should facilitate and encourage its use.

Recommendation 9-13: States should strengthen efforts to prevent and detect use of false identification by minors to make alcohol purchases. States should:

- **prohibit the production, sale, distribution, possession, and use of false identification for attempted alcohol purchase;**

- issue driver licenses and state identification cards that can be electronically scanned;
- allow retailers to confiscate apparently false identification for law enforcement inspection; and
- implement administrative penalties (e.g., immediate confiscation of a driver's license and issuance of a citation resulting in a substantial fine) for attempted use of false identification by minors for alcohol purchases.

Penalties

The overriding purpose of prescribing and enforcing penalties against underage youth for possession of or attempted purchase of alcohol, and using a false ID for this purpose, is to serve as a deterrent. The deterrent effect of the penalties is affected by their severity, the probability of their imposition, and the swiftness with which they are imposed (e.g., Ross, 1982). Severe, criminal penalties for minors in possession of alcohol or attempting to purchase alcohol are seldom enforced and thus generate, at best, only a modest deterrent effect (Hafemeister and Jackson, in press), and the limited deterrent effects most likely affects the location of drinking (e.g., drinking in public places, which is more likely to be detected) than its occurrence. Arrest of minors appears to be rare for these offenses (Wagenaar and Wolfson, 1994), in part because of the burden of prosecuting them as criminal violations and the reluctance of law enforcement officials and courts to enforce criminal penalties in such cases (Little and Bishop, 1998; Wolfson et al., 1995). This reluctance stems from a widespread belief that giving a young person a criminal record for drinking or possessing alcohol is excessive and unfair. Moreover, because criminal proceedings are often lengthy and removed in time from the infraction, the punishment is seldom swift or certain (Hafemeister and Jackson, in press).

In the committee's view, a less severe sanction would be more likely to be enforced and would generate a greater deterrent than an under-enforced criminal penalty. Possession, consumption, and attempted purchase of alcohol by minors, and use of false IDs for this purpose, should be treated as noncriminal infractions punishable by fines, community service, and similar sanctions, and should not lead to a criminal record that may ruin the life chances of a young person. Moreover, alcohol infractions should be handled administratively through citations issued at the time of apprehension, without requiring court appearances. The size of the fines and length of community service should be sufficiently substantial to register social disapproval and to generate a meaningful deterrent effect. Models for designing sanctions for such noncriminal transgressions are available, including youth-only offenses punishable in juvenile courts and the civil penalties created in some states for possession of marijuana (Bonnie, 1977).

Recommendation 9-14: States should establish administrative procedures and noncriminal penalties, such as fines or community service, for alcohol infractions by minors.

States might also want to consider immediate administrative driver license revocation, not just for driving-related alcohol infractions, but also for consumption, possession, or attempted purchase of alcohol by minors. However, the use of license revocation as a penalty for offenses unrelated to driving raises constitutional concerns and also would be accompanied by higher litigation costs than other penalties (see Hafemeister and Jackson, 2004).

In summary, the committee believes that state access restrictions, and their enforcement, should be strengthened, with existing ambiguities clarified, and loopholes removed. At the same time, however, the penalties for violations by underage drinkers should be reduced, thereby facilitating the use of less costly procedures and more widespread and consistent enforcement. Overall, this approach should be welcomed by parents because it will solidify and clarify the legal prohibitions, while removing the fear of excessive punishment.

10

Youth-Oriented Interventions

I n 1994 the Institute of Medicine proposed a framework for prevention of mental health illnesses that included three broad classes of prevention strategies—universal measures, selective measures, and indicated preventive measures: that framework is instructive in considering the approaches outlined in this chapter. Although developed in the context of mental health, the framework is applicable to most public health problems not caused primarily by biological agents.

Consistent with the population health orientation of the overall strategy, the approaches discussed in this chapter are predominately universal measures—those that are appropriate and cost-effective for a broad population (e.g., all adolescents who might use alcohol). Media messages that encourage young people to avoid alcohol use are an example of a universal measure: if the media message has been demonstrated to have the desired effect of dissuading young people from using alcohol, it would be cost-effective and appropriate to deliver to all adolescents in the U.S. population.

Selective preventive measures are desirable for the population subgroup whose risk of developing a certain health problem is greater than that for the general population. In the context of alcohol problems, a selective preventive measure would target a population known to be at greater risk for experiencing alcohol-related problems. An example would be a subset of college students who are white, male, fraternity members under the age of 24 who have a tendency to socialize, characteristics that research has shown to be associated with heavy drinking. The third intervention approach, indicated preventive measures, applies to "individuals who are found to manifest a risk factor, condition, or abnormality that identifies them, individually, as being at high-risk for the future development of a disease" (Institute of Medicine, 1994b, p. 21). For example, a young person who during an interview with a physician (or through some other screening method) indicates having used alcohol at a very young age (e.g., at 11 or 12) may not yet have a problem with alcohol (i.e., is not yet in need of treatment) but because of the risks associated with early onset of use would be a candidate for an intervention that deters further alcohol use. Thus, selective measures focus on a subgroup of the population that has an increased risk of mental health problems and indicated measures focus on individuals who clearly demonstrate a specific risk factor.

The approaches outlined in this chapter, consistent with the committee's overall task of developing a strategy to reduce underage drinking across a wide range of youth populations, are by and large universal measures. We discuss the possible value of a youth-oriented media campaign aimed at changing youth drinking behaviors; school-based approaches; approaches at residential colleges and universities; and potential opportunities in other settings, including healthcare and faith-based institutions, the workplace, and the military. We do not discuss the literature regarding family-based interventions, although we recognize the importance of family involvement in the interventions mentioned above and in responses developed by communities to address community-specific problems.

We also do not discuss other selective and targeted interventions with specific subsets of youth who may be at increased risk of developing alcohol problems, with two exceptions: interventions on residential campuses and treatment for adolescents. The underage drinking problem on residential campuses has been well documented and a cause of public concern for years. Given the unique concentration of underage youth and the major problems of underage drinking, residential campuses are a necessary target for intervention. Our discussion of treatment recognizes that some youths have developed or will develop alcohol abuse and dependence problems. While we believe the emphasis should be on prevention, some attention must be paid to those youths.

A YOUTH-FOCUSED MEDIA CAMPAIGN

A key element of the committee's charge was to assess the potential effectiveness of a youth-focused media campaign built on the models of the youth components of the anti-drug campaign of the Office of National Drug Control Policy or of the American Legacy Foundation's Truth™ Campaign. For that reason, we consider in some detail what such a youth-focused campaign would involve and the available evidence about the potential effectiveness of such a campaign.

Supporting Evidence

We begin with evidence favoring such a campaign. There is good evidence that youth who disapprove of heavy alcohol use and who see great harm in alcohol use are less likely to drink. For example, among twelfth-grade students in the Monitoring the Future (MTF) Survey in 1998, about half said that there is "great risk" of physical or other harms in having five or more drinks once or twice each weekend. Of those who said there was great risk, about 16 percent said they had had five or more drinks at least once in the previous 2 weeks. Of those who said there was only a moderate, slight, or no risk, 48 percent said they had had five or more drinks in this time frame. This finding leads to the hypothesis that a campaign to convince more youth that there is great risk in heavy drinking would result in a reduction in the amount of heavy drinking. This argument is less relevant regarding any use of alcohol: few youth of any age believe that "any use" of alcohol carries great risk (12 percent of eighth and tenth graders and 8 percent of twelfth graders). Thus, on its face, it would seem quite difficult to convince most youth that such drinking carries great risk.

Support for a youth-focused approach also comes from the latest results from the MTF Survey in 2002, which shows a decline in drinking between 2000 and 2002 for eighth and tenth graders (see Chapter 2). For example, for tenth graders, heavy drinking in the past 30 days declined from 24 percent to 18 percent. Until the past 2 years there had been stability in both any drinking and heavy drinking at all age levels. The recent decline raises the possibility that youth are reconsidering drinking behavior and might be open to further persuasion. This hypothesis might be supported by the idea that it is easier to ride with the current (reinforcing a trend already under way) than to row against it (trying to suppress an emerging or established behavioral trend).

A third support for directly addressing youth and persuading them not to drink comes from the positive evidence from antismoking efforts by individual states and by the American Legacy Foundation. There has been a substantial decline in the prevalence of youth smoking, with 30-day prevalence among twelfth graders declining from a high of 37 percent in 1997 to the 2002 level of 27 percent. There is credible although not definitive evidence that the mass media campaigns have been a substantial force in this decline (Siegel and Biener, 2000; Sly et al., 2001; Siegel, 2002). If it worked for tobacco, why wouldn't it work for alcohol? (We return to this issue below.)

Contrary Evidence

Although there is a substantial logic favoring a youth campaign approach, there are also some contrary arguments. First, the hypothesis that increasing the proportion of youths who perceive great risk in heavy drinking will reduce heavy drinking among youths by an equivalent amount may be unfounded. The hypothesis rests on the assumption that the oft-demonstrated relationship between risk perception for heavy drinking and actual heavy drinking is a causal one. However, since most of the available data are cross-sectional, one cannot be confident of that causal relationship. Not being a drinker and not perceiving increased risk are correlates, but neither may "cause" the other; to some extent, at least, they are both manifestations of an underlying set of causal influences that tend to produce both decisions about drinking and positive or negative attitudes toward alcohol use. Thus, to the extent that a youth-focused campaign would aim mainly to increase perception of drinking-related risks, it might not rest on a strong foundation.

A second, and related, concern is that the recent survey data may not be as persuasive as they seem in supporting a risk-oriented campaign. Although the recent decline in drinking is worth attention, the decline may be merely an anomaly (see Chapter 5). And even if the decline is real, it may not reflect the influence of changes in perceived harmfulness. Indeed, the data about harmfulness of heavy drinking do not show a consistent parallel improvement (Johnston et al., 2003). Thus, any decline in behavior may reflect the influence of changes in the environment around drinking, rather than a change in underlying beliefs about drinking.

Strikingly, the long-term stability in heavy drinking rates contrasts with the sharp reduction in one form of harm associated with such behavior—fatal alcohol-related crashes among teenage drivers. The Centers for Disease Control and Prevention reports that such crashes have declined by nearly 60 percent for 16- to 17- year-olds and 55 percent for 18- to 20-year-olds between 1982 and 2001. However, the decline ended in 1997. Since that time the levels are stable or perhaps rising slightly (Elder and Shults, 2002). These data suggest that preventing alcohol-related harms may have more potential to be effective than those aiming to discourage drinking (or even heavy drinking) per se. This finding parallels the evidence for adult drinking and adult drinking and driving.

The lack of any longer-term downward trend in drinking or heavy drinking, despite the presence of a wide variety of public efforts to address these issues, is then one concern about initiating a major campaign against youth alcohol use, though not by itself sufficient to reject such an effort. If there have been negative alcohol messages directed toward youth, they likely pale before the pro-alcohol onslaught that surrounds youth (see Chapter 7). Perhaps the lack of a longer-term downward trend reflects the competition between positive and negative alcohol messages, which has turned into a standoff. Perhaps a focused and substantially larger effort would better counterbalance the positive alcohol-related messages.

A third concern about launching a youth-directed campaign arises from the few specific efforts that have been evaluated. There is some evidence for effects of designated driver campaigns directed to youth (DeJong and Hingson, 1998). However, there are very few studies of youth-focused media campaigns that deal with alcohol consumption as the main outcome variable for evaluating results, particularly for youths not yet in college. The evaluation of the Australian National Alcohol Campaign measured consumption before and after its focused launch and booster campaigns; it did not find consistent evidence of reduced consumption (Ball et al., 2002). The teen-focused part of the Winners Campaign had a quite weak evaluation component (with only 100 respondents per city); it, too, did not detect behavioral effects (Wallack, 1979; Wallack and Barrows, 1982). Some successful programs, like Project Northland (Perry et al., 2002) and the Midwestern Prevention Project (Pentz et al., 1989) made use of community media as part of a multifaceted campaign, but one cannot separate the effects of media from other components of the strategy. There are two additional field trials now approaching completion, each of which has incorporated a discrete mass media component, but those results have not yet been published (Robert Hornik personal communications with Michael Slater and Brian Flynn, 2003). As of this writing, the committee does not have evidence of success in reducing youth alcohol use from any evaluated campaign (excluding limited evidence on specific college campuses). There is no alcohol-focused program that can be used as a prototype for a youth-focused national mass media campaign effort.

Comparisons with the Anti-Tobacco and Anti-Drug Campaigns

Our fourth concern relates to whether the apparently successful anti-tobacco effort can be used as a prototype. In contrast to that success, there are, thus far, problematic results from the National Youth Anti-drug Media Campaign. Since 1999, the White House Office of National Drug Control Policy (ONDCP) has sponsored this campaign to reduce youths' use of illegal drugs, particularly marijuana. The program has spent close to $1 billion on mass media advertising and other outreach programs, both to youth and their parents. Results through mid-2002 do not show positive effects on youth. Indeed, some evidence suggests that the campaign might be having an unfavorable effect, with the youth most exposed to the campaign messages more likely than others to form attitudes and intentions favoring marijuana use (Hornik et al., 2002). This effect is sometimes called a boomerang effect. At the end of 2002, the message focus of the anti-drug campaign was redefined with additional attention to the negative consequences of marijuana use. The effectiveness of that new campaign focus is not yet known. There are published results, based on a much earlier period of the anti-drug campaign sponsored by the Partnership for a Drug-Free America, which show positive effects (Block et al., 2002), and there is also evidence of success for a field experimental anti-drug campaign in Kentucky (Palmgreen et al., 2001). Thus, the appropriate conclusion is that the national ONDCP-sponsored campaign has not been successful, through mid-2002, not that the general approach is always unsuccessful.

If the anti-tobacco efforts are a positive model and the anti-drug efforts are not encouraging, wouldn't it be possible to model a campaign against youth alcohol use on the first and avoid the mistakes of the second? This question requires a careful consideration of how the tobacco and drug campaigns were different from one another and how the behaviors they addressed are different from alcohol use.

The expenditures for advertising expenditures for the youth parts of both national campaigns were in the range of $60 to 100 million per year. But there are a number of important differences in the two campaigns. First, the styles of the two campaigns have been quite different. The anti-tobacco campaigns have focused on a variety of messages, but a particularly striking set focused on anti-industry arguments—the tobacco industry kills people and is trying to manipulate you. The anti-drug messages focused (through the end of 2002) on positive alternatives to drug use— "What's your anti drug?"—and on the negative consequences of drug use.

Second, the American Legacy Foundation's anti-tobacco advertising has adopted an edgy style, with youth apparently in control. The anti-drug advertising has had a more conventional style, with clear sponsorship by ONDCP and the Partnership for a Drug-Free America.

Third, the tobacco messages were launched in the context of broad media coverage of tobacco issues as Congress and the states' attorneys general struggled with the tobacco industry toward legislation and the eventual master settlement of 1997. In contrast, anti-drug general media coverage was likely declining during the period of the national anti-drug campaign directed toward youth.

Fourth, there were important changes in the environment surrounding youth tobacco use that were complementary to campaign efforts, including price changes related to tax increases, increasing public concern with second-hand smoke, and increased restrictions on where smoking was permitted. There also was substantial change in public norms about the acceptability of smoking. While these other changes do not completely account for the reduction in tobacco use among youth, they had some direct effects and likely reinforced the media messages about smoking. In contrast, there is little parallel environmental change around the use of drugs (or alcohol).

It is tempting to point to the anti-tobacco campaign and call it a good model for an anti-underage drinking campaign. However, the differences between an anti-tobacco campaign and a campaign against youth alcohol use are too substantial too ignore. Even if some of the lessons about edgy, youth-controlled message development could be borrowed from the anti-tobacco campaigns, other lessons could not: no campaign against youth alcohol use, much less a federally sponsored one, could successfully replicate the anti-industry tactics that have been the hallmark of the California, Florida, and Legacy Foundation campaigns, not only because moderate alcohol use is widely accepted among adults, but also because the claims about industry duplicity and misrepresentation are rooted in the tobacco industry's unique history.

There are other important differences as well. The context of broad media coverage in which the anti-tobacco campaigns have been mounted would not likely be matched by a campaign against youth alcohol use. Similarly, the complementary changes in the normative, legal, and regulatory environments around tobacco do not apply to an effort aimed at youthful alcohol consumption. In addition, the sharp contrast in the nature of the behaviors would remain. The ban on underage drinking struggles with its nearly universal trial use among youth, the majority view that moderate daily use is not high-risk, and acceptability for use among adults. Tobacco use contrasts with alcohol use on each of these points.

Next Steps

These observations do not show that a youth-focused media campaign would surely fail, only that it would be premature to mount one given what is known today. It would certainly not be sensible to mount a large campaign, at significant cost, based on wishful thinking. It is tempting to suggest going ahead with a modest campaign on the grounds that it cannot hurt but the example of the anti-drug campaign and its possible boomerang effects raises doubts about this idea. The most sensible course, at this time, is to begin to test a serious prototype for a youth-focused campaign. One possible model for this exploratory effort would be to fund one or more campaigns in geographically well-defined areas, put substantial resources both into message development and transmission, sustain them for 2 to 4 years, and evaluate them carefully.

The appropriate message focus for such prototype campaigns would need to be researched, developed, and carefully tested before launch. At a minimum, a campaign would have to focus on the specific messages that can convince youths of the high risk of heavy drinking. This research would balance epidemiological evidence about the risks with evidence from research with vulnerable youth as to what risks are of concern. There are a variety of other possible focuses, including beliefs about the outcomes of drinking, social norms about drinking, and skills to avoid drinking. The potential for each of these approaches would likely vary with age and other characteristics of the target populations. The most promising strategy, as well as the best ways to implement it, would have to be developed through intensive formative research with the target populations. Care must be taken to avoid a boomerang effect of any campaign that is mounted. A particular concern would be if heavy exposure to messages about the risks of alcohol use carried with them the implied idea that many youths are using alcohol. It is possible that a resulting increase in the "descriptive norm" could lead youths to feel it was okay to use alcohol since large numbers of young people do so (Cialdini et al., 1990; see Chapter 4).

In considering the development of a campaign against youth alcohol use, whether as part of the larger societywide campaign the committee recommends or as a stand-alone program, careful research and development should be at the core of these efforts. These efforts should be conceived as similar in logic to the efforts to develop in-school or community interventions that have been effective. Multiple efforts have been funded with the recognition that only some of them were likely to be effective. A similar approach would need to be taken with the development of underage drinking communication interventions. Some interventions should focus on reducing heavy drinking and some on discouraging all underage drinking; some interventions should focus on perceived risk and negative consequences, while others should focus on changing perceived norms or increasing skills at resisting peer pressure to drink. Some interventions will incorporate more than one of these elements. The National Institute on Alcohol Abuse and Alcoholism (NIAAA) and National Institute on Drug Abuse have funded some of these types of test programs but there need to be enough of them and with sufficient resources to really learn how to construct youth-focused campaigns that will address underage alcohol use successfully. Once the evidence is in, assuming that one or more successful approaches have been identified, it might be possible to launch a large-scale national campaign with a good expectation for success.

Recommendation 10-1: Intensive research and development for a youth-focused national media campaign relating to underage drinking should be initiated. If this work yields promising results, the inclusion of a youth-focused campaign in the strategy should be reconsidered.

SCHOOL-BASED APPROACHES

School-based approaches designed to prevent substance use among students are common in the United States (see Hansen and Dusenbury, 2004, for descriptions of specific programs). Delivery of such programming through schools offers the benefits of reaching a wide (and captive) audience, as most young people (especially elementary and middle-school-aged children) are enrolled in school. In addition, schools offer the potential to ensure that intervention programs are institutionalized and run by trained staff members and that boosters to initial exposure to programs are delivered at specific developmental intervals. School-based intervention programs represent an important opportunity to prevent and reduce alcohol use among youth.

Overall Results

Meta-analyses of school-based interventions (e.g., Gottfredson and Wilson, 2003) have shown that they vary widely in their ability to effect alcohol-related outcomes. Positive effects are small to modest. Research has shown, however, that some school-based approaches are more effective than others at reducing youth alcohol use. The goal of delaying the onset of alcohol use is most effective with students who have not yet begun drinking, and given that American adolescents tend to have their first drink between ages 12 and 14, education with this age group and those slightly younger is sensible (Paglia and Room, 1999). Programs (and evaluations of these programs) that seek to affect students who are already drinking are somewhat less common. In addition, the objectives for this population are less clear—should one try to encourage them to abstain (which may be difficult to achieve), get them to engage in less risky drinking behaviors (e.g., fewer episodes of heavy drinking), or minimize the harm from alcohol use (e.g., no driving after drinking)? Further research on school-based interventions with students already using alcohol is needed.

Programs relying on provision of information alone, fear tactics, or messages about not drinking until one is "old enough" have consistently been found to be ineffective in reducing alcohol use and, in some cases, produce boomerang effects (Botvin, 1995; Swisher and Hoffman, 1975; D'Emidio-Caston and Brown, 1998; Gottfredson and Wilson, 2003; Tobler, 1992). Many early drug education curricula that relied on factual information about alcohol and other drugs, including information on the negative consequences of use, or fear arousal were based on the theory that adolescents who used alcohol and drugs had insufficient knowledge about the consequences of use and that increased information would make them more likely to decide not to use drugs. While these types of interventions may increase knowledge, they do not affect behavior. There are several possible explanations: information-only approaches focusing on risks and dangers may arouse curiosity; fear tactics that overemphasize the potential negative consequences of drinking may be viewed as alarmist and lacking in credibility; moral lecturing can backfire with rebellion-oriented youths who are seeking to establish independence; and messages that tell youth to wait until they are "old enough" may serve to make alcohol a symbol of maturity and independence (Paglia and Room, 1999).

Strategies focused on increasing self-esteem also have not proven to be effective, perhaps because of the low correlation between self-esteem and alcohol use or the lack of a specific focus on substance use (Donaldson et al., 1995; Gottfredson and Wilson, 2003; Hawthorne et al., 1995; Paglia and Room, 1999; Tobler, 1992). Programs that focus on strategies to resist peer pressure have also not been demonstrated to be effective (Donaldson et al., 1994). Although among some peer groups alcohol use may represent a social norm, it is less common for peers to directly pressure each other to use alcohol; peer influence is more likely to be subtle. As a result, strategies to resist direct pressure may not be very helpful (Paglia and Room, 1999). Many of these strategies have been long used in prevention programming; since research has shown them to be ineffective, they should not be continued.

It has been a common practice to identify youths who have problems with alcohol use and other high-risk behaviors and put them together in groups. Results of studies of such programs, usually done for the purposes of simplifying interventions, have met with mixed results (Eggert et al., 1994). Some research has indicated that high-risk behaviors have actually increased among such groups (Dishion and Andrews, 1995). It is possible that in such circumstances, deviant norms become established and youth inadvertently adopt those norms rather than learn about and adopt positive norms.

School-based interventions that use normative education to undermine youth beliefs that alcohol use is prevalent among their peers and that their peers universally approve of this behavior appear to have promise. Efforts to establish nonuse norms—implemented in conjunction with a critical look at both alcohol advertising and media and other cultural messages that make alcohol use symbolic of qualities youth want to attain (e.g., maturity, independence, popularity)—may also be promising. Gottfredson and Wilson (2003), Tobler (1992), Tobler and Stratton (1997), and Botvin et al. (1995) have found that programs using such approaches, especially when they are delivered in an interactive manner, may produce reductions in alcohol use for several years after the initial program delivery. In addition, there is some evidence that these approaches may be effective with a broad range of youths, including ethnic minorities (Perry and Kelder, 1992). A limited number of studies (Austin and Johnson, 1997a, 1997b) have shown some positive effects of media literacy programs aimed at affecting perceptions of alcohol advertising and alcohol norms, but there is insufficient evidence to make conclusions about the application of this approach in the context of underage alcohol use.

Approaches that have been demonstrated to reduce youth alcohol use have many program elements in common. However, similar to other approaches recommended in this report, the committee believes that education-oriented interventions should be implemented in the context of a comprehensive approach.

Attributes of Effective Interventions

A considerable amount of research (Gottfredson and Wilson, 2003; Hansen and Dusenbury, 2004; Tobler and Strattan, 1997), primarily in primary and secondary schools, has identified several critical elements of successful school-based educational interventions. In addition, research on communitywide alcohol prevention programming (see Chapter 11), such as Project Northland and family-based approaches like the Michigan State University Multiple Risk Outreach Program, offer additional critical elements that can make education interventions more effective (Williams et al., 1999; Nye et al., 1995). Research on such interventions offers a number of lessons about what educational strategies are important for preventing alcohol use and alcohol problems among minors. These lessons, or critical elements, offer a starting place for innovative education interventions and for developing priorities about what kinds of education interventions should be funded. The interventions need to be multicomponent and integrated; sufficient in "dose" and follow-up; establish norms that support nonuse; stress parental monitoring and supervision; be interactive; be implemented with fidelity; include limitations in access; be institutionalized; avoid an exclusive focus on information and avoid congregating high-risk youth; and promote social and emotional skill development among elementary school students.

Multicomponent and Integrated Schools provide a captive population for the delivery of prevention programs and effects can last for 3 to 4 years. Similarly, family and community-based interventions have also produced reductions in the prevalence and intensity of alcohol use. However, prevention effects are maximized when all of these venues are used in concert in a coordinated and mutually supporting manner. For example, meta-analyses (Gottfredson and Wilson, 2003; Tobler et al., 2000) revealed that systemwide change interventions were most effective. Project Northland (see Chapter 11), which included school-based education programs, community activities and outreach, and environmental strategies that reduced the availability of alcohol to youth, is regarded as a highly effective program (Perry et al, 1996; Williams and Perry, 1998). These interventions use a community component involving family and other community leaders (e.g., teachers, counselors) or may strive to change the school or community environment. Communities should adopt prevention interventions that include school, family, and community components.

Sufficient in Dose and Follow-Up Significant developmental changes occur during adolescence. For educational interventions to be effective, they must be delivered throughout this period. Educational and family programs usually focus most heavily on the first part of adolescence. The increased use of boosters and multiyear programs should be encouraged. Community interventions also tend to focus on discrete portions of the adolescent years. However, a combined and consistently implemented approach to prevention has been shown to yield stronger results.

Norms That Support Nonuse Extensive research demonstrates that establishing norms that support nonuse is a key component of approaches to prevent alcohol use and misuse. During adolescence, it is common for youth who engage in inappropriate drinking behaviors to grossly overestimate the prevalence and acceptability of alcohol use among peers. As a result, these young people choose to use alcohol in a manner that matches these misperceived norms. Establishing beliefs in conventional norms among students—or, in other words, making young people's estimates about their peers' alcohol use more realistic—has significant potential to reduce alcohol use among young people. For example, the normative education element in interventions like the Adolescent Alcohol Prevention Trials significantly deterred use of alcohol, tobacco, and marijuana among middle and high school students (Hansen and Graham, 1991).

Parental Monitoring and Supervision Parents are a powerful source of influence on their children, and, using the right practices, parents can significantly decrease the likelihood that their children will drink. Research on prevention with families consistently demonstrates that parental monitoring of children—including monitoring their free time and time with friends and actively supervising them by being present during youth activities—is highly effective as a strategy for preventing the onset of alcohol use and misuse (Dusenbury, 2000; Vicary et al., 2000). Monitoring can make gaining access to alcohol more difficult and can help to reinforce family rules and policies prohibiting the use of alcohol. Programs can provide parents with skills and motivation for actively monitoring and supervising their children.

Interactive Educational programs demonstrated to reduce alcohol use and abuse have all been highly interactive. That is, they did not rely on didactically presented messages, but used teaching techniques that encouraged participants to be actively engaged in the process of forming social norms. Meta-analyses (Gottfredson and Wilson, 2003; Tobler et al., 2000) revealed that interactive programs that delivered more hours of programming were more effective than interactive programs that delivered fewer hours. This trend was not evident among noninteractive programs.

Implemented with Fidelity There is strong evidence that the quality of program delivery is highly related to successful outcome (Dusenbury et al., 2003). Training for providers is crucial. It is also essential for providers to have sufficient time to become fluent in delivering the program. On their initial attempt, program providers typically focus on understanding the mechanics of a program. It is only after they have mastered the mechanics of program delivery that they are able to focus on underlying psychological and sociological constructs that define quality implementation.

Access Limitations Family and community interventions that have been shown to be effective included a focus on limiting youth access to alcohol (see also Chapter 9). Such approaches need to include not only the adoption of laws and ordinances, but also their enforcement and the development of a strong social norm that supports the intent of such legislation. For example, Project Northland (Komro et al., 1994), Day One Community Partnership (Rohrbach et al., 1997), Communities Mobilizing for Change (CSAP model program), and Community Trials Intervention to Reduce High-Risk Drinking (a model program of the Substance Abuse and Mental Health Services Administration [SAMHSA]) all included efforts to reduce underage access to alcohol, and in each case these efforts were found to have significant effects on reducing drinking (see also Chapter 11).

Institutionalized Institutionalization is crucial for prevention to realize its full potential. It can ensure that new social norms in a community are perpetuated by exposing new community members (e.g., every fifth grade class in a school) to the norms, that well-trained professionals facilitate the intervention, and that programs are regularly evaluated and adjusted to meet the changing needs of the community. This kind of consistency and rigor has the potential to ensure that programs shown to reduce underage drinking can have long-lasting effects. However, schools and communities are often funded to implement these programs through temporary mechanisms and often at a level that does not allow sustained implementation.

Avoiding a Focus on Information and on Congregating High-Risk Youth As discussed above, programs with an exclusive focus on information are ineffective at changing behavior and programs that congregate high-risk youth have had mixed and, in some cases, negative effects.

Social and Emotional Skill Development There has been limited research on alcohol prevention among preschool and elementary school children. Norm-setting approaches, discussed above, are promising for older elementary school students (Donaldson et al., 1995). In addition, there is evidence that good academic achievement and such characteristics as good school climate, cooperative learning, and strong bonds between children and school have the potential to help prevent subsequent alcohol use (Battistich et al., 1996; Hawkins et al., 1999). Research has clearly shown that the causes of early alcohol use are related to the failure to develop social and personal competencies. These competencies include the ability to make good decisions and solve problems, set and achieve goals, effectively manage emotions and stress, communicate effectively, and build relationships that support a positive peer group.

In sum, although more research on education interventions is needed, these programmatic elements can be adopted with confidence. In addition, there are some programmatic elements that have not shown desired effects (e.g., didactic information sessions and scare tactics) and in some cases produce boomerang effects. Programs that rely heavily on these elements should not be funding priorities.

Recommendation 10-2: The U.S. Department of Health and Human Services and the U.S. Department of Education should fund only evidence-based education interventions, with priority given both to those that incorporate elements known to be effective and those that are part of comprehensive community programs.

These funding priorities should promote the key elements of prevention described in the principles of effectiveness defined by the Department of Education. Namely, funding decisions should be based on (1) demonstrated need, (2) defined behavior change goals, (3) clear objectives for how behavior change will be accomplished, and (4) the adoption of approaches with demonstrated effectiveness. As part of this approach, the Department of Education and SAMHSA list of evidence-based programs should be reviewed and revised annually. Funding should give priority to programs that have been independently demonstrated to be effective at deterring the onset of alcohol use and misuse or having an effect on other meaningful outcomes.

Regional conferences should be held for program developers, evaluators, schools currently using programs, and potential grantees to bridge the gap between research and practice. In addition, funds should be provided to support independent local and national evaluations that should include both the assessment of self-reports of alcohol consumption and assessments of changes in key outcomes of successful alcohol prevention, such as truancy, motor vehicle accidents, and academic performance. A specific, uniform percent of grant funding should be earmarked for local evaluation. Additional funding, equal perhaps to 10 percent of all local awards, should be provided for a national evaluation. A consortium of evaluators should be established to inform the Departments about the impact of programs on alcohol prevalence and consumption.

Identifying and selecting model programs are only part of the process in launching a successful education strategy. Experience over the past two decades reveals that most schools do not implement research-based programs as intended or do not continue to use them over time. Failure to institutionalize interventions is likely to prevent them from realizing their full potential. Federal and state policies are needed to encourage and support the institutionalization of research-based programs. Most research and funding has been conducted in secondary/middle schools; additional focus should be directed at primary and high schools. In addition, funding is needed to support program champions at the school and district level who provide the organizational memory as well as the necessary training resources to sustain prevention intervention. Finally, additional research is needed to determine how schools, families, and communities can be supported as they implement promising strategies and how effective strategies in these areas can be institutionalized.

RESIDENTIAL COLLEGES AND UNIVERSITIES

Educational interventions with underage drinkers at colleges and universities present a unique set of challenges. By the time they reach college, the majority of students have tried alcohol, and the majority of students who report current use also drink heavily (Flewelling et al., 2004). Furthermore, 31 percent of college students meet diagnostic criteria for alcohol abuse and 6 percent meet criteria for alcohol dependence; these data suggest that individual-based strategies for screening and intervention or referral may need to be a component of a comprehensive college based approach (Knight et al., 2002).

All residential college and university students should be exposed to alcohol education interventions—indeed, the transition to college offers an important opportunity in which expectations about alcohol use and nonuse on campus can be established and in which young people may be more receptive to messages about nonuse and harm reduction (Pandina, 2003). Recent studies suggest that working with parents and students, rather than with students alone, regarding transition difficulties at college is an effective approach (Wintre and Sugar, 2000). However, in addition to universal prevention approaches, interventions that selectively target heavy drinkers have the potential to reduce harm to the individual, the college community, and the neighborhood in which the college resides (NIAAA, 2002). According to NIAAA's recent report on college drinking, programs that target heavy drinkers through unified education interventions that include cognitive behavioral skills, norm clarification, and motivational enhancement interventions in conjunction with environmental and policy changes is the approach most likely to be effective at addressing college student drinking (NIAAA, 2002).

Interventions focused on students who drink heavily may have significant positive effects on the health and well-being of students and the quality of the college environment (Knight et al., 2002; Park, 1967; Perkins et al., 1980). Nationally, only one in five students report frequent heavy drinking, yet this group accounts for two-thirds of all the alcohol consumed by college students, more than half of all the alcohol-related problems other students experience, and more than 60 percent of all the reported injuries, vandalism, and problems with the police (Wechsler et al., 1998).

Despite public concern and media attention describing the problems associated with college student alcohol consumption, there is a relative lack of well-developed and evaluated intervention programs designed to assist college service providers. The Center for the Advancement of Public Health (CAPH) at George Mason University, based on data from their annual College Alcohol Survey, has created a sourcebook of strategies used by colleges across the United States, as well as recommendations for future college endeavors. Although CAPH notes that a number of campuses have developed innovative approaches for addressing college drinking, few strategies are applied on campuses with fidelity or consistency, and rarely are these approaches evaluated (CAPH, 2001).

Although a majority of colleges and universities have established campus alcohol prevention programs (Wechsler et al., 1999), survey data from the past decade show that the rates of heavy drinking on college campuses have not declined in the past 10 years. Part of this may be the lack of evaluations of college-based interventions and lack of dissemination about programs that are effective. Other deficiencies related to university alcohol policy and intervention may also contribute to the ineffectiveness of current programs (Wechsler, 1996; Cohen and Rogers, 1997; Ziemelis, 1998; Black and Coster, 1996; Smith, 1989), including:

• lack of data intended to identify specific campus problems for the "rational planning" of services;

- inconsistent enforcement of university policies and codes for student conduct;
- continued institutional reliance on informational approaches as a primary prevention strategy;
- limited student exposure to prevention activities;
- lack of use of counseling and treatment resources by students who may need those services the most; and
- failure to screen and provide services for students through regular physician visits to college health clinics and emergency room visits, and for students who violate alcohol policies.

Research does provide guidance to colleges' approaches to alcohol use on their campuses.

Education-Based Intervention Strategies

As with school-based programs, research on college-based programs demonstrates that programs primarily using information-only and scare tactic strategies concerning alcohol consequences and local laws and policies are ineffective or are insufficient on their own (Larimer and Cronce, 2002; Wechsler et al., 2002; Perry et al., 1996; Moskowitz, 1989; NIAAA, 2002). The NIAAA report on college drinking also found that values clarification about alcohol, when used alone and when providing blood alcohol content feedback to students, were ineffective.

Interventions with High-Risk Heavy Drinkers

Three education approaches—cognitive-behavioral skills, norm clarifications, and motivational enhancement interventions—have been found to be effective with heavy alcohol users on campus (NIAAA, 2002). The skills training approach uses a cognitive behavioral model to address problem or heavy alcohol use by altering beliefs associated with alcohol use. This approach may also involve general life-skills development, including assertiveness training and stress management training. The goal of this approach is to change an individual's expectations about alcohol's effects, monitor alcohol use over time, and develop effective coping techniques. Alcohol expectancies have been found to predict drinking behavior among college students (Christiansen et al., 1989; Stacy et al., 1990), and research suggests that interventions that challenge the behaviors students expect to result from drinking can decrease alcohol consumption (Darkes and Goldman, 1998), at least for some students.

Normative feedback or norm challenging is a strategy designed to address an individual's misperceptions regarding the rates of alcohol use on campus, as well as perceptions regarding the role of alcohol on campus (Schroeder and Prentice, 1998; Baer et al., 1991). In such interventions, a student's alcohol use patterns are assessed, and the student is provided feedback regarding the rates of alcohol use by his or her peers. Often, the student is also provided information regarding the prevalence of his or her alcohol use pattern. Prevention strategies have used different modalities to provide this feedback, including one-on-one interviews, small groups, and such media as online web-based programs (Marlatt et al., 1995; Borsari and Carey, 2000). The variety of modalities through which this approach can be delivered may make it a viable option for wide use on campuses, rather than only with identified heavy drinkers. Additional research in this area, especially concerning the comparative effectiveness of different modes of delivery, is needed.

Motivational interviewing techniques associated with alcohol use are designed to provide an assessment of student use and provide nonjudgmental feedback regarding a person's alcohol consumption and the negative consequences associated with use. Such techniques also often include normative feedback on peer alcohol use rates. Such interventions are designed to initiate an individual's desire to change behavior (Miller et al., 1992). Brief motivational enhancement interventions have been found to affect problems associated with alcohol consumption, including driving after drinking, riding with an intoxicated driver, and injuries (Marlatt et al., 1998; Monti et al., 1999). Opportunities for motivational interviews are available when heavy drinkers are identified through the campus judicial system or through screening at campus health care facilities. Few campuses have programs that link heavy drinkers—even when they are identified through campus systems—to such interventions.

The integration of skills training, normative feedback, and motivational interviewing techniques has been applied to one-on-one and small group interventions in order to reduce drinking rates. These education strategies may be applied in a universal fashion with a general student population, such as first-year students who may be forming ideas (and misperceptions) about how alcohol fits into college life. In addition, these education approaches could be incorporated into programs that specifically target groups at risk for heavy drinking and individuals who, through the college judicial system or screening provided through university health care systems (see below), are identified as heavy drinkers. Research has demonstrated that this general integrated approach also reduces the negative consequences of alcohol use (Baer et al., 2001; Larimer and Cronce, 2002; Marlatt et al., 1998).

Broad Interventions

One educational approach that has received considerable attention and that is directed at a general college population (rather than just heavy drinkers) is the social norms approach. A fundamental premise of this approach is that a majority of college students do not accurately perceive the rates of alcohol use on campus and may drink to the level of this misperception in order to fit in. Perceptions regarding the amount and frequency of substance use on campus are often greater than actual use (Perkins and Berkowitz, 1986; Perkins, 2002). Several institutions have reported reduction in high-risk drinking over a relatively short time using such approaches (Berkowitz, 1997; DeJong and Linkenbach, 1999; Haines and Spear, 1996; Johannessen et al., 1999, 2002).

Research on social norms campaigns has indicated some promise, although research has generally been limited to case studies of individual campuses, generally without appropriate comparison or control groups, and they often do not control for other interventions aimed at reducing drinking problems. Given the limitations of social norms evaluations, such interventions should be further evaluated. If implemented, social norms approaches should be one component of a comprehensive effort and should not be used as a single strategy.

Environmental Factors On and Off Campuses

A growing body of evidence points to the importance of addressing the multiple environmental contributors to alcohol use and abuse, both on and off campus. Research has demonstrated that changes in the normative environment within which students reside can influence drinking behavior. Specific environmental elements on campus—including fraternity or sorority participation, living on campus, and the ready availability of alcoholic beverages—have been identified as the most important determinants of drinking and heavy drinking among college students (Chaloupka and Wechsler, 1996). Research has demonstrated the importance of several environmental factors: access (Wechsler et al., 2002; Weitzman et al., 2003; Bormann and Stone, 2001); cost (Williams et al., 2002; Clapp, 2001); exposure to high-use residential climates (Sher et al., 2001); contextual factors that are predictive and protective of heavy drinking (Clapp and Shillington, 2001); and alcohol policies and enforcement procedures (Eigen, 1991; Palmer et al., 2001). Examples of protective measures include new campus alcohol policies (e.g., no kegs at on-campus parties), legal regulations, alcohol server training programs, and the restriction of low-cost alcohol promotions or "happy hours." Some studies have shown that college policies affecting access to alcohol on campus—for instance, whether a residence hall is wet or dry and whether a college has an alcohol ban on the campus—generally decrease the frequency of student alcohol use, heavy drinking, and frequent heavy drinking (Wechsler et al., 2001a, 2001c; Weitzman et al., 2003a).

Consistent Policy Enforcement and Application of Sanctions

Research investigating student sentiment toward alcohol policies and laws consistently documents support for policies that control underage drinking (Wechsler et al., 2002). Within the college environment there are multiple agents for enforcement, including campus police and safety officers, residence housing personnel, residence-based student paraprofessionals, athletic team coaches, academic advisers, sponsors of student organizations, and fraternity and sorority advisers. Despite these multiple opportunities for intervention, enforcement is often left to one or two of these groups (e.g., campus police, residential life professional staff), or enforcement occurs only among some staff within a group. Often these individuals are hesitant to hold college students accountable for their behavior, as they may view the university sanctioning process as punitive or inconsistent with their roles as mentors and advisers for students. Such a circumstance creates inconsistent enforcement of policies and sends mixed messages to students.

Colleges should pursue strategies to strengthen linkages between policy and enforcement. The judicial process on many college campuses offers an important—and underutilized—opportunity to send consistent messages to students and ensure that intervention programs reach students whose drinking has become a problem for the campus. Interventions based upon motivational enhancement, skill development, and normative clarification can promote values that are consistent with the values already found within the university culture.

Parental Notification

The Higher Education Amendments of 1998 provide assistance to colleges and universities in their efforts to address student alcohol and other drug use. Section 952 clarified that institutions of higher education are allowed (but not required) to notify parents if a student under the age of 21 at the time of notification commits a disciplinary violation involving alcohol or a controlled substance. The U.S. Department of Education's final regulations issued in 2000 further clarified the intent of the 1998 amendment, stating that campus officials may notify parents whenever they determine that a disciplinary violation has occurred and that those determinations can be made without conducting a formal disciplinary proceeding or hearing.

Research has begun to document the extent of parental notification practices used by colleges. One survey (Palmer et al., 2001) involving 189 colleges and universities found that 58 percent of the colleges indicated having parental notification policies (77 percent of private institutions and 43 percent of public institutions). An additional 24 percent were considering integrating parental notification as part of their sanctioning process. Of the campuses reporting they use parental notification as a sanction, 59 percent use mail correspondence as the vehicle to notify parents. This survey also reported that campus officials rated the response of parents who received notification of their child's alcohol or drug violation as very supportive (72 percent) and supportive (6 percent).

Although no well-controlled research has been conducted, the campuses that use parental notification procedures report reductions of more than one-half in the number of alcohol violations following implementation of the parental notification policies. Several colleges, such as the University of Delaware, have adopted parental notification within a comprehensive approach to prevention. The integration of parental notification as part of a system to increase the monitoring, enforcement, and publicity associated with the institution's alcohol and other drug polices, has resulted in fewer suspensions, a decrease in disciplinary cases, less vandalism, and reductions in high-risk drinking behavior.

If the notification of parents is integrated into the institution's sanctioning process, the notification response should be one of several approaches serving to deter student misbehavior. A comprehensive approach needs to involve education, screening, and intervention. Ongoing publicity of a parental notification policy may be necessary in order for this sanction to be applied as an effective deterrent. Information regarding the goals of the parental notification response and how and when it is to be used should be clearly articulated before implementation. The institution should also develop means to consider issues that may warrant exceptions for the use of parental notification (for example, students who may experience undue hardship, history of abuse in the family, or students who do not have dependent status). Students should also be provided the opportunity to discuss the incident with their parent prior to the institution's contact.

Availability of Alcohol-Free Social Activities

Several universities offer alcohol-free social and recreational activities, often on Friday and Saturday nights, when students often consume alcohol. These activities cover a broad range, including late-night intramural tournaments, concerts, theatrical performances, movie showings, dances, ice skating, trivia bowls, and laser tag. These activities are developed and offered by student activities departments and by student organizations. Although such approaches have not been evaluated, alcohol-free, late-night activities are an alcohol prevention strategy with theoretical promise.

Screening for High-Risk and Heavy Drinkers

Research on college student subcultures has identified specific student groups that accept and promote heavy substance use among their members (Astin, 1993; Dean, 1982). If a campus can identify these groups, selective prevention programming could be targeted to these subcultures as a way to reduce underage drinking.

College health service agencies and the judicial discipline system are two primary contact points for substance abuse screening and intervention on college campuses. These systems are positioned to link students who are heavy drinkers or show signs of early alcohol dependence to intervention programming and, in some cases, needed treatment.

The university's judicial response to violations in alcohol policy is also part of the educational lesson the institution can provide to students (Smith, 1989). By providing a network through which university alcohol policies are clearly communicated and consistently applied to student misconduct by all parts of the university community, then addressed through a screening and brief intervention, a university can provide students an effective and efficient response to high-risk drinking and associated behaviors. This system simultaneously allows students to evaluate their alcohol use and its role in their lives while holding them accountable for their behavior. Brief motivational interventions may be the best response for policy infractions. It has been proven to effectively reduce high-risk behaviors associated with alcohol consumption, is sensitive to the developmental and psychological characteristics found among traditionally aged college students (18 to 22 years of age), provides a supportive, personally reflective, and educational opportunity for students, and has values that are consistent with the values found within institutions of higher education (NIAAA, 2002).

The challenge for the judicial process is in balancing responsibilities in several different areas—enforcing the university's policy, encouraging health-promoting behavior, and protecting the rights of students who drink moderately or choose not to drink at all. Research has noted that effective early intervention strategies rely on consistent enforcement of policies on the campus, which is essential to the quality of the educational environment (Wechsler and Davenport, 1999).

The active involvement of college student healthcare professionals in alcohol prevention is supported by the *Guidelines for Adolescent Preventive Services* (Elster and Kuznets, 1994), which recommend that healthcare providers ask all adolescent patients annually about their alcohol and other drug use as part of routine care. Given the prevalence of drinking among 18- to 20-year-olds, it is reasonable to also expect college healthcare professionals to conduct similar screening with their patients. Like the campus judicial process, healthcare services offer an important and underutilized opportunity to link services for heavy alcohol users to students who could benefit from such interventions.

While an overwhelming majority of colleges and universities indicate they have an alcohol and other drug prevention program (Wechsler et al., 1999), very little data exist on the organizational characteristics of these programs, the scope of their prevention efforts, their financial support, and the financial resources needed to effectively implement the empirically validated and multiple prevention strategies recommended in this document and by NIAAA (2002). There also is inadequate evaluation of approaches, such as social norms marketing, parental notification, interventions in healthcare settings, and other innovative approaches. Future research should also consider institutional characteristics associated with alcohol outcomes, including the effects of size of student enrollment, type of institution (2- or 4-year college, residential or commuter), location in either an urban or rural setting, and organizational properties of colleges, including affiliations such as historically black or women's institutions.

> **Recommendation 10-3:** Residential colleges and universities should adopt comprehensive prevention approaches, including evidence-based screening, brief intervention strategies, consistent policy enforcement, and environmental changes that limit underage exposure and access to alcohol. They should use universal education interventions, as well as selective and indicated approaches with relevant populations.

> **Recommendation 10-4:** The National Institute on Alcohol Abuse and Alcoholism and the Substance Abuse and Mental Health Services Administration should continue to fund evaluations of college-based interventions, with a particular emphasis on targeting of interventions to specific college characteristics, and should maintain a list of evidence-based programs.

OTHER INTERVENTION OPPORTUNITIES

Research on educational approaches has focused on primary and secondary schools and college settings. Faith-based organizations and health care settings have frequent contact with young people and may offer important intervention opportunities. Similarly, many young people either join the military or enter the labor maker rather than attending college or finishing school. However, interventions with youth in these settings, and evaluation of the few interventions that do exist, are scarce.

Available research does not allow recommendation of particular approaches in these settings. However, future strategies would benefit from the development and evaluation of interventions in these areas (see Chapter 12). Research on educational approaches in schools, colleges and communities may offer some lessons that may reasonably be applied to these settings.

Faith-Based Interventions

Research on the effectiveness of faith-based initiatives for preventing alcohol use and alcohol problems is very limited. However, family involvement in faith-based institutions, religiosity, and spirituality all have been shown in research to reduce the risk for adolescent substance use. According to Miller (1998), there is a consistent effect of commitment to religion and reduced alcohol use. Young people whose families are active in religious activities are less likely to drink beer and distilled alcohol (Hardesty and Kirby, 1995).

Interventions delivered through faith-based organizations represent a new area of exploration for prevention research. Such research might include examining what faith-based groups currently do that addresses alcohol, with the goal of understanding how involvement in faith-based institutions moderates alcohol use and developing and evaluating innovative strategies for alcohol prevention in faith-based settings. However studies of faith-based interventions must be carefully designed to account for the possibility that selection bias, rather than program effects, accounts for any positive outcomes (Miller, 1998; Hardesty and Kirby, 1995).

The Department of Health and Human Services should apply the same standards for providing care and determining the effectiveness of faith-based interventions as has been established for school- and community-based interventions. Innovative approaches should be independently evaluated using standard approaches for documenting effectiveness.

Health System Interventions

Doctors are viewed as authorities for all health issues by adolescents and parents (Mullen and Katayama, 1985) and therefore should be actively involved in assisting with prevention. There are national guidelines for physicians' provision of comprehensive preventive services to adolescent patients. In general, these clinical guidelines recommend that all adolescents have an annual, confidential, preventive services visit during which they are screened, educated, and counseled on a number of biomedical, emotional, and sociobehavioral topics, including alcohol use (e.g., Werner, 1995). There is a growing interest in drawing healthcare providers into alcohol and substance abuse prevention with youth, and healthcare systems and providers represent an as yet untapped resource in prevention programming. Cavanaugh and Henneberger (1996) reported that more than nine out of ten parents in their study thought that pediatricians should discuss alcohol with their children during routine visits. Research also suggests that adolescents are more willing to disclose information about alcohol use to physicians who assure them of complete confidentiality (Ford et al., 1997).

In spite of the existing guidelines, physicians do not screen or educate the majority of their adolescent patients regarding alcohol. Only 25 percent of physicians educate their patients on the basis of the standards established by the American Medical Association for screening (Millstein and Marcell, 2003). Even when physicians do counsel adolescents regarding alcohol use, they predominantly use ineffective interventions (Millstein and Marcell, 2002). Although, on average, physicians report screening 70 percent of their adolescents about alcohol use, only 47 percent of patients are asked about drinking and driving (Halpern-Felsher et al., 2000). Furthermore, only about half of patients are educated about the risks of alcohol use.

Emerging research suggests that physicians' rates of screening adolescents for alcohol use can be improved (from an average of 59 percent to 76 percent) by training physicians on the knowledge, attitudes, and skills that are necessary to create behavior change (Lustig et al., 2001). Ozer et al. (2001) also showed that physicians' alcohol-related screening and counseling rates could increase significantly following training, the implementation of charting forms, and if an on-site health educator is available. Preliminary data are beginning to suggest that implementing preventive services does reduce adolescents' risk behavior (Ozer et al., 2003).

Healthcare facilities have significant and promising, but as yet unproven, potential to influence alcohol use and alcohol problems among adolescents. Interventions using a variety of media might be developed for patients to be implemented during time spent in the waiting room and during follow-up visits. Future research should promote the development and evaluation of innovative interventions that target adolescents in healthcare settings. Additional research and evaluation are needed to determine whether interventions implemented by physicians or other healthcare professionals are effective with adolescents and whether and how training can enhance effectiveness.

Workplaces

Young people who work full or part time while attending school are more likely than their peers to use alcohol and drink heavily (McMorris and Uggen, 2000; Mortimer and Johnson, 1998), and most heavy drinkers of any age are in the workforce (Cook and Schlenger, 2002). A full- or part-time job provides discretionary money that young people may choose to spend on alcohol. Workplace social norms may facilitate drinking behavior and additional exposure to adults who are of the legal drinking age may provide a mode of access for underage drinkers to procure alcohol.

There are compelling reasons to expand workplace prevention programming. Workplaces may offer a key site in efforts to reduce underage drinking because of the potential to interrupt the relationship between employment and youth alcohol use. Such interventions may also serve to reach a population of young people who are not exposed to school-based interventions.

Workplace alcohol prevention programs have existed for the past 50 years, no doubt because alcohol use and abuse can result in accidents, lost productivity, and worker turnover. Workplace drug testing and prevention programs have become more prevalent in the past 10 years, as has research evaluating the effectiveness of primary prevention strategies. There is some evidence to suggest that workplace drug testing has helped to reduce drug use but additional research on effectiveness is needed. In addition, it is not clear if a deterrent effect extends beyond the drugs tested for to a substance like alcohol.

Although little research has been conducted on workplace prevention programs with underage youth, at least two program characteristics appear to have the potential to have positive effects (Cook and Schlenger, 2002; National Research Council and Institute of Medicine, 1994). First, programs that seek to change workplace culture and social norms around alcohol use may be particularly effective in work settings that support or have a permissive culture around drinking. A second characteristic is that intervention programs must avoid the stigma of alcohol abuse in order to encourage worker participation. For example, a workshop on alcohol abuse is not likely to be well attended, but a stress management program that addresses alcohol use as a part of its curriculum may be appealing to employees. There are likely other characteristics that will contribute to the design and implementation of effective workplace interventions.

Unfortunately, the available research about prevention programs does not include any program that specifically targets or seeks to address the needs and concerns of underage workers. In fact, the committee is unaware of any workplace programs that address the specific needs of underage employees.

Workplace prevention programming has the potential to disrupt the relationship between youth employment and drinking and may reach young people who would not otherwise be reached. More evaluations of existing general workplace programs are needed, including whether underage employees participate in such programs, the factors that influence their participation, and whether the programs meet the needs and concerns of young workers. Other creative new programs specifically targeting underage populations also should be developed and evaluated. Employers with large concentrations of workers under age 21 are one possible venue for testing intervention approaches.

The Military

Alcohol use in the military has historically been widespread and commonly accepted, provided that it did not result in irresponsible behavior or harm. A study by Ames et al. (2002) suggests that the military environment does not serve as a protective factor for heavy drinking. Over the past several decades, the military has increased efforts to test for drug and alcohol use, developed interventions aimed at decreasing risky health behaviors, including alcohol use, and increased efforts to provide treatment for those with identified drug and alcohol problems. For example, the navy began drug testing in 1981. At that time, 50 percent of enlisted personnel tested positive; by 1984, only 5 percent tested positive. Yet many employers who instituted drug testing also initiated other prevention programs at a similar time—this was certainly true of the navy's approach to substance abuse prevention—and research has not been conducted to separate the relative influence of the effects of drug testing and other programming (Cook and Schlenger, 2002).

Most military-based interventions have focused on the military audience at large and have not had a specific focus on the underage, primarily enlisted, audience. Though approaches aimed at changing the military culture around drinking have value, more attention should be paid to approaches that specifically target underage personnel. Such approaches will admittedly face unique challenges in terms of the inconsistency between policies that allow young men and women to be put in harm's way but do not allow them to drink, as well as their living in countries that may have minimum legal drinking age policies that differ from those in the United States. Nonetheless, the military setting provides an important opportunity for exploring prevention interventions with underage personnel.

Prevention programs at colleges offer resources from which the military can develop innovative interventions with underage personnel but these programs would need to be adapted to the specific context and culture of the military. One program—PREVENT (Personal Responsibility and Values: Education and Training)—developed for and implemented in the navy, has a number of components that parallel college programs and that make use of some of the known critical elements (see Chapter 11). PREVENT is a multifaceted education curriculum that seeks to link knowledge of health behaviors and risks to behavioral changes. It addresses a number of issues (drug and alcohol use, decision-making, and financial management) and builds knowledge and skills.

An interesting element to this program is that it uses values traditionally associated and promoted by the military (e.g., personal responsibility, integrity, minimizing risk to other sailors, mission readiness) as a way to encourage sailors to reduce alcohol use and alcohol-related consequences. This element capitalizes on military culture for health promotion and alcohol prevention—something that might be uniquely possible in the military. Based on reports issued by the U.S. Navy, PREVENT appears to be a promising program. For example, graduates reported a 45 percent reduction in heavy drinking days per month and an 82 percent decrease in driving after drinking. Costs associated with alcohol-related incidents and lack of readiness were also decreased (U.S. Navy, 2003). Additional evaluations of military-based programs, including the extent to which they reach underage populations, are warranted.

TREATMENT PROGRAMS

Despite efforts to prevent underage drinking, some youth will drink at a level that requires clinical treatment. Findings from the National Household Survey on Drug Abuse indicate that about 10 percent of 12- to 17-year-olds (about 2.3 million) are heavy users of alcohol. The proportion of users who are clinically dependent is not known, but it is believed to be unacceptably high. Treatment for underage alcohol dependency is scarce. The juvenile justice system is the major route through which most adolescents get into treatment. Although estimates of the cost-effectiveness of early treatment are speculative, research suggests that early treatment has the potential to be cost-effective, especially in comparison with incarceration or treatment for a long-term alcohol abuse problem. For instance, cost-benefit research on drug and alcohol treatment generally (Office of National Drug Control Policy, 2001) suggests that the range of savings is between $2.50 and $9.60 for every dollar spent on treatment. Although these savings were calculated on the basis of adult treatment, and included drugs as well as alcohol, it is reasonable to assume that savings for effective youth alcohol treatment would be at least this high. Unfortunately, only one person in seven who would qualify for treatment was admitted to treatment in 1999 (National Institute on Drug Abuse Community Epidemiology Work Group, 1999). The proportion of youth who are admitted to treatment is undocumented but believed to be even smaller.

Research on treating underage alcohol abusers reveals that nine elements are crucial to success: matching treatment to needs; comprehensive and integrated treatment; family involvement; developmental appropriateness; recognition of gender and cultural differences; continuing care; and assessment (Hansen and Dusenbury, 2004).

Matching Treatment to Needs Assessment is important to determine the type of treatment approach to which an adolescent may respond (Pickens and Fletcher, 1991; Bergmann et al., 1995; Jainchill et al., 1995; Werner, 1995). Because the severity of adolescents' alcohol use varies considerably, matching the severity of their problem to intensity of treatment is important (Jenson et al., 1995). Treatment formats range in intensity and include:

- brief intervention, typically delivered by physicians, counselors, or others who do not specialize in drug and alcohol abuse treatment per se;
- outpatient treatment, which includes programs that can range from 2 to 20 hours per week;
- day treatment or partial hospitalization, including professionally directed treatment after school, in the evenings, or on weekends, often combining individual, group, and family therapy;
- inpatient treatment; and
- detoxification, a 3- to 5-day period of intensive medical monitoring and management that is often part of a 28-day intensive inpatient treatment program.

Comprehensive and Integrated Treatment is more effective if it is fully integrated into all aspects of an adolescent's life—school, home, family, peer group, and workplace. For example, treatment programs should actively help students keep up with their schoolwork and feel integrated in the school environment.

Involvement of Families Family development research clearly supports the need for understanding an adolescent's relationship with his or her family and including families in therapy wherever possible. Families can be either a source of strength or a risk for continued alcohol abuse. For instance, family involvement can be particularly important in retaining teenagers in treatment, while alcohol problems among other family members can influence youths to continue engaging in heavy drinking. Family involvement usually includes education about treatment and how families can support the treatment process. Families sometimes need intervention in order to change the environment or structure they provide to the underage drinker in treatment (Spoth et al., 2001). In addition, family interventions need to be prepared to address familial alcoholism, which represents a significant risk factor for youth alcohol use and future dependence.

Developmental Appropriateness Program models specifically designed for adolescents are more effective than programs based on adult regimens. Adolescent treatment needs to emphasize maturational issues, psychological issues, and emotional and sexual issues. Treatment programs should be tailored to the different cognitive abilities of older and younger adolescents and deal differently with concrete versus abstract styles of thinking.

Retention Underage drinkers are often less motivated than adults to participate in treatment. They are often referred through delinquent acts at school or through the criminal justice system; they rarely self-refer. Programs need to develop strategies that engage and retain teenagers in treatment. Retaining underage abusers in treatment often requires the application of age-appropriate sanctions and rewards.

Gender and Cultural Issues It is important to recognize issues that are particular to some groups. For instance, there is a correlation between childhood trauma and substance abuse for girls and women. Often, female substance abusers have been sexually abused. For these reasons, it is contraindicated to put girls in a coed setting for treatment. Other differences along race and ethnicity must also be considered and attended to as a part of treatment. Alcohol use is often defined as part of a cultural context and certain cultural attitudes may affect use patterns as well as how an adolescent understands his or her alcohol use. Treatment programs that can attend to these differences may have greater potential to produce successful outcomes compared to those that do not.

Continuing Care Continuing care is crucial to achieving positive long-term outcomes (McKay et al., 2002). Underage drinkers who require intense treatment will also require intense continuing care. Currently, continuing care for adolescent drug and alcohol problems is rarely available. There is little research on continuing care to provide guidance regarding what kinds of continuing care are the most effective for these adolescents. Additional research in this area would be useful.

Assessment of Outcomes Most adolescent treatment programs have not been rigorously evaluated, though many keep track of outcome data and are able to provide statistics that suggest the effectiveness of the treatment and recovery strategies (SAMSHA, 2000; Pickens and Fletcher 1991; Bergmann et al., 1995; Jainchill et al., 1995; Werner, 1995). One of the challenges for treatment providers is that evaluation of treatment programs is costly and difficult (Kaminer and Bukstein, 1989; Milby, 1981). However, evaluation not only validates effective approaches, it also provides information that is essential for improving treatment strategies (Kaminer and Bukstein, 1989).

It is crucial to the success of adolescent treatment that referral to service is coordinated within communities. Strategies that increase coordination among institutions in the community including schools, workplaces that employ teenagers, law enforcement, courts, faith-based institutions, and public and private treatment providers that may refer teens to treatment should be developed, disseminated, and evaluated. Training should be provided for key individuals all of these institutions about indicators of risk and procedures for referral.

> **Recommendation 10-5: The U.S. Department of Health and Human Services and states should expand the availability of effective clinical services for treating alcohol abuse among underage populations and for following up on treatment. The U.S. Department of Education, the U.S. Department of Health and Human Services, and the U.S. Department of Justice should establish policies that facilitate diagnosing and referring underage alcohol abusers and those who are alcohol dependent for clinical treatment.**

Adolescents often enter alcohol treatment through the criminal justice system. The Department of Justice should facilitate the development of a coordinated approach that encourages the use of effective approaches for dealing with adjudicated youth. In addition, these approaches should also be designed in a manner that will allow them to address alcohol use when it occurs in conjunction with other drug use. The criminal justice system should establish policies that ensure that referral to alcohol treatment is appropriate and accomplished systematically.

Schools do not yet systematically identify and refer students in need of diagnosis and treatment for alcohol problems. State agencies should encourage schools, health care providers, and other professionals to access state-of-the-art resources to help them identify youth who may need help and make referrals to appropriate agencies for diagnosis and treatment. In addition, policies and programs should support screening and referral that matches the needs of adolescent alcohol abusers with appropriate treatment options.

11

Communities

In a democratic society, the mobilization of communities in civic life is in and of itself of significant value. Democratic life relies on civic participation and an active, informed citizenry. Community-based groups facilitate the formation of diverse constituencies and support their work with organizational, material, technical, financial, and training assistance. Coalitions also enhance dialogue and cooperation by bringing together stakeholders for strategy development and mobilization on critical issues.

Although most community coalitions have not been rigorously evaluated, several community trials provide evidence that community coalitions can affect alcohol-related outcomes and also document the elements that make community initiatives successful. In addition, numerous case studies and substantial qualitative research attest to the effectiveness of community coalitions. On the basis of this evidence, combined with the strong logical reasoning behind the value of community-level interventions, the committee concludes that community mobilization specific to underage drinking is an attractive complement to national- and state-level interventions. Future evaluations should continue to refine the critical elements of these initiatives.

COMMUNITY-BASED ACTIVITIES

While community mobilization has been studied as an intervention in itself, it also provides a context within which interventions can occur, thereby increasing the likelihood that those interventions will succeed. It is a tool that can be used to implement and support various interventions, especially those that target community-level policies and practices. It can help to create the political will and organizational support for developing and implementing proven strategies for decreasing underage drinking (such as minimum age drinking laws, zero tolerance laws, and measures to reduce physical availability and outlet concentration). It can help to change the normative climate surrounding the acceptability of underage drinking, and create greater awareness of, and publicity about, enforcement activities, such as random breath testing and sting operations. It also helps establish the idea that alcohol and other drugs are a community problem that local people can solve, thereby increasing the likelihood that people will support and sustain efforts they help create.

There is a long and varied history of community mobilization around alcohol problems in the United States, dating back to the nineteenth century. In recent years, community mobilization has been recognized, documented, and evaluated in efforts to reduce alcohol-related problems, including underage drinking. Case studies have documented how communities have organized and used the news media to support changes in alcohol availability, reductions in outdoor advertising of alcohol, increased compliance checks on retailers regarding service and sales of alcohol to minors, keg registration laws, and campaigns to eliminate alcohol sponsorship from ethnic holiday events.

It is important for communities to rely on scientifically based strategies to reduce underage drinking. For example, research shows that positive outcomes can be achieved by combining environmental and institutional change with theory-based health education programs (Hingson and Howland, 2002). Community-based prevention research points to the importance of broad efforts to reshape the physical, social, economic, and legal environment affecting alcohol use. Promising evidence suggests that coalitions can effectively address youth access to alcohol and high-risk behaviors associated with alcohol consumption (Hingson and Howland, 2002; Manger et al., 1992).

Concerns about the prevalence and effects of alcohol use by underage youth have led to a large proliferation of community-based coalitions across the country (Butterfoss et al., 1996; Lerner and Miller, 1993; Robert Wood Johnson Foundation, 1993). These coalitions have engaged community residents, advocacy groups, representatives of nongovernmental organizations, government agencies, and universities in collaborative activities to address youth risk behaviors, particularly those associated with alcohol and other drug use (Fawcett et al., 1997; Hawkins et al., 1992; Mansergh et al., 1996). Having the flexibility to choose one's partners has been an important ingredient in the success of many effective coalitions. Some coalitions have included local alcohol retailers, while others have limited their membership to public health, safety, and other noncommercial organizations. There is some evidence that coalition partners with strong ties to alcohol producers may not support effective environmental interventions. Government agencies may or may not play a major role.

Community-driven initiatives should be tailored to the specific problems and resources in a community. Different communities will therefore have different priorities based on their particular needs. For example, some research suggests that minority communities may be targeted by some alcohol advertisers (Alaniz and Wilkes, 1995; Altman et al., 1991; Hackbarth et al., 2001) and that outlet density in these communities is particularly high (LaVeist and Wallace, 2000; Gorman and Spear, 1997). Although a specific relationship between advertising and underage drinking has not been shown, recent cross-sectional research has shown a correlation between outlet density and underage drinking. For example, outlet density has been associated with increased incidence of youth driving under the influence (Treno, Grube, and Martin, 2003), ease of alcohol purchase (Freisthler et al., 2003) and heavy and frequent drinking and alcohol problems (Weitzman et al., 2003a). Similarly, Wechlser and Wuethrich (2002) suggest that controlling outlet density can help alleviate market pressures that result in discounted pricing, a factor in underage drinking.

Research has also shown that while newly arrived immigrants have lower rates of alcohol use than others, their consumption increases and they develop more liberal attitudes toward drinking as they become more acculturated (National Institute on Alcohol Abuse and Alcoholism, 1994; National Women's Health Information Center, 2002). Communities should consider the variety of factors that may affect underage drinking, as well as the specific characteristics of underage drinking in their communities in developing community-specific strategies.

In large states, such as California, local coalitions have sometimes had greater success than statewide efforts. Other successful coalition efforts across the United States have been supported by statewide organizations or systems. States have organized regional coalitions consisting of representatives from institutions of higher education, city and state political officials, liquor control and licensing officials, state and local law enforcement officials, restaurant and tavern proprietors, state health officials, and researchers to support the development and implementation of broad and comprehensive strategies. The National Highway Traffic Safety Administration (2002) recently sponsored a project by the Pennsylvania Liquor Control Board to develop a manual to help alcohol beverage control (ABC) agencies identify opportunities and initiatives to reduce underage drinking.

Statewide initiatives can begin in a number of ways. Some are the result of the leadership of state agencies, such as the state department of public health or the state liquor control board. Others emerge through college and university administrations or statewide college task forces, as found in the states of Missouri and California. Still others may be the result of grassroots organizations from a number of localities realizing that they have common interests at the state level, and banding together for coordinated and more effective action.

> **Recommendation 11-1: Community leaders should assess the underage drinking problem in their communities and consider effective approaches—such as community organizing, coalition building, and the strategic use of the mass media—to reduce drinking among underage youth**

SUCCESSFUL COMMUNITY COALITIONS: TWO PORTRAITS

Successful community coalitions include the use of multiple program strategies, such as education programs, community organization, environmental policy changes, strategic use of the news media, and heightened enforcement of existing policies (Hingson and Howland, 2002). Strategic use of the mass media by communities is an important component of community mobilization and can support other interventions. It can be an effective vehicle for publicizing new or existing policies and gaining public support for alcohol control policies and increased enforcement efforts (Casswell and Gilmore, 1989; Stewart and Casswell, 1993). Skillful use of media resources can support community organization and public education about successful strategies, as well as influence those who have the power to make changes in enforcement practices or in policies. Community groups that have developed the skills to use the news media strategically to support their objectives for changes in the environments contributing to public health problems can influence public opinion and public policy (Wallack et al., 1996; Wallack, 2000; Seevak, 1997).

Two examples of coalition-building in communities comprised primarily of racial and ethnic minority groups provide instructive lessons. Oakland, California, achieved successful alcohol policy outcomes through the work of a single coalition consisting primarily of professionals and government officials. The central focus of the coalition was to develop legislation that would tax all alcohol outlets in the city to provide funds for improving neighborhood safety and beautification. The major strategy relied much more on skillful use of the media than on grassroots organizing. The "Deemed Approved Ordinance," enacted by the city in 1993, charged alcohol outlets an annual fee of $600 for monitoring establishments. At the same time, the city also enacted a 1-year moratorium on new licenses and required a 1,000-foot separation between alcohol outlets citywide except for the downtown area. A year later, in 1994, Oakland received a $100,000 grant from the state alcoholic beverage control agency to hire a police officer and other personnel to deal specifically with alcohol-related enforcement; they became known as the alcohol beverage action team (ABAT). ABAT set up many decoy operations with minors to buy alcohol and cigarettes, which put retail establishments on notice. The police also built a closer relationship with the ABC agency, building records against problem alcohol outlets and sending that information to the agency. Community respondents also reported that working together on these alcohol-related issues has led to more general improvements on community life and personal empowerment.

Los Angeles provides another instructive example. For 20 years, public concern has focused on the proliferation of alcohol outlets and the role they played in the city's well-known neighborhood and social problems, especially the drug trade. The Community Coalition for Substance Abuse Prevention and Treatment began in the early 1990s conducting research on the problem, initiating a community dialogue, and highlighting a history of alcohol activism in the city. These efforts were invigorated by the overnight destruction of almost a third of the alcohol outlets in the infamous south central area during the riots following the Rodney King decision. The coalition relied on grassroots community organizing, which led to the involvement of city council members, as well as networking with decision makers and other activists at the state level. Their efforts led to state legislation permitting local control of alcohol outlets. Coalition efforts also decreased the number of retail outlets operating in south central Los Angeles, improved environmental standards for outlet operation, increased awareness of alcohol policy issues at the local level, and increased empowerment and participation of neighborhood residents in the process of local governance.

EVIDENCE OF EFFECTIVENESS

The effectiveness of community activities to combat underage drinking has been a focus of national and international efforts since the early 1980s. One rigorous evaluation provides lessons about what does not work. Evaluation of a demonstration project investigating the effectiveness of a comprehensive coalition-building model in reducing alcohol and other drug problems, the Fighting Back Initiative funded by the Robert Wood Johnson Foundation, found little positive effect on youth or adult substance use. However, two flaws may have doomed the project from the start. First, the coalition organizers sought to include all major community stakeholders, including those who were members of or closely aligned with commercial interests in alcohol production or sales. Controversial interventions, such as those affecting the availability of alcohol, were not even considered almost from the start in many of the coalitions. Second, the interventions used had not been proven to be effective. The easiest interventions to achieve politically are often the least effective in reducing alcohol-related problems. Reliance on the scientifically proven interventions though potentially more difficult to implement can prevent years of wasted effort.

Examples of What Works

In contrast, four other major experimental studies of community mobilization have demonstrated what does work. Project Northland in Minnesota was a randomized community trial implemented in 24 communities with a study population in early adolescence and in the final years of high school. There were three phases. In the early phase, the project's interventions included school curricula, parent involvement, peer leadership, and community task forces. During the second phase, there were no interventions. In the third phase, the interventions were classroom curriculum, parent education, a print media campaign, and youth development and community organizing. The evaluation measured the tendency to use alcohol, to drink heavily, and to obtain alcoholic beverages. The project had its greatest success in the early years; the progress eroded during the period of no intervention and showed modest success in the final phase. The failure of the project to maintain its effectiveness during the interim phase demonstrates the importance of intervention throughout adolescence, and it also points to the significance of community-level policy and other actions that change community norms around youthful drinking (Perry et al., 2002). The Project Northland team has increased their focus on community-level change in a replication of the program that is currently under way in 61 schools and communities in the Chicago area.

A 5-year community alcohol trauma prevention trial, the Community Trials Program, involving a quasi-experimental design with three experimental communities and matched controls in California and in South Carolina, used community mobilization and strategic use of the mass media. It addressed all alcohol use, not only that of underage youth. Two of three communities were composed primarily of ethnic minority residents, which may have implications for implementing prevention efforts in other minority communities. The program had five mutually reinforcing components:

1. Community mobilization addressed support for public policy interventions by increasing general awareness, knowledge, and concern about alcohol-related trauma. Program initiatives were jointly planned by project organizers and local residents and implemented by the residents.

2. The responsible beverage service component sought to reduce sales to intoxicated patrons and increase enforcement of local alcohol laws by

working with restaurants, bar and hotel associations, beverage wholesalers, the Alcohol Beverage Control Commission, and local law enforcement.

3. Another component sought to decrease driving after drinking by increasing the number of DWI (driving while intoxicated) arrests through a combination of special officer training, deployment of passive alcohol sensors, and the use of sobriety checkpoints. News coverage publicized these activities.

4. A component directed toward underage drinking sought to reduce alcohol sales to minors by enforcing underage sales laws; the training of sales clerks, owners, and managers to prevent sales of alcohol to minors; and the strategic use of the news media to bring media attention to the issue of underage drinking.

5. Local zoning and other municipal powers that determine alcohol outlet density were used to reduce availability of alcohol.

This multicomponent approach resulted in a 43 percent decline in alcohol-related assault admissions to hospitals and decreases in heavy drinking. There was strong support for the efficacy of a coordinated, comprehensive community-based intervention to reduce high-risk alcohol consumption and alcohol-related trauma, although frequency of drinking did not change and there was a slight increase in the number of persons who reported any drinking in the intervention communities (Holder et al., 2000).

Intermediate outcomes also indicated success, including decreases in alcohol outlet sales to underage-appearing pseudo-patrons without identification. Local regulations of alcohol outlets and public sites for drinking were changed in all three experimental communities. Changes in the Northern California intervention city were typical. The city council implemented a proposal to eliminate special land use conditions for alcohol outlets, adopted restrictions on the availability of alcohol in city parks, denied a new alcohol license, revoked a retailer's conditional use permit because of liquor sales violations, and instituted a citywide ordinance requiring new owners of offsite and onsite alcohol outlets to complete a responsible server course. In addition, the Hispanic Chamber of Commerce voted to make its annual festival alcohol free.

The DWI reduction component resulted in an increase in news coverage of DWI arrests, additional police enforcement, greater use of breathalyzer equipment, and increased public perceptions of risk of arrest for DWI. Alcohol-related crash involvement as measured by single vehicle night crashes declined 10 to 11 percent more among program than comparison communities.

Communities Mobilizing for Change on Alcohol (CMCA) was a 6-year project designed to test creative approaches to reducing drinking by young people. The project was implemented in seven small to mid-sized communities in Minnesota and Wisconsin in 1993; eight other communities in the region served as a control group. CMCA emphasized environmental factors that affect the supply of alcohol to youth and used a community organization approach to achieve policy changes among local institutions. The community coalitions included a variety of citizens with differing connections to the community and the issue: parents, youth involved in school service activities, and social service workers, as well as law enforcement officers and politicians. Adults and young people in each community identified and promoted a variety of issues designed to change the local environment in ways that made alcohol more difficult to obtain and made underage drinking less acceptable (Wagenaar et al., 1999, 2000a, 2000b).

The specific objectives of the project were to change community policies and procedures to reduce: access to alcohol by underage youth, whether through retail sales to youth or purchase or provision by parents, other adults, or older youth; number and proportion of alcohol outlets selling to underage individuals; youth and adult support for or tolerance of underage purchase and consumption of alcohol; prevalence, quantity, and frequency of alcohol consumption among youths aged 15 to 20; and incidence of alcohol-related health and social problems among youths aged 15 to 20 (Wagenaar and Perry, 1994).

Outcomes included increases in intervention communities of age identification checking by retailers and reduced sales to minors, especially in on-sale establishments. Young people aged 18 to 20 reduced their propensity to provide alcohol to other teens and were less likely to try to buy alcohol, drink in a bar, or consume alcohol. However, there were no effects on drinking by high school seniors (Wagenaar et al., 1999, 2000a).

Additional analyses of arrest and traffic crash data indicated that DUI violations declined in the intervention communities. Again, this effect was most marked for college-age youth and only approached significance for youth aged 15 to 17. There were no differences in arrests for disorderly conduct or traffic crashes for either age group. Collectively, findings from the CMCA project indicate that a community-organization approach to limiting youth access to alcohol can be effective for college-age youth (18- to 20-year-olds) (Wagenaar et al., 1999, 2000a, 2000b).

The Massachusetts Saving Lives Program (Hingson et al., 1996) sought to reduce drunk driving and speeding through community mobilization. Communities introduced media campaigns, drunk driving checkpoints, business information programs, speeding and drunk driving awareness days, speed watch telephone hotlines, police training, high school peer-led education, Students Against Drunk Driving chapters, college prevention programs, alcohol-free prom nights, beer keg registration, and increased liquor outlet surveillance by police to reduce underage alcohol purchase. To increase pedestrian safety and safety belt use, program communities conducted media campaigns and police checkpoints, posted crosswalk signs warning motorists of fines for failure to yield to pedestrians, added crosswalk guards, and offered preschool education programs and training for hospital and prenatal staff. Coordinators engaged in numerous activities designed to help local news outlets move beyond reporting only the specifics of motor vehicle crash injuries and deaths to explaining trends in local traffic safety problems and strategies communities were implementing to reduce traffic injury and death (Hingson et al., 1996).

During the 5 years of the program, the proportion of drivers under age 20 who reported driving after drinking in random-digit dial telephone surveys declined from 19 percent during the final year of the program to 9 percent in subsequent years. The proportion of vehicles observed speeding (through use of radar from unmarked cars) was cut in half, and safety belt use increased from 22 percent to 29 percent. (Differences between intervention and comparison communities were statistically significant.) Alcohol-related traffic deaths declined 42 percent more in the program cities than in cities in the rest of the state during the 5 years of the program, when compared with the previous five years. This decline was also seen among 16- to 25-year-olds, many of whom may have been college students (Hingson et al., 1996).

Ingredients of Success

Assessments of public awareness of problems related to underage drinking, and of existing support for policies and programs to reduce those problems, can provide measures of baseline community knowledge as well as readiness for change. To maximize the effects of limited human and financial capital, previous community-based efforts have emphasized the importance of conducting assessments of community needs and resources to help develop coalition goals and strategies (Mills and Bogenschneider, 2001). This approach was used in the three successful community mobilization projects discussed above.

Support for effective strategies may in fact be higher than is often assumed by organizers at the outset of community mobilization efforts. For instance, research investigating student sentiment toward alcohol policies and laws consistently documents support for policies that control underage drinking (Wechsler et al., 2002). In a 1998 national opinion poll on how to control alcohol-related problems in the United States, the Robert Wood Johnson Foundation reported that 69 percent of young adults said they did not want to see the minimum drinking age lowered from 21 to 19. It appears that the true level of support for alcohol policies that have been shown to be effective (e.g., the minimum drinking age, alcohol excise taxes to pay for programs designed to prevent underage drinking) is significantly underestimated by students, as well as by administrators and other key members of college communities. Most college students support more strict and consistent enforcement of existing policies, as well (DeJong et al., 2001).

A clear mission is critical to the success of community mobilization efforts. Different objectives may lead to different compositions of community coalitions. For instance, successful adoption of server training requires the cooperation and collaboration of local alcoholic beverage retailers. This constituency, however, may oppose keg registration. Having the flexibility to build coalitions or implementation teams on the basis of the goals is important to success. Strategic planning of coalition initiatives may also include establishing measurable objectives, creating target timelines, clearly defining member responsibilities, and developing leadership to maintain coalition efforts and membership involvement.

Qualitative results from an evaluation of the 37 colleges across Ohio involved in the Ohio College Initiative to Reduce High Risk Drinking indicate that strong, well-trained leadership, active involvement of key campus leaders, and committed resources are the components sustaining organized efforts to change attitudes and behaviors. Turnovers in leadership appeared to have a negative affect on sustainability: coalitions were twice as likely to be sustained when there were no leadership turnovers (Peters, 2002), although it is difficult to determine to what extent leadership stability as opposed to other factors contributed to success. Project directors and coalition chairs from participating institutions indicated being a member of the Ohio College Initiative to Reduce High-Risk Drinking was helpful through the initiative's provision of training, technical assistance and a forum for exchange of information. Training (see recommendation five below) in the environmental model was identified as critical to the success of implementation of environmental management strategies. Coalition longevity was also closely associated with the number of designated staff, both full and part time, working on the prevention effort.

Grassroots participation is essential to the success of some community mobilization efforts. It is important for ensuring that local community interests are represented, thereby enhancing the acceptability and feasibility of implementing prevention efforts. Youth development and behavior may be shaped by factors that are unique to a specific environment, including the structure and dynamics of a family, neighborhood, community, and culture (Lerner, 1995). Community participants provide essential knowledge of their environment that can yield the most accurate assessments of the problem and a menu of possible solutions that are sensitive to local conditions (Mills and Bogenschneider, 2001). Such a locally driven process also gives the local participants a vested interest in developing resources to support coalition initiatives, and strengthens their commitment to and support for coalition initiatives.

Finally, the involvement of gatekeepers and key community leaders and institutions is an important aspect of adopting and implementing successful community mobilization strategies. The role of key leaders is to develop support for and cooperation with different institutional components of interventions (e.g., cooperation between law enforcement, educators, city council members, and retailers) on strategies to enforce existing laws regarding eliminating sales to minors. For instance, the involvement of college officials and presidents (see below) is also important in communicating the importance of policy enforcement. Involvement of key community leaders can be an essential ingredient for success, provided that they have access to training and information regarding approaches to reducing underage drinking whose effectiveness has been scientifically demonstrated. Strong key leaders combined with substantial grassroots support can provide the community and social capital necessary to undertake effective interventions.

Collaboration Between Communities and Colleges

Institutions of higher education can play a critical role in community mobilization efforts. Comprehensive college-based approaches to address underage alcohol consumption and high-risk drinking should be predicated on a model of student drinking that incorporates the environment and student campus culture, as well as individual factors (Presley et al., 2002) (see also Chapter 10). Building a coalition between campus and community is a vital component of effective alcohol and other drug prevention efforts of colleges (Wechsler, 1996; Presidents Leadership Group, 1997; DeJong et al., 1998; DeJong and Langford, 2002) and is a promising vehicle for promoting environmental change (DeJong et al., 1998). College campuses and local communities have a reciprocal influence on one another in relation to college student alcohol use. Communities within the immediate proximity of college campuses are more likely to report a lowered quality of neighborhood life due to alcohol related behaviors, including noise, public disturbance, and vandalism (Wechsler et al., 1995). Similarly, effective restrictions on underage access to alcohol in a community may be severely undermined by the ease of alcohol access in the campus living communities. The reverse is also true: even a substantial campus-based alcohol prevention strategy cannot succeed if it is surrounded by a community with easy access to alcohol.

Institutions of higher education influence the local environment, with a potential to offer either a positive or adverse climate regarding underage alcohol consumption. Colleges working with local police can enhance the consistency of enforcement efforts by notifying one another of alcohol-related incidents and by seeking timely and meaningful sanctions. Shared initiatives require few university resources, but they can lead to policy reforms and changes in enforcement that can significantly change the drinking environment.

A campus and community partnership can substantially affect relationships overall, improving the coordination between student affairs offices and local police or other agencies related to student concerns (Gebhardt et al., 2000). Three elements are critical to the development, maintenance, and success of community and university partnerships: (1) the development of consistent support, with associated financial and human resources, (2) the identification of goals and focused planning efforts based on an assessment of local needs and problems and available resources, and (3) the application of assessment and evaluation to measure the effect of partnership activities.

Resource identification and development is often the central challenge of health-based prevention efforts. Needed resources include not only financial support, but also human capital, community capital, in-kind contributions, and partnerships among groups and agencies. Previous college-community coalition initiatives have relied on regionally based assessment, planning, and training in order to effectively address local needs (Gebhardt et al., 2000).

The inclusion of colleges and universities as members of local or state-wide coalitions may offer significant contributions in terms of leadership, organization, and resources. Colleges and universities can assist in the development of financial resources, the locality or state, and they can also be a valuable partner in the pursuit of grant and foundation resources. Institutions of higher education may also provide research and evaluation resources for the assessment of partnership efforts. Program evaluation functions as an important component in monitoring the implementation and impact of coalition efforts. College-community coalitions may also function as the best instrument to support recommendations from the National Institute on Alcohol Abuse and Alcoholism associated with future research, including the implementation of a national surveillance and data system for all U.S. colleges and universities and the evaluation of the effectiveness of joint campus-community coalitions.

New laws and regulations that affect the general community will also affect college student alcohol use, making institutions of higher education natural allies for coalition efforts. The coalition model not only allows colleges and universities in any one region or state the opportunity to pool and share resources, but also provides a venue for campuses to make a clear statement that underage drinking and high-risk alcohol use are not confined to any single campus. Issues associated with alcohol use are shared problems that require a collaborative effort to generate shared solutions. Given the increased media attention often gained by both statewide efforts and college student alcohol consumption, this high visibility can help raise awareness of the issue and mobilize additional support in a community or state for the coalition's initiatives.

To develop financial support, coalition partnerships can cosponsor fundraising events and develop joint grant proposals. The development of partnerships between multiple groups allows for the effective coordination of resources. Such partnerships can provide a sharing of resources, facilities, and personnel. Interagency cooperation also allows for the pooling of resources to provide opportunities for sponsoring joint programs and for technical assistance and training. Community partnerships help to identify and express common goals, resulting in consistent and unified messages within the community.

College students may benefit from communitywide efforts. Several coalition efforts have been designed to address underage alcohol use (Hingson et al., 1996; Hingson and Howland, 2002; Gebhardt et al., 2000; Saltz and Stanghetta, 1997). These community efforts have led to reductions in underage alcohol use and alcohol-related problems. College students are not the primary focus of these coalitions, but are likely to benefit from the broader, communitywide aspects of the program designed to reduce such behaviors as drinking and driving and sales to minors. The Higher Education Center for Alcohol and Other Drug Prevention, a primary national resource center for institutions of higher education funded by the United States Department of Education, recommends a comprehensive approach to prevention that includes strategies designed to change the campus and community environment in which students make decisions about alcohol use (DeJong et al., 1998). The Higher Education Center has reported more than 42 statewide coalition efforts that include institutions of higher education in varying degrees of development and activity.

Ongoing efforts in this arena include the Ohio College Initiative to Reduce Underage Drinking, the Memorandum of Understanding Program recently undertaken by the campuses of California State University, the Committee on Community and University Relations begun in 1990 by the State University of New York at Albany, and the Matter of Degree Program developed by the American Medical Association and the Robert Wood Johnson Foundation. Based in part on the findings of the original Harvard School of Public Health College Alcohol Study (Wechsler et al., 1994), the ultimate goals of this 8-year, $10 million national demonstration project are to reduce heavy episodic drinking rates and to test the public health model on which the program is based, as well as to share the lessons learned with other colleges and universities. The Harvard School of Public Health is conducting an evaluation of the program to identify successful interventions and to track reductions in alcohol consumption. Program interventions include: (1) controlling the proliferation of bars and other alcohol outlets in proximity to campuses; (2) working with neighborhood associations, law enforcement, and landlords to address loud house parties and the disruption they create; (3) eliminating alcohol-industry sponsorship of athletics and other campus social events; (4) limiting tailgate parties to pregame time only, creating alcohol-free tailgate zones, and restricting alcohol sales at concerts and other campus events; and (5) establishing higher standards—including academic achievement, community service, and compliance with campus and community alcohol policies—for fraternities and sororities and linking rush privileges to their adherence.

The early achievements (Weitzman et al., 2003a, 2003b) of some of the campuses involved in the program to date point to the potential of such interventions (Alcohol Policy Solutions, n.d.):

- The University of Nebraska saw a decline in heavy episodic drinking rates from 64 percent in 1997 to 55 percent in 2001, and more students are drinking less when they choose to drink; in 2001, 71 percent said they drank four or fewer drinks per occasion, compared with 53 percent in 1997.
- Lehigh University has reported a dramatic reduction in alcohol-related crimes on campus. Overall, crime is down 51 percent—from 418 reports in 1998-1999, to 204 in 2000-2001. The percentage of Lehigh students negatively affected by high-risk drinking is declining: students reporting that they got into a fight with a student using alcohol dropped 21 percent, and the percentage of students who had study or sleep interrupted dropped 13 percent.
- The University of Colorado and the city of Boulder banned beer sales in the university's football stadium, which has resulted in a 69 percent reduction in fans being kicked out of the stadium and a 75 percent decline in arrests.
- Georgia Institute of Technology and the city of Atlanta supported a successful statewide effort to create a keg registration law, to help reduce underage access to alcohol. The campus has seen a 9 percent reduction in heavy episodic drinking, and 12 percent fewer students report driving after drinking.
- The University of Iowa and Iowa City succeeded in preventing a landmark soda fountain near campus from becoming a liquor store, and the city council enacted an ordinance to improve the enforcement of state laws regarding sales to minors and intoxicated persons. The new law also prohibits some drink specials, such as free alcohol, 2-for-1, and all-you-can-drink specials.

- The University of Wisconsin prohibited alcohol sales in the university's Kohl Center, representing a forfeiture of $500,000 in alcohol revenues every hockey season. The project worked with the Madison Alcohol License Review Committee to allow new liquor licenses in the campus area only if the establishment generates at least 50 percent of its revenue from food, effectively prohibiting large-capacity "drinking barns."
- Florida State University and the city of Tallahassee eliminated alcohol advertising on campus and developed a strategic plan to reduce the effects of high-risk drinking in the community, including suspension of driver's licenses for underage drinking and providing incentives to owners of bars and other alcohol outlets to maintain responsible business practices.
- The University of Delaware and the city of Newark are members of the Mayor's Alcohol Commission, which has developed policy recommendations on the sale and consumption of alcohol in the community, particularly in the areas of law enforcement, land use, and zoning.
- The University of Vermont and the city of Burlington led the effort to develop a responsible alcohol beverage service training for bar owners, managers, and servers, which is now part of the city's alcohol licensing review process.
- Louisiana State University (LSU), the LSU Campus-Community Coalition for Change, and the Baton Rouge Metropolitan Council unanimously agreed to restrict underage house parties, which members expect will reduce high-risk drinking at off-campus rental properties, which essentially operate as uncontrolled "bars" for underage students.

Reviews of campus and community coalition efforts have identified several strategies that contribute success of both on and off campus: (1) control of alcohol availability for underage youth, (2) increase in the level and consistency of policy and law enforcement and the development of new policies, and (3) attention to the irresponsible sale, promotion, and marketing of alcohol.

FUNDING

Just as community mobilization provides an essential context for effective interventions to reduce underage drinking, a strong and ongoing commitment on behalf of public and private funders to provide resources for community mobilization is critical to the success of the overall strategy recommended in this report.

One existing model of federal support is the Drug Free Communities Program, originally authorized by Congress in 1997 and reauthorized in 2001. This national initiative awards a maximum of $100,000 per year in federal funds directly to community anti-drug coalitions in the United States to combat youth substance abuse. After 5 years of the program, annual national competitions have awarded 531 grants to coalitions in 50 states, the District of Columbia, Puerto Rico, and the U.S. Virgin Islands. These coalitions work to reduce substance abuse among youth and strengthen collaboration among organizations and agencies in both the private and public sectors.

The Drug-Free Communities Program (DFC) represents a collaborative effort involving the White House Office of National Drug Control Policy, the Department of Justice's Office of Juvenile Justice and Delinquency Prevention, and the Department of Health and Human Services' Center for Substance Abuse Prevention. An 11-member expert advisory commission appointed by the president provides guidance.

DFC coalitions are required to include members from various sectors of the community working on multiple community prevention strategies. Members include youths, parents, businesses, the media, schools, youth organizations, law enforcement, religious or fraternal organizations, civic groups, health care, state, local or tribal governmental agencies, and other organizations. The DFC program represents a useful model for a national program to reduce underage drinking.

Recommendation 11-2: Public and private funders should support community mobilization to reduce underage drinking. Federal funding for reducing and preventing underage drinking should be available under a national program dedicated to community-level approaches to reducing underage drinking, similar to the Drug Free Communities Act, which supports communities in addressing substance abuse with targeted, evidence-based prevention strategies.

12

Federal and State Governments

The federal and state governments have several roles to play in implementing the proposed strategy. However, as emphasized throughout this report, responsibility for preventing and reducing underage drinking lies with everyone, as a national community. For example, although minimum drinking age laws enacted and enforced by government underpin society's efforts, their effectiveness depends on the active support of parents and other adults, businesses, and many other organizations in every community. In addition to their roles in enacting and enforcing pertinent laws, federal and state governments have many other important opportunities to stimulate and solidify the strategy. They can fund statewide or national media campaigns, provide financial support and other assistance to communities to help them mobilize to reduce underage drinking, set up the necessary apparatus to monitor trends in underage drinking and the effectiveness of efforts to reduce it, and support necessary research. In this chapter we lay out the roles for the federal and state governments in the overall strategy. Two of these roles are to coordinate and monitor the various components, including providing the data and research needed to assess and improve the strategy. The third role is to increase alcohol excise taxes to both reduce consumption and provide funds to support the strategy. There is strong and well-documented evidence of the effects of raising taxes on consumption, particularly among youth.

FEDERAL AND STATE ACTIVITIES

Federal Programs

Multiple federal agencies play a role in preventing underage drinking. According to a recent report by the U.S. General Accounting Office (GAO) (2001) that reviewed federal funding targeted at preventing underage drinking, the U.S. Departments of Justice, Health and Human Services, Transportation, Labor, Defense, Treasury, Agriculture, and Interior, as well as the Executive Office of the White House and the Corporation for National Service funded efforts that include underage alcohol use within broader mandates that target alcohol and other drug use. Of the total amount reported ($1.09 billion), almost all ($1.01 billion) included alcohol as part of a larger undifferentiated category relating to alcohol and other drug use; thus, it was not possible to determine what portion of the funds were targeted specifically to alcohol prevention activities. A relatively small proportion—less than 7 percent of the total amount–in three federal departments both had a specific focus on alcohol and identified youth or youth and the broader community as the specific target population.

Specifically, the Departments of Justice, Health and Human Services (HHS), and Transportation reported a combined $71.1 million focusing on alcohol and youth or alcohol and youth and the broader community. According to the GAO report, within HHS, resources are split between the National Institute on Alcohol Abuse and Alcoholism (NIAAA), the Substance Abuse and Mental Health Services Administration (SAMHSA), and the Centers for Disease Control and Prevention (CDC). The majority of HHS resources that specifically target underage drinking are in NIAAA, (part of the National Institutes of Health) that "conducts and supports biomedical and behavioral research in order to provide science-based approaches to the prevention and treatment of alcohol abuse and alcoholism (General Accounting Office, 2001, p. 11)." The GAO report provides no specific information about how these funds are used to prevent underage drinking; NIAAA staff report that the preponderance of their resources are used for research. Research is primarily investigator-initiated and includes such topics as the effectiveness of various media campaigns; education interventions, and environmental strategies, as well as research on the epidemiology and causes of underage drinking.

NIAAA also has supported two notable efforts to influence local action. The first is a comprehensive effort to review approaches to drinking on college campuses, which resulted in the publication of *A Call to Action: Changing the Culture of Drinking at U.S. Colleges* (NIAAA, 2002) which outlines strategies for addressing drinking on college campuses. NIAAA is currently in the process of conducting regional meetings to disseminate the report's findings nationwide. NIAAA also is one of the leading funders, with SAMHSA and the Robert Wood Johnson Foundation, of Leadership to Keep Children Alcohol Free, a major national effort involving governors' spouses to reduce alcohol use among children aged 9 to 15. SAMHSA staff reported funding a wide variety of interventions including initiatives aimed at education and awareness, supporting community-based initiatives, developing guides and toolkits, and furthering research objectives. Several of these initiatives involve collaboration with other HHS agencies (e.g., NIAAA, CDC).

The largest single targeted program included in the GAO report is in the Department of Justice's Office of Juvenile Justice and Delinquency Prevention (OJJDP). According to the report (U.S. GAO, 2001, p. 12), OJJDP funds "retail compliance initiatives, prevention programs, and fostering a juvenile justice system that, among other things, provides appropriate sanctions, treatment and rehabilitative services based on the needs of the individual juvenile." OJJDP's Enforcing the Underage Drinking Laws Program is "designed to reduce the availability of alcoholic beverages to minors and prevent the consumption of alcoholic beverage by minors." The funds are distributed through block and discretionary grants. A national training and technical assistance center, the Center for Enforcing the Underage Drinking Laws Program is funded through this program.

A relatively small program at the National Highway Traffic Safety Administration (NHTSA) funds interventions that "address the problems of drunk and drugged driving and prevention programs targeting zero tolerance for alcohol and drug use among youth. They administer a formula and incentive grant program, award discretionary grants and contracts and enter into cooperative agreements with other entities (U.S. GAO, 2001, p. 14)." Formula grants to states fund highway safety programs, which may include underage drinking programs.

Several agencies also provide resources to advance efforts to prevent underage drinking. Both NIAAA and SAMHSA have published several technical assistance documents highlighting various aspects of underage drinking and approaches to reducing underage drinking and have multiple mechanisms in place to disseminate this information. OJJDP provides both training and technical assistance through its Center for the Enforcement of Underage Drinking Laws. NHTSA has published several documents aimed at reducing drinking and driving. In addition, the Department of Education, through its Higher Education Center for Alcohol and Other Drug Prevention, provides training and technical assistance related to reducing drinking on college campuses. However, there is no coordinated, central mechanism for disseminating research findings or providing technical assistance to grantees or others interested in developing strategies that target underage drinking.

In sum, numerous federal agencies fund multiple research, intervention, and technical assistance efforts to reduce underage drinking. Although coordination mechanisms are in place for specific initiations, and agency staff report regular staff-level communication, the committee is not aware of any ongoing effort to coordinate all of the various federal efforts either within or across departments. The multitude of agencies and initiatives involved suggests the need for an interagency body to provide national leadership and provide a single federal voice on the issue of underage drinking.

Recommendation 12-1: A federal interagency coordinating committee on prevention of underage drinking should be established, chaired by the secretary of the U.S. Department of Health and Human Services.

Membership on the coordinating committee should include senior officials from each of the agencies included in the GAO report. The coordinating committee also should periodically consult with the range of national nongovernmental organizations—including National Alcohol Beverage Control Association, Mothers Against Drunk Driving, Students Against Destructive Decisions, Distilled Spirits Council of the United States, Century Council, National Beer Wholesalers Association—who sponsor initiatives aimed at preventing underage drinking to facilitate a coordinated, research-based approach by all key players. Once the recommended nonprofit foundation is established, the foundation should also be regularly consulted.

The committee recommends that the secretary of HHS chair the coordinating committee for several reasons. First, HHS plays the federal government's lead role in the prevention of substance abuse. Although other agencies have programs that target underage drinking, their primary missions are not related to substance abuse. The initiatives funded by and evaluated by HHS have the widest scope. HHS also administers the major national surveys that are likely to be used to monitor changes in the prevalence or intensity of youth drinking and has the greatest resources available to fund the research necessary for continued improvement of the strategy. Which HHS agency should have operational responsibility for the coordinating committee should be determined by the secretary.

Recommendation 12-2: A National Training and Research Center on Underage Drinking should be established in the U.S. Department of Health and Human Services. This body would provide technical assistance, training, and evaluation support and would monitor progress in implementing national goals.

To the greatest possible extent, interventions aiming to prevent or reduce underage drinking should be science based. In addition, as discussed in Chapter 11, community efforts are most likely to succeed if they have strong and informed leadership. For this reason, resources are needed for training and leadership development for coalition and task force members as well as key decision makers. The recommended center would complement HHS's existing activities on underage drinking.

This report sets forth a comprehensive set of recommendations for the reduction of underage drinking, and community mobilization will provide the context for many of these interventions. Thus the mission of the new center would include the provision of technical assistance and training in community assessment, leadership development, policy development, community organizing, strategic use of the news media, and community-based evaluation to support the program of action laid out in this committee's recommendations.

Currently the federal government does not report regularly on activities across the various agencies that fund targeted underage drinking activities, and evaluating the effect of those activities, as it does for illegal drugs through an annual report issued by the Office of National Drug Control Policy.

Recommendation 12-3: The secretary of the U.S. Department of Health and Human Services should issue an annual report on underage drinking to Congress summarizing all federal agency activities, progress in reducing underage drinking, and key surveillance data.

At a minimum, this report should include

- amount and sources of funds targeted at underage drinking;
- activities funded;
- results of activities funded;
- data on key indicators of underage drinking to monitor progress in reaching stated objectives (discussed below);
- data on brand preferences and source of alcohol (discussed below);
- data on the extent to which alcohol advertising or entertainment with alcohol content reaches underage populations (discussed below); and
- future planned activities and modifications in strategy.

State Programs

Numerous state-level agencies are also involved in administering programs to reduce underage drinking. The precise role of various agencies and their relative contributions vary from state to state. However, in most states, the health or human service, transportation, and criminal justice departments play some role. Those roles include administration of a variety of federal block grants that target underage drinking. In addition, in states that control the sale and distribution of alcohol, the state alcohol beverage control (ABC) body likely plays an important role.

Currently, each state and Washington, D.C., receives a block grant under OJJDP's Enforcing the Underage Drinking Laws Program for activities related to preventing underage drinking. According to OJJDP staff, these funds are administered by a variety of agencies, including those for health and human services, traffic safety, criminal justice, and law enforcement, ABC agencies and other agencies. Each state also receives block grants that include underage drinking from HHS (substance abuse prevention and treatment) and from the Department of Transportation (highway safety and drunk driving). The diversity of agencies involved in administering the OJJDP block grant illustrates the fact that there is no clear lead agency across the states. In the committee's view, the identity of the lead agency is unimportant as long as there is one within each state.

Recommendation 12-4: Each state should designate a lead agency to coordinate and spearhead its activities and programs to reduce and prevent underage drinking.

Coordinating the efforts of all the participating state agencies is particularly important to local communities that are trying to create strong coalitions. The committee also suggests that states be encouraged to produce annual reports on their activities and progress based on those activities.

SURVEILLANCE AND MONITORING

In order to assess the overall public health effects of the strategy proposed by the committee—to reduce underage drinking and the harms it causes—the strategy must include an adequate surveillance and monitoring system. Such a system can provide a significant portion of the information necessary to make informed policy decisions. In the context of this report, a surveillance system should include information on:

- the onset and prevalence of underage drinking;
- the patterns and consequences of underage drinking;
- the amounts and types of alcohol products consumed by underage populations; and
- the availability of alcohol to underage populations and the exposure of this population to messages regarding alcohol in alcohol advertising and in the entertainment media.

National Indicators

There are three national surveys commonly used to report on the prevalence of underage drinking: the National Survey on Drug Use and Health (NSDUH, formerly the National Household Survey on Drug Abuse, NHSDA), the Youth Risk Behavior Survey (YRBS), and Monitoring the Future (MTF). The NHSDA was an annual household-based survey of individuals 12 and older funded by SAMHSA. YRBS and MTF are school-based surveys. YRBS, conducted in conjunction with the states on a voluntary basis, and funded by CDC, surveys high school students (grades 9-12) on a biannual basis. MTF, a survey of eighth, tenth, and twelfth-graders, has been conducted annually since 1975 by the University of Michigan, funded by the National Institute on Drug Abuse.

Differences in the estimates produced by these various surveys have been publicly acknowledged and widely debated. There has been no consensus, however, on the preferable survey to use or the best set of questions to include. In fact, a recent series of articles (Harrison, 2001; Fendrich and Johnson, 2001; Fowler and Stringfellow, 2001; Cowan, 2001) analyzing differences in the surveys generally concluded that each has merit in its own right and did not recommend one over the other. The articles did report, however, that while the overall trends are generally consistent across the three surveys, the NHSDA tended to provide the lowest estimates and may underestimate youth consumption. One unique aspect of the NHSDA was the inclusion of adults in the sample, which allows comparison of adult and youth consumption patterns. The NSDUH is continuing the format.

Recommendation 12-5: The annual report of the secretary of the U.S. Department of Health and Human Services on underage drinking should include key indicators of underage drinking.

The key indicators should include:

- (average) age of first use;
- prevalence of (current) use among pertinent age groups;
- intensity (frequency and quantity) of drinking among pertinent age groups; and
- harmful consequences of alcohol use among pertinent age groups.

The committee does not believe it matters which data source is used for these indicators, provided it is used consistently over time.

Quantity Consumed and Brand Preferences

As discussed in Chapter 3, none of the major surveys currently include adequate items on the amount (number of drinks) and type of alcohol (beer, wine, liquor) consumed on specific occasions or during specific time periods to allow direct estimates of quantity of underage consumption. Moreover, there are currently no national data on the brands of alcohol consumed by youth. MTF data provides general evidence that youth tend to consume beer more often than other types of alcohol, but the data do not allow more in-depth analysis. For alcohol, MTF does not collect information on the preferred brand. In contrast, MTF asks respondents the brand of cigarette usually smoked which revealed that three cigarette brands account for nearly all teen smoking and that one of those brands alone accounts for the majority of the underage tobacco market (Johnston et al., 1999). While a logical hypothesis is that a small number of brands also account for the underage drinking market, available monitoring systems do not provide the data necessary to make this conclusion.

> **Recommendation 12-6: The Monitoring the Future (MTF) Survey and the National Household Survey on Drug Use and Health (NSDUH) should be revised to elicit more precise information on the quantity of alcohol consumed and to ascertain brand preferences of underage drinkers.**

Although questions could be added to any of the three relevant national surveys, the committee recommends that parallel questions be added to the MTF survey and the NSDUH. The MTF survey already includes a question on type of beverage, and the administrators of the survey have experience developing a similar question related to preferred tobacco brands, so the MTF should be able to serve as a model in developing a consistent approach across the two surveys. Questions should be added to the NSDUH as well as MTF to include underage drinkers not in school and allow comparisons to adults.

Groups that represent alcohol producers consistently emphasize their commitment to reducing underage drinking. This new data would help target industry efforts toward specific producers. The monitoring of specific brands, coupled with information on advertising and marketing by specific producers, would also provide the public and policy makers with information necessary to hold alcohol producers accountable for profits made from persons who are illegally using their product.

Monitoring of Advertising and Entertainment Media

As discussed in Chapter 7, abundant evidence shows that alcohol advertising and other promotional activities now reach large underage audiences, and it is reasonable to expect more aggressive self-regulatory efforts by the alcohol industry to restrain marketing practices that tend to encourage underage drinking, even in the absence of clear evidence that such exposures cause underage drinking. Similarly, Chapter 8 shows that movies, television, video, and musical recordings are awash with images appealing to youth. Although research does not indicate that these media have a causal impact on underage drinking, the entertainment industries also share a social responsibility to refrain from glamorizing alcohol use. The committee believes that standards to minimize underage exposure should be implemented on a voluntary basis, similar to the alcohol industry. However, some independent oversight of these standards is warranted. In both contexts, the committee believes that the most promising strategy is to promote industry accountability by facilitating public awareness of industry practices. Accordingly, the committee recommends that DHHS be authorized and funded to monitor these media practices and report to Congress and the public.

EXCISE TAXES

As discussed in Chapter 1, one approach to reducing underage consumption is to reduce the overall level of alcohol consumption in the society. Although such an approach has its advocates, the committee decided that primary reliance on such a strategy would not be compatible with the congressional mandate to which this report responds. Instead, we took the view that broad interventions (those that would tend to affect overall consumption rather than underage consumption alone) should be included in the strategy only if they could be expected to have a particularly strong effect on the harms associated with underage consumption.

We have concluded that there is one such intervention—increasing alcohol excise taxes. There are three arguments for higher taxes to combat underage drinking. First, underage drinking imposes particularly high average social costs, as discussed below. Second, raising excise tax rates, and hence prices, is a strategy that has strong and well-documented prevention effects on underage drinking. Third, a designated portion of the funds generated by the taxes can be earmarked for preventing and reducing underage drinking.

Around the world, historically and currently, alcoholic beverages have been singled out for special taxes. Indeed, the first inland-revenue measure enacted by the first U.S. Congress was a tax on whiskey. Currently, special excise taxes are imposed on alcoholic beverages by the federal and all state governments. The federal tax rates are at $2.14 per 750 milliliter bottle of 80 proof spirits, $0.33 per six-pack of beer, and $0.21 per bottle of table wine.

By the standards of recent history, current tax rates are low; see Figure 12-1. Congress has not legislated increases in these taxes, so their real costs have been eroded by inflation. Restoring the federal excise tax on beer to its

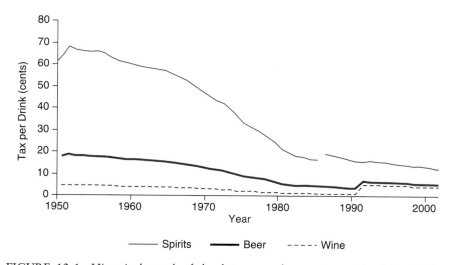

FIGURE 12-1 Historical trends, federal taxes on beer, wine, and spirits 1950-2002, with tax per drink in 2002 dollars.
SOURCE: Adapted from the Bureau of Alcohol, Tobacco, and Firearms web site (2003) and the Bureau of Labor Statistics web site (2003).

value in, say, 1960, would require that it be increased by a factor of three. The same lack of adjustment to inflation has occurred at the state level. One result was a long steep slide in the prices of distilled spirits relative to the price of other goods. Beer prices also declined in inflation-adjusted terms until the early 1980s. Alcohol prices have kept roughly even with overall inflation since then. Overall, alcoholic beverages are far cheaper today than they were in the 1960s and 1970s.

Current excise taxes and prices are low not only by historical standards, but also and more importantly by the standard that prices (inclusive of tax) should reflect the full social cost of production and consumption: if an item is underpriced, then too much will be purchased and consumed. A much-cited study of the costs of heavy drinking by Willard Manning and his associates documented this gap between social cost and price (Manning et al., 1989). They used the economists' normative framework, distinguishing between internal costs (those that are borne by the drinker and therefore presumably taken into account in the drinking decision) and external costs (inflicted by drinkers on bystanders and not therefore taken fully into account in the drinking decision). If the principle of consumer sovereignty is accepted, they argue, then it is only the external costs that are relevant for tax-policy purposes. On the basis of data from the mid-1980s, they found that the external cost per ounce of ethanol consumed was about 48 cents, double the average combined state and federal tax per ounce that was then in place. Much of the external costs of alcohol consumption are borne by victims of intoxicated drivers. A subsequent study amplified this conclusion by noting that Manning and colleagues had failed to account for nonfatal highway injuries (Miller and Blincoe, 1994); including injuries increased the estimate of external costs to 63 cents per ounce.

Such cost-per-drink numbers are averages over all consumption. The social costs for drinks consumed by teenagers are higher than for older drinkers. While there are no estimates for teen drinking that are directly comparable to those cited above, there is a more recent and comprehensive estimate (Pacific Institute for Research and Evaluation, 1999), discussed in Chapter 3. According to that estimate, the total social costs of underage drinking are $53 billion. Given that underage youths account for at least 10.8 percent of total consumption, that works out to $0.91 per ounce of ethanol.[1] One explanation for the high social costs per drink is the abusive style of teen drinking. By one estimate, based on the National Household Survey on Drug Abuse, 91 percent of all drinks consumed by teenagers are consumed by those who drink heavily (Biglan et al., 2003). Furthermore, alcohol abuse amplifies what tend to be high baseline (that is, when sober) rates of risky and harmful activity, including reckless driving, violent crime, and unsafe sex. Of course, as discussed in Chapter 1, these are precisely the arguments that support minimum drinking age laws and accompanying restrictions on youthful access to alcohol: the social costs of drinking by youths are unacceptably high.

Higher taxes would bring alcohol prices closer to the average social costs of consumption by youths (and others) and create an incentive for youths to consume less alcohol. Despite various arguments that alcohol is somehow the exception to the economists' principle of downward-sloping of demand (that is, that for any commodity, the quantity consumed is inversely related to price) the empirical evidence demonstrates that alcoholic beverages are not exceptional in this respect (Chaloupka, 2004; Cook and Moore, 2002). The overall quantities of beer, wine, and distilled spirits that are sold respond to changes in price in the expected way. The extensive published research on youthful drinking is quite consistent in reporting that the prevalence of drinking by underage youths, and the prevalence of heavy

---

[1]This figure is not directly comparable with the cost figures in the preceding paragraph, which are for a different year and which omit costs incurred by the drinker. One reason to include the internal costs is that the principle of consumer sovereignty is less applicable to adolescents than adults—that some degree of adult control is appropriate for those with such limited experience—so that the *internal* damage from youthful drinking should be included in the calculation of social cost.

drinking, are responsive to even small changes in tax rates (Chaloupka, 2004; Cook and Moore, 2002). The evidence also supports a conclusion that an increase in alcohol excise taxes leads to a reduction in alcohol-related harms (Coate and Grossman, 1988; Kenkel, 1998; Saffer and Grossman, 1987; Chesson et al., 1997).

One interesting question is whether youthful drinking is more or less responsive to changes in price than adult drinking. Responsiveness is usually measured by the price elasticity of demand, defined as the percentage reduction in alcohol consumed in response to a 1 percent increase in price. A typical estimate of the overall price elasticity of demand for beer, for example, is –0.3, which is to say that beer purchases decline by about 0.3 percent in response to a 1 percent increase in price. Estimated elasticities for wine and spirits are higher than for beer (Cook and Moore, 2000). In a state in which excise taxes (federal and state combined) constitute 10 percent of the average price of a six-pack, doubling the tax would increase the average price by about 10 percent, which would result in a 3 percent reduction in sales.

There are reasons to believe that underage drinking is more responsive to price changes than adult drinking: youths tend to have less discretionary income, and they are more likely to buy their drinks from package stores rather than at bars and restaurants (where the large mark-up makes the excise tax proportionately less important). Although there are a range of estimates for the price elasticity for youths and adults, there are no studies that provide evidence on the relative elasticities using comparable data and methods. However, on the basis of evidence available for other goods, including tobacco (Chaloupka and Warner, 2001), it seems highly likely that youthful drinking is more responsive to price changes, in a proportional sense, than adult drinking.

There is stronger evidence on the effects of excise taxes (reflecting presumed differences in price) on the *harms* associated with youthful alcohol abuse. An analysis of state-level highway fatality rates during the 1980s (Chaloupka et al., 1993, pp. 161-162) concluded that "significant increases in alcoholic beverage excise taxes are among the most effective policies for reducing drinking and driving in all segments of the population, with the largest reductions occurring among teens and young adults." This result was confirmed by Ruhm (1996)[2] and is in accord with studies of survey

---

[2]Ruhm used annual state-level data for the contiguous 48 states for the period 1982-1988. In Table 4, he reports the results of four different regression specifications. All include fixed effects for the states, and motor vehicle miles driven. The specifications differ with respect to which socioeconomic variables are included, but the estimated coefficients on beer tax are quite consistent. They are –0.3462, –0.4231, –0.4258, and –0.4398. We have used the value –0.40 in our calculations.

data on self-reported drinking and driving (Kenkel, 1993; Chaloupka and Laixuthai, 1997). Other studies have documented the influence of alcohol excise taxes on such predominantly youthful activities as robbery, rape, and the transmission of gonorrhea through unprotected sex (Chaloupka, 2004).

A focus on the beer excise tax is warranted by the fact that beer is the most popular form of alcoholic beverage with underage drinkers by a wide margin. The fact that the federal excise tax on beer is less than half that on distilled spirits (per ounce of ethanol) reflects a traditional belief that more dilute beverages (beer) are less harmful than "hard" liquor. But, the predominant beverage of use and abuse by youths is beer.

Of course the conventional reason to raise tax rates is to increase tax revenues. Alcohol excise taxes contribute $12 billion to the federal and state treasuries, and raising the rates would lead to a near-proportional increase in that revenue, despite the fact that higher tax rates will reduce consumption. The arithmetic here is simple. If, as in the example presented earlier, the combined state and federal beer excise rate is doubled, beer sales would decrease by about 3 percent, and tax revenue would almost double. These calculations depend to some extent on the mark-up applied to tax increases by beer sellers—a large mark-up would result in a somewhat larger reduction in sales and a correspondingly smaller increase in revenue. Under commonsense assumptions about the mark-up (i.e. that the mark-up is about 20 percent), it remains true that a doubling of the tax will result in a near-doubling of revenue.

The committee concludes that state and federal excise taxes are potentially important instruments for preventing underage drinking and its harmful consequences and for generating revenue to fund a broad prevention strategy. We believe the long downward slide in the actual cost of these taxes to consumers has considerably exacerbated the underage drinking problem. Raising these tax rates at both the federal and state level is justified by established principles of public finance, by public health considerations, and by the specific goals of Congress in creating this committee. Of course, the amount of any increase is not a scientific question; rather it is a policy question.

Recommendation 12-7: Congress and state legislatures should raise excise taxes to reduce underage consumption and to raise additional revenues for this purpose. Top priority should be given to raising beer taxes, and excise tax rates for all alcoholic beverages should be indexed to the consumer price index so that they keep pace with inflation without the necessity of further legislative action.

RESEARCH AND EVALUATION

The committee believes that rigorous research and evaluation is necessary to ensure that any national strategy is based on the most effective approaches.

> **Recommendation 12-8: All interventions, including media messages and education programs, whether funded by public or private sources, should be rigorously evaluated, and a portion of all federal grant funds for alcohol-related programs should be designated for evaluation.**

To ensure that activities are adequately evaluated and that interventions are research based, the committee recommends that a specific standard portion, perhaps 15 percent, of grant funds be set aside for independent evaluations. Currently, the proportion set aside for evaluation varies from program to program. There is an obvious tension between the need for resources to fund services and the need for evaluation. Both SAMHSA and the Department of Education have demonstrated a commitment to funding research-based interventions. The committee believes that this interest, and the effectiveness of funded programs, would be enhanced by a standard evaluation expectation across all funded programs. Programs also need to be provided with tools for conducting research and evaluation.

Chapter 6 outlines the need for prototype development for the proposed adult media campaign. This research activity is a core component of the strategy outlined in this report. There are several other approaches discussed throughout this report that may have promise, but where the evidence is insufficient to make definitive recommendations. We therefore recommend several areas for continued research.

Youth Media Messages

As discussed in Chapter 10, careful research should be conducted to identify specific messages to use in a youth-oriented media campaign that would demonstrate the risks of alcohol use, especially of heavy drinking. In the short-term, this should include testing a serious prototype for a youth-focused campaign. For example, the research design might include funding one or more 2- to 4-year campaigns in geographically focused areas, with substantial resources both in message development and transmission and in careful evaluation. The appropriate message focus for such prototype campaigns would need to be researched, developed, and tested before launching the campaigns.

Access

Numerous interventions have been designed to reduce underage access to alcohol. Some have not yet been extensively evaluated and could be further improved by continued research. States and the federal government should study the effect of a range of access-oriented interventions on underage drinking and drinking problems:

- dram shop liability laws;
- shoulder tap and similar programs;
- keg registration laws;
- social host liability laws;
- conditional use permits; and
- sobriety checkpoints.

Youth-Oriented Interventions

Further research and evaluation is necessary to identify successful approaches for reaching populations generally not included in school-based education approaches and refine assessments of interventions on college campuses.

Recommendation 12-9: States and the federal government—particularly the U.S. Department of Health and Human Services and the U.S. Department of Education—should fund the development and evaluation of programs to cover all underage populations.

Such programs should consider a wide range of issues:

- preschool, early elementary, and high school strategies for preventing alcohol use, and, for high school, additional emphasis on programs targeted at individuals with apparent drinking problems;
- characteristics of colleges and universities that may be associated with intervention effectiveness, including the size of student enrollment, type of institution (e.g., 2- or 4-year college, residential or commuter campus, single gender), and urban versus rural setting;
- effectiveness of social norms approaches, parental notification, and other college-based interventions;
- continuing care approaches for treatment;
- interventions implemented within healthcare settings (including campus-based health care) and whether and how training for health professionals can enhance effectiveness of screening and referral for underage populations;
- faith-based approaches to prevention and treatment;

- workplace-based and military-based interventions that target underage populations;
- interventions with youth who are currently drinking; and
- research to further refine understanding of the multiple interrelated factors that affect underage drinking and long-term outcomes.

COSTS AND COST-EFFECTIVENESS OF THE STRATEGY

Some of the committee's recommendations, especially those in Chapters 7 and 8, are addressed to the private sector; they do not entail any public expenditure and, for the most part, require little more than commercial self-restraint. Similarly, some of the recommendations directed to the government in this chapter do not involve significant new expenditures. The data collection and monitoring needed to implement the overall strategy are unlikely to entail substantial new costs, although the proposed data collection efforts may require consideration of the value and opportunity costs of the data proposed in comparison with the data that are currently collected. Similarly, the committee's recommendation (in Chapter 10) that resources for school-based programs be explicitly targeted at programs with elements of proven effectiveness will entail a shift of funding rather than significant new expense. And the committee's recommendations for research are an effort to identify policy-relevant priorities for research funding agencies, both private and public, and do not necessarily involve new funding.

Several components of the proposed strategy will require new investment, at the federal, state, or community levels: the adult-centered media campaign (Chapter 6); improved enforcement of existing laws at the state and local levels (Chapter 9); community mobilization grants (Chapter 11); funding for prevention and treatment of adolescent alcohol use and abuse (above); and resources for HHS to monitor adolescent exposure to alcohol messages in advertising and entertainment media (above). Responsibility for funding the strategy could be shared by the federal and state governments and the industry-funded nonprofit foundation envisioned by the committee (Chapter 7). The necessary government contribution could be offset by revenue generated by increased federal and state alcohol excise taxes (above).

Available data do not allow the committee to make specific estimates of the costs of developing and implementing individual components of the strategy or the strategy as a whole. However, the actual costs of similar programs provide a starting point for gauging the likely cost of some components. For example, the Office of National Drug Control Policy's anti-drug campaign and the American Legacy Foundation's anti-tobacco campaign each cost approximately $100 million per year for production and advertising for a single audience[3] during full implementation. The campaign proposed in this report is likely to be larger and to entail more outreach work than either of these campaigns, but the 3-year developmental phase is likely to be less costly since it will not require national media time.

A possible model for new community mobilization grants that are specific to underage drinking is the Drug-Free Communities Support Program, which provides grants to community coalitions of up to $100,000 per year with a dollar-for-dollar match from nonfederal sources. The number of such grants would depend, of course, on the strength of the proposals as well as the availability of funds. The committee is not aware of a model on which to base an estimate of the cost for HHS to monitor alcohol advertising messages and entertainment media. The Center on Alcohol Marketing and Youth, a private organization, receives foundation funding to conduct similar activities, but its mandate is broader than what the committee has proposed. We do not anticipate that the monitoring will be necessary on an annual basis, however, or that it will continue to be necessary over the long term.

The level of new expenditure required for state and local enforcement activities (e.g., compliance checks) and substance abuse prevention and treatment will vary, depending on how much is currently spent on those activities and how those resources are used. States currently receive block grant funds and some states receive discretionary funds targeted at enforcing the underage drinking laws through the Department of Justice, but there is wide variability in how those funds are used. States also receive block grant funds for substance abuse prevention and treatment through the Department of Health and Human Services, but there is no information on how much of this is spent on youth-specific activities. These block grant funds are often supplemented with other state, local, or private resources. For example, state alcohol beverage control agencies often dedicate resources to such activities as compliance checks to enforce underage drinking laws. It is worth emphasizing, however, that the committee anticipates that much of the effort to promote compliance will be undertaken though education and communication approaches rather than direct enforcement activities.

The lack of precise data with which to determine program costs, to predict the level of effects, or to quantify likely outcomes also preclude a prospective determination of the cost-effectiveness of the proposed strat-

---

[3]The ONDCP campaign included both a parent and a youth component, with about half spent on each: the $100 million figure is an estimate of the single-audience cost since the committee's proposed campaign is for an adult audience only.

egy. Nonetheless, the committee believes that the proposed strategy, if adequately implemented, could reasonably be expected to achieve a significant reduction in underage drinking and the associated social costs. The exact decrease that could be expected is speculative. Available information on the social costs of underage drinking is a starting point for gauging the potential cost-effectiveness of the recommended strategy. If annual social costs attributable to underage drinking (conservatively estimated to be $53 billion per year in 1996; most likely higher now due to inflation) were reduced by only 2 percent after 10 years, or if a 1 percent reduction were sustained for 2 years, an expenditure of approximately $1 billion over that period would be economically justified. If social costs were reduced by 5 or 10 percent after 10 years, the economically justifiable cost would be significantly higher. While the committee believes that the enormous social costs of underage drinking warrant an investment in the proposed strategy, specific efforts to collect cost data and to quantify the proposed outcome measures should be built into strategy implementation in order to obtain more precise measures of cost-effectiveness.

References

Aas, H., and Klepp, K.I. (1992). Adolescents' alcohol use related to perceived norms. *Scandinavian Journal of Psychology, 33*(4), 315-325.

Abbey, A., Ross, L.T., McDuffie, D., and McAuslan, P. (1996). Alcohol and dating risk factors for sexual assault among college women. *Psychology of Women Quarterly, 20*, 147-169.

Ajzen, I. (1991). The theory of planned behavior. *Organizational Behavior and Human Decision Processes, 50*, 179-211.

Alaniz, M.L, and Wilkes, C. (1995). Reinterpreting Latino culture in commodity form: The case of alcohol advertising in the Mexican American community. *Hispanic Journal of Behavioral Sciences, 17*(4), 430-451.

Alcohol Policy Solutions. (2003). *A matter of degree: The national effort to reduce high-risk drinking on college campuses, creating solutions by changing environments.* Available: http://www.alcoholpolicysolutions.net/bi_amod.htm [October, 2003].

Allen, J.P., and Hauser, S.T. (1996). Autonomy and relatedness in adolescent-family interactions as predictors of young adults' states of mind regarding attachment. *Development and Psychopathology, 8*(4), 793-809.

Altman, D.G., Schooler, C., and Basil, M.D. (1991). Alcohol and cigarette advertising on bill boards. *Health Education Research, 6*(4), 487-490.

American Academy of Pediatrics. (1995). Children, adolescents, and advertising. *Pediatrics, 95*, 295-297.

Ames, G.M., Cunradi, C.B., and Moore, R.S. (2002, June). Alcohol, tobacco, and drug use among young adults prior to entering the military. *Prevention Science, 3*(2), 135-144.

Anderson, D.S., and Cohen, A.Y. (2001, June). *A technology-based intervention for preventing college alcohol abuse: Evaluation of the alcohol 101 program.* Fairfax, VA: George Mason University.

Anderson, R.N. (2002, September). Deaths: Leading causes for 2000. *National Vital Statistics Report, 50*(16), 1-85.

Arnett, J., and Balle-Jensen, L. (1993). Cultural bases of risk behavior: Danish adolescents. *Child Development, 64*(6), 1842-1855.

Ary, D.V., Tildesley, E., Hops, H., and Andrews, J. (1993). The influence of parent, sibling, and peer modeling and attitudes on adolescent use of alcohol. *International Journal of the Addictions, 28*(9), 853-880.

Astin, A. (1993). *What matters in college? Four critical years revisited.* San Francisco, CA: Jossey-Bass.

Atkin, C. (1987). Alcoholic-beverage advertising: Its content and impact. In H. Holder (Ed.), *Control issues in alcohol abuse prevention: Strategies for states and communities* (pp. 267-287). Greenwich, CT: JAI Press.

Atkin, C. (1995). Survey and experimental research on effects of advertising. In S.E. Martin (Ed.), *The effects of the mass media on the use and abuse of alcohol* (pp. 39-68). Bethesda, MD: National Institute on Alcohol Abuse and Alcoholism.

Atkin, C. (2004). Media intervention impact: Evidence and promising strategies. In National Research Council and Institute of Medicine, *Reducing underage drinking: A collective responsibility, background papers.* [CD-ROM]. Committee on Developing a Strategy to Reduce and Prevent Underage Drinking, Division of Behavioral and Social Sciences and Education. Washington, DC: The National Academies Press.

Atkin, C.K., and Block, M. (1981). *Content and effects of alcohol advertising* (Report No. PB-82-123141). Washington, DC: Bureau of Tobacco, Alcohol, and Firearms.

Atkin, C.K., Hocking, J., and Block, M. (1984). Teenage drinking: Does advertising make a difference? *Journal of Communication, 28,* 71-80.

Austin, E.W., and Johnson, K.K. (1997a). Effects of general and alcohol-specific media literacy training on children's decision making about alcohol. *Journal of Health Communication, 2*(1), 17-42.

Austin, E.W., and Johnson, K.K. (1997b). Immediate and delayed effects of media literacy training on third graders' decision making for alcohol. *Health Communication, 9*(4), 323-349.

Austin, E.W., and Nach-Ferguson, B. (1995). Sources and influences of young school-age children's general and brand-specific knowledge about alcohol. *Health Communications, 7,* 1-20

Bachman, J.G., and Schulenberg, J. (1993). How part-time work intensity relates to drug use, problem behavior, time use, and satisfaction among high school seniors: Are these consequences or just correlates? *Developmental Psychology, 29,* 220-235.

Bachman, J.G., Wadsworth, K.N., O'Malley, P.M., Johnston, L.D., and Schulenberg, J.E. (1997). *Smoking, drinking, and drug use in young adulthood: The impacts of new freedoms and new responsibilities.* Mahwah, NJ: Lawrence Erlbaum.

Baer, J.S., Stacey, A., and Larimer, M. (1991). Biases in the perception of drinking norms among students. *Journal of Studies on Alcohol, 52,* 580-586.

Baer, J.S., Barr, H.M., Bookstein, F.L., Sampson, P.D., and Streissguth, A.P. (1998). Prenatal alcohol exposure and family history of alcoholism in the etiology of adolescent alcohol problems. *Journal of Studies on Alcohol, 59*(5), 533-543.

Baer, J.S., Kivlahan, D.R., Blume, A.W., McKnight, P., and Marlatt, G.A. (2001). Brief intervention for heavy-drinking college students: 4-year follow-up and natural history. *American Journal of Public Health, 91*(8), 1310-1316.

Ball, J., Barbir, N., Carroll, T., Lum, M. (2002). *Evaluation report for the Launch and Booster Phases of the National Alcohol Campaign.* Prepared for the Department of Health and Ageing by the Research and Marketing Group, Population Health Division, Sydney, Australia.

Balmforth, D. (1999). *National survey of drinking and driving, attitudes and behavior: 1997.* (DOT HS 808 844). Washington, DC: U.S. Department of Transportation, National Highway Traffic Safety Administration.

Bandura, A. (1986). *Social foundations of thought and action: A social cognitive theory.* Englewood Cliffs, NJ: Prentice Hall.

Bandura, A. (1997). *Self-efficacy: The exercise of self-control.* New York: W.H. Freeman.

Barnes, G.M., Farrell, M.P., and Banerjee, S. (1995). Family influences on alcohol abuse and other problem behaviors among black and white Americans. In G.M. Boyd, J. Howard, and R.A. Zucker (Eds.), *Alcohol problems among adolescents.* Hillsdale, NJ: Lawrence Erlbaum.

Barnes, G.M., Reifman, A.S., Farrell, M.P., and Dintcheff, B.A. (2000). The effects of parenting on the development of adolescent alcohol misuse: A six-wave latent growth model. *Journal of Marriage and the Family, 62*(1), 175-186.

Basch, C.E., DeCicco, I.M., and Malfetti, J.L. (1989). A focus group study on decision processes of young drivers: Reasons that may support a decision to drink and drive. *Health Education Quarterly, 16,* 389-396.

Battistich, V., Schaps, E., Watson, M., and Solomon, D. (1996). Prevention effects of the Child Development Project: Early findings from an ongoing multisite demonstration trial. *Journal of Adolescent Research, 11,* 12-35.

Bauman, K.E., Fisher, L.A., and Koch, G.G. (1989). External variables, subjective expected utility, and adolescent behavior with alcohol and cigarettes. *Journal of Applied Social Psychology, 19,* 789-804.

Baumeister, R.F., and Muraven, M. (1996). Identity as adaptation to social, cultural, and historical context. *Journal of Adolescence, 19,* 405-416.

Beck, K.H., and Lockhart, S.J. (1992). A model of parental involvement in adolescent drinking and driving. *Journal of Youth and Adolescence, 21,* 35-51.

Beck, K.H., and Treiman, K.A. (1996). The relationship of social context of drinking, perceived social norms, and parental influence to various drinking patterns of adolescents. *Addictive Behaviors, 21*(5), 633-644.

Beck, K.H., Scaffa, M., Swift, R., and Ko, M. (1995). Survey of parent attitudes and practices regarding underage drinking. *Journal of Youth and Adolescence, 24*(3), 315-334.

Bell, R.M., Ellickson, P.L., and Harrison, E.R. (1993). Do drug prevention effects persist into high school? How Project ALERT did with ninth graders. *Preventive Medicine: An International Journal Devoted to Practice and Theory, 22,* 463-483.

Benthin, A., Slovic, P., and Severson, H. (1993). A psychometric study of adolescent risk perception. *Journal of Adolescence, 16,* 153-168.

Bergmann, P.E., Smith, M.B., and Hoffman, N.G. (1995). Adolescent treatment: Implications for assessment, practice guidelines, and outcome management. *Pediatrics Clinical North America, 42,* 453-472.

Berkowitz, A. (1997). From reactive to proactive prevention: Promoting an ecology of health on campus. In P. Rivers, E. Shore (Eds.), *Substance abuse on campus: A handbook for college and university personnel* (pp. 119-139). Westport, CT: Greenwood Press.

Beyth-Marom, R., Austin, L., Fischhoff, B., and Palmgren, C. (1993). Perceived consequences of risky behaviors: Adults and adolescents. *Developmental Psychology, 29,* 549-563.

Biddle, B.J., Bank, B.J., and Marlin, M.M. (1980). Parental and peer influence on adolescents. *Social Forces, 58,* 1057-1079.

Bierness, D.J., Foss, R.D., Wilson, R.J., and Mercer, G.W. (2000, May). *Roadside breath testing surveys to assess the impact of an enhanced DWI enforcement campaign in British Columbia.* Presented at the International Conference of Alcohol, Drugs and Traffic Safety (ICADTS), Stockholm, Sweden.

Biglan, A., Ary, D.V., Smolkowski, K., Duncan, T., and Black, C. (2000). A randomized controlled trial of a community intervention to prevent adolescent tobacco use. *Tobacco Control, 9,* 24-32.

Biglan, A., Brennan, P.A., Foster, S.L., Holder, H.D., Miller, T.L., Cunningham, P.B. (2003). *Multiproblem youth: Prevention, intervention, and treatment.* New York: Guilford.

Black, D.R., and Coster, D.C. (1996). Interest in a stepped approach model (SAM): Identification of recruitment strategies for university alcohol programs. *Health Education Quarterly, 23*(1), 98-114.

Blanton, H., Gibbons, F.X., Gerrard, M., Conger, K.J., and Smith, G.E. (1997). Role of family and peers in the development of prototypes associated with substance use. *Journal of Family Psychology, 11*(3), 271-288.

Block, L.G., Morwitz, V.G., Putsis, W.P., Jr., and Sen, S.K. (2002). Assessing the impact of antidrug advertising on adolescent drug consumption: Results from a behavioral economic model. *American Journal of Public Health, 92*(8), 1346-1351.

Boase, P., and Tasca, L. (1998). *Graduated licensing system evaluation: Interim report '98.* Toronto: Ministry of Transportation of Ontario.

Bogenschneider, K., Wu, M.-Y., Raffaelli, M., and Tsay, J.C. (1998). "Other teens drink, but not my kid": Does parental awareness of adolescent alcohol use protect adolescents from risky consequences? *Journal of Marriage and the Family, 60*, 356-373.

Bonnie, R. (1977). Decriminalizing the marijuana user: A drafter's guide. *Michigan Journal of Law Reform, 11*, 3-50.

Bonnie, R. (1982). Discouraging the use of alcohol, tobacco and other drugs: The effects of legal controls and restrictions. In N.K. Mello (Ed.), *Advances in substance abuse research, Volume II* (pp. 145-184). Greenwich, CT: JAI Press.

Bonnie, R. (1985). Regulating conditions of alcohol availability: Possible effects on highway safety. *Journal of Studies on Alcohol, 29*(Supp. #10), 129-143.

Bonnie, R. (1986). The efficacy of law as a paternalistic instrument. In G. Melton (Ed.), *Nebraska symposium on motivation, 1985, volume 33: The law as a behavioral instrument* (pp. 131-211). Lincoln, NE: University of Nebraska Press.

Boots, K., and Midford, R. (1999). "Pick-a-Skipper": An evaluation of a designated driver program to prevent alcohol-related injury in a regional Australian city. *Health Promotion International, 14*, 337-345.

Bormann, C.A., and Stone, M.H. (2001). The effects of eliminating alcohol in a college stadium: The Folsom Field beer ban. *Journal of American College Health, 50*(2), 81-88.

Borsari, B., and Carey, K.B. (2000). Effects of a brief motivational intervention with college student drinkers. *Journal of Consulting and Clinical Psychology, 68*, 728-733.

Botvin, G.J., Baker, E., Dusenbury, L., Botvin, E.M. and Diaz, T. (1995). Long-term follow-up results of a randomized drug abuse prevention trial in a white middle-class population. *Journal of the American Medical Association, 273*(14), 1106-1112.

Brannigan, R., Falco, M., Dusenbury, L., and Hansen, W.B. (2004). Teen treatment: Addressing alcohol problems among adolescents. In National Research Council and Institute of Medicine, *Reducing underage drinking: A collective responsibility, background papers.* [CD-ROM]. Committee on Developing a Strategy to Reduce and Prevent Underage Drinking, Division of Behavioral and Social Sciences and Education. Washington, DC: The National Academies Press.

Brody, G.H., and Forehand, R. (1993). Prospective associations among family form, family processes, and adolescents alcohol and drug-use. *Behaviour Research and Therapy, 31*(6), 587-593.

Brooks II, J.H., and DuBois, D.L. (1995). Individual and environmental predictors of adjustment during the first year of college. *Journal of College Student Development, 36*(4), 347-360.

Brown, B.B., Mory, M., and Kinney, D.A. (1994). Casting adolescent crowds in relational perspective: Caricature, channel, and context. In R. Montemayor, G.R. Adams, and T.P. Gullotta (Eds.), *Advances in adolescent development: Vol. 6. Personal relationships during adolescence.* Newbury Park, CA: Sage.

Brown, S.A., and Tapert, S.F. (2004). Health consequences of adolescent alcohol involvement. In National Research Council and Institute of Medicine, *Reducing underage drinking: A collective responsibility, background papers.* [CD-ROM]. Committee on Developing a Strategy to Reduce and Prevent Underage Drinking, Division of Behavioral and
Social Sciences and Education. Washington, DC: The National Academies Press.

Brown, S.A., Tapert, S.F., Granholm, E., and Delis, D.C. (2000). Neurocognitive functioning
of adolescents: Effects of protracted alcohol use. *Alcoholism: Clinical and Experimental
Research, 24*(2), 164-71.

Buka, S.L., and Birdthistle, I.J. (1999). Long-term effects of a community-wide alcohol server
training intervention. *Journal of Studies on Alcohol, 60,* 27-36.

Bureau of Alcohol, Tobacco, and Firearms. (2003). *Historical tax rates—alcoholic beverages.*
Available: http://www.ttb.gov/alcohol/stats/historical.htm [August 5, 2003].

Bureau of Labor Statistics. (2003). *Consumer price index rate for urban consumers since
1913.* Available: http://www.bls.gov/cpi/home.htm#data [August 5, 2003].

Butterfoss, F.D., Goodman, R.M., and Wandersman, A. (1996). Community coalitions for
prevention and health promotion: Factors predicting satisfaction, participation, and planning. *Health Education Quarterly, 23*(1), 65-79.

Caetano, R., and Clark, C.L. (1998). Trends in alcohol consumption patterns among whites,
blacks, and Hispanics: 1984-1995. *Journal of Studies on Alcohol, 59*(6), 659-668.

Calfee, J.E., and Scheraga, C. (1994). The influence of alcohol advertising on alcohol consumption: A literature review and econometric analysis of four European nations. *International Journal of Advertising, 13,* 287-310.

Cameron, L.A. (1999). Understanding alcohol abuse in American Indian/Alaskan Native
youth. *Pediatric Nursing, 25*(3), 297-300.

Cameron, M., and Newstead, S. (1996). Mass media publicity supporting police enforcement
and its economic value. In *Proceedings of the symposium on mass media campaigns in
road safety, Scarborough Beach, Western Australia.* Medlands: Road Accident Prevention Unit, Department of Public Health, University of Western Australia.

Carlson, J.M., Chudley, Werch, C.E., Owen, D.M., Moore, M.J., Kolomeyer, I., Jobli, E.C.,
and Provencher, L. (2001). *Recruitment and retention in a longitudinal study to prevent
binge drinking among residential college students.* Jacksonville: Center for Drug Prevention and Health Promotion, University of North Florida.

Casswell, S., and Gilmore, L. (1989). An evaluated community action project on alcohol.
Journal of Studies on Alcohol, 50(4), 339-346.

Casswell, S., and Zhang, J.F. (1998). Impact of liking for advertising and brand allegiance on
drinking and alcohol-related aggression: A longitudinal study. *Addiction, 93,* 1209-
1217.

Cavanaugh, R.M., and Henneberger, P.K. (1996, February). Talking to teens about family
problems: An opportunity for prevention. *Clinical Pediatrics, 35*(2), 67-71.

Center for Science in the Public Interest. (2002). *Alcohol policies project, alcohol advertising:
Are our kids collateral or intended targets?* Washington, DC: Author.

Center for the Advancement of Public Health. (2001). *Sourcebook 2001. Promising Practices:
Campus Alcohol Strategies.* Fairfax, VA: Author, George Mason University.

Center on Alcohol Marketing and Youth. (2002a). *Overexposed: Youth a target of alcohol
advertising in magazines.* Washington, DC: Author, Georgetown University.

Center on Alcohol Marketing and Youth. (2002b). *Television: Alcohol's vast adland.* Washington, DC: Author, Georgetown University.

Center on Alcohol Marketing and Youth. (2003). *Drops in the bucket: Alcohol industry
"responsibility" advertising on television in 2001.* Washington, DC: Author, Georgetown
University.

Centers for Disease Control and Prevention. (2001). *Injury statistics query and reporting system (WISQARS)*. Atlanta, GA: National Center for Injury Prevention and Control, Centers for Disease Control and Prevention (producer). Available: http://webapp.cdc. gov/sasweb/ncipc/leadcaus10.html [September, 2003].

Century Council. (2001). *Promising practices sourcebook 2001: Campus alcohol strategies*. Washington, DC: Author.

Chaloupka, F.J. (2004). The effects of price on alcohol use, abuse, and their consequences. In National Research Council and Institute of Medicine, *Reducing underage drinking: A collective responsibility, background papers*. [CD-ROM]. Committee on Developing a Strategy to Reduce and Prevent Underage Drinking, Division of Behavioral and Social Sciences and Education. Washington, DC: The National Academies Press.

Chaloupka, F.J., and Laixuthai, A. (1997). Do youths substitute alcohol and marijuana? Some econometric evidence. *Eastern Economic Journal, 23*(3), 253-276.

Chaloupka, F.J., and Warner, K.E. (2001). The economics of smoking. In J.P. Newhouse and A.J. Cuyler (Eds.), *The handbook of health economics* (pp. 1539-1627). New York: North-Holland, Elsevier Science.

Chaloupka, F.J., and Wechsler, H. (1996). Binge drinking in college: The impact of price. *Contemporary Economic Policy, 14*, 112-124.

Chaloupka, F.J., Saffer, H., and Grossman, M. (1993). Alcohol control policies and motor vehicle fatalities. *Journal of Legal Studies, 22*, 161-186.

Chen, M.J., Grube, J.W., and Madden, P.A. (1994). Alcohol expectancies and adolescent drinking: Differential prediction of frequency, quantity, and intoxication. *Addictive Behaviors, 19*(5), 521-529.

Chesson, H.W., Harrison, P., and Kassler, W.J. (1997). Alcohol, youth, and risky sex: The effect of beer taxes, and the drinking age on gonorrhea rates in teenagers and young adults. Working Paper. Atlanta: CDC.

Christensen, P.G., Henriksen, L., and Roberts, D.F. (2000). *Substance use in popular primetime television*. Washington, DC: Office of National Drug Control Policy.

Christiansen, B.A., and Smith, G.T. (1991). Alcoholism and memory: Broadening the scope of alcohol-expectancy research. *Psychology Bulletin, 110*, 137-146.

Christiansen, B.A., Goldman, M.S., and Inn, A. (1982). Development of alcohol-related expectancies in adolescents: Separating pharmacological from social-learning influences. *Journal of Consulting and Clinical Psychology, 50*(3), 336-344.

Christiansen, B.A., Roehling, P., Smith, G., and Goldman, M. (1989). Using alcohol expectancies to predict adolescent drinking behavior after one year. *Journal of Consulting and Clinical Psychology, 57*(1), 93-99.

Chudley E.W., Pappas, D.M., Carlson, J.M., and DiClemente, C.C. (2000). *Longitudinal effects of a tailored alcohol preventive*. Jacksonville: Center for Drug Prevention and Health Promotion, University of North Florida.

Cialdini, R.B., Reno, R.R., and Kallgren, C.A. (1990). A focus theory of normative conduct: Recycling the concept of norms to reduce littering in public places. *Journal of Personality and Social Psychology, 58*, 1015-1026.

Clapp, J.D. (2000). Deconstructing contexts of binge drinking among college students. *The American Journal of Drug and Alcohol Abuse, 26*(1), 139.

Clark, D.B., Kirisci, L., and Moss, H. (1998). Early adolescent gateway drug use in sons of fathers with substance use disorders. *Addictive Behavior, 49*(2), 115-121.

Clark, D.B., Neighbors, B.D., Lesnick, L.A., Lynch, K.G., and Donovan, J.E. (1998). Family functioning and adolescent alcohol use disorders. *Journal of Family Psychology, 12*(1), 81-92.

Cloninger, C.R. (1991). *Personality traits and alcoholic predisposition.* Paper presented at the conference of the National Institute on Drug Abuse, University of California at Los Angeles.

Coate, D., and Grossman, M. (1988). Effects of alcoholic beverage prices and legal drinking ages on youth alcohol use. *Journal of Law and Economics, 31*(1), 145-171.

Cohen, D.A., Mason, K., and Scribner, R.A. (2001). The population consumption model, alcohol control practices, and alcohol-related traffic fatalities. *Preventive Medicine, 34,* 187-197.

Cohen, D.A., Richardson, J., and LaBree, L. (1994). Parenting behaviors and the onset of smoking and alcohol use: A longitudinal study. *Pediatrics, 94*(3), 368-375.

Cohen, F., and Rogers, D. (1997). Effects of alcohol policy change. *Journal of Alcohol Drug Education, 42*(2), 69-82.

Community Anti-Drug Coalitions of America and Center for Science in the Public Interest. (n.d.). *Alcohol advertising: Its impact on communities, and what coalitions can do to lessen that impact.* Alexandria, VA: Community Anti-Drug Coalitions of America.

Connell, J.P., and Halpern-Felsher, B.L. (1997). How neighborhoods affect educational outcomes in middle childhood and adolescence: Conceptual issues and an empirical example. In J. Brooks-Gunn, G. Duncan, and J.L. Aber (Eds.), *Neighborhood poverty volume I: Context and consequences for children* (pp. 174-199). New York: Russell Sage Foundation.

Connell, J.P., Halpern-Felsher, B.L., Clifford, E., Crichlow, W., and Usinger, P. (1995). Hanging in there: Behavioral, psychological, and contextual factors affecting whether African-American adolescents stay in high school. *Journal of Adolescent Research, 10,* 41-63.

Connor, J.P., Young, R.M., Williams, R.J., and Ricciardelli, L.A. (2000). Drinking restraint versus alcohol expectancies: Which is the better indicator of alcohol problems? *Journal of Studies on Alcohol, 61*(2), 352-359.

Cook, P.J. (1981). The effect of liquor taxes on drinking, cirrhosis, and auto fatalities. In M. Moore and D. Gerstein (Eds.), *Alcohol and public policy: Beyond the shadow of prohibition* (pp. 255-285). Washington, DC: National Academy Press.

Cook, P.J. (1991). The social costs of drinking. In *The expert meeting on the negative social consequences of alcohol abuse.* Oslo: Norwegian Ministry of Health and Social Affairs.

Cook, P.J., and Ludwig, J. (2000). *Gun violence: The real costs.* New York: Oxford University Press.

Cook, P.J., and Moore, M.J. (1993a). Economic perspectives on alcohol-related violence. In S.E. Martin (Ed.), *Alcohol-related violence: Interdisciplinary perspectives and research directions* (pp. 193-212). NIH Publication No. 93-3496. Rockville, MD: National Institute on Alcohol Abuse and Alcoholism.

Cook, P.J., and Moore, M.J. (1993b). Drinking and schooling. *Journal of Health Economics, 12,* 411-429.

Cook, P.J., and Moore, M.J. (2000). Alcohol. In A.J. Culyer and J.P. Newhouse (Eds.), *Handbook of health economics* (pp. 1629-1673). New York: Elsevier.

Cook, P.J., and Moore, M.J. (2001). Environment and persistence in youthful drinking patterns. In J. Gruber (Ed.), *Risky behavior among youths: An economic analysis.* Chicago: The University of Chicago Press.

Cook, P.J., and Moore, M.J. (2002). The economics of alcohol abuse and alcohol-control policies. Price levels, including excise taxes, are effective at controlling alcohol consumption: Raising excise taxes would be in the public interest. *Health Affairs, 21*(2), 120-133.

Cook, P.J., and Tauchen, G. (1982). The effect of liquor taxes on heavy drinking. *Bell Journal of Economics, 13*(2), 379-390.

Cook, P.J., and Tauchen, G. (1984). The effect of minimum drinking age legislation on youthful auto fatalities, 1970-77. *Journal of Legal Studies, 13,* 169-190.

Cook, R., and Schlenger, W. (2002). Prevention of substance abuse in the workplace: Review of research on the delivery of services. *Journal of Primary Prevention, 31*(1), 115-142.

Cowan, C.D. (2001). Coverage, sample design, and weighting in three federal surveys. *Journal of Drug Issues, 31*(3), 12-239.

Crews, F.T., Braun, C.J., Hoplight, B., Switzer III, R.C., and Knapp, D.J. (2000). Binge ethanol consumption causes differential brain damage in young adolescent rats compared with adult rats. *Alcoholism, Clinical and Experimental Research, 24*(11), 1712-1723.

Csikszentmihalyi, M., and Larson, R. (1984). *Being adolescent.* New York: Basic Books.

Curry, C., Trew, K., Turner, I., and Hunter, J. (1994). The effect of life domains on girls' possible selves. *Adolescence, 29*(113), 133-150.

Dalton, M.A., Sargent, J.D., Beach, M.L., Titus-Ernstoff, L., Gibson, J.J., Ahrens, M.B., Tickle, J.J., and Heatherton, T.F. (2003). Effect of viewing smoking in movies on adolescent smoking initiation: A cohort study. *The Lancet, 362*, July 26.

Darkes, J., and Goldman, M.S. (1998). Expectancy challenge and drinking reduction: Process and structure in the alcohol expectancy network. *Experimental and Clinical Psychopharmacology, 6*(1), 64-76.

Dean, J. (1982). Approaches to alcohol abuse prevention. In J. Dean and W. Bryan (Eds.), *Alcohol programming for higher education* (pp. 82-84). Carbondale, IL: ACPA Media Southern Illinois University Press.

De Bellis, M.D., Clark, D.B., Beers, S.R., Soloff, P.H., Boring, A.M., Hall, J., Kersh, A., and Keshavan, M.S. (2000). Hippocampal volume in adolescent-onset alcohol use disorders. *American Journal of Psychiatry, 157*(17), 737-744.

DeJong, W., and Hingson, R. (1998). Strategies to reduce driving under the influence of alcohol. *Annual Reviews Public Health, 19*, 359-378.

DeJong, W., and Langford, L.M. (2002). A typology for campus-based alcohol prevention: Moving toward environmental management strategies. *Journal of Studies on Alcohol, 14*, 140-147.

DeJong, W., Langford, L.M., and Pryor, J.H. (2001). College students' support for tougher alcohol policies: A silent majority. *Alcohol, Tobacco, and Other Drugs Spring, 16*(2), 9-12.

DeJong, W., and Linkenbach J. (1999). Telling it like it is: Using social norms marketing campaigns to reduce student drinking. *American Association for Higher Education Bulletin, 32*(4), 11-16.

DeJong, W., Vince-Whitman, C., Colthurst, T., Cretella, M., Gilbreath, M., Rosati, M., and Zweig, K. (1998). *Environmental management: A comprehensive strategy for reducing alcohol and other drug use on college campuses* (HEC 113). Newton, MA: Higher Education Center for Alcohol and Other Drug Prevention.

D'Emidio-Caston, M., and Brown, J.H. (1998). The other side of the story: Student narratives on the California Drug, Alcohol, and Tobacco Education Programs. *Evaluation Review, 22*, 95-117.

DiClemente, R.J., Wingood, G.M., Crosby, R., Sionean, C., Cobb, B.K., Harrington, K., Davies, S., Hook III, E.W., and Oh, M.K. (2001). Parental monitoring: Association with adolescents' risk behaviors. *Pediatrics, 107*(6), 1363-1368.

Dishion, T.J., and Andrews, D.W. (1995). Preventing escalation in problem behaviors with high-risk young adolescents: Immediate and 1-year outcomes. *Journal of Consulting and Clinical Psychology, 63*, 538-548.

Dishion, T.J., Kavanagh, K., Schneiger, A., Nelson, S., and Kaufman, N.K. (2002). Preventing early adolescent substance use: A family-centered strategy for the public middle school. *Prevention Science, 3*(3), 191-201.

Donaldson, S.I., Graham, J.W., and Hansen, W.B. (1994). Testing the generalizability of intervening mechanism theories: Understanding the effects of adolescent drug use prevention interventions. *Journal of Behavioral Medicine, 17*(2), 195-216.

Donaldson, S.I., Graham, J.W., Piccinin, A.M., and Hansen, W.B. (1995). Resistance-skills training and onset of alcohol use: Evidence for beneficial and potentially harmful effects in public schools and in private Catholic schools. *Health Psychology, 14*(4), 291-300.

Donohew, R.L., Hoyle, R.H., Clayton, R.R., Skinner, W.F., Colon, S.E., and Rice, R.E. (1999). Sensation seeking and drug use by adolescents and their friends: Models for marijuana and alcohol. *Journal of Studies on Alcohol, 60*(5), 622-631.

Dresser, J., and Gliksman, L. (1998). Comparing statewide alcohol server training systems. *Pharmacology, Biochemistry, and Behavior, 61,* 150.

Dunn, M.E., and Goldman, M.S. (1996). Empirical modeling of an alcohol expectancy memory network in elementary school children as a function of grade. *Experimental and Clinical Psychopharmacology, 4*(2), 209-217.

DuRant, R.H., Rome, E.S., Rich, M., Allred, E., Emans, S.J., and Woods, E.R. (1997). Tobacco and alcohol use behaviors portrayed in music videos: A content analysis. *American Journal of Public Health, 87,* 1131-1135.

Durkin, K.F., Wolfe, T.W., and Phillips III, D.W. (1996). College students' use of fraudulent identification to obtain alcohol: An exploratory analysis. *Journal of Alcohol and Drug Education, 41,* 92-104.

Dusenbury, L. (2000). Family-based drug abuse prevention programs: A review. *Journal of Primary Prevention, 20,* 337-352.

Dusenbury, L., Brannigan, R., Falco, M., and Hansen, W.B. (2003). A review of research on fidelity of implementation: Implications for drug abuse prevention in school settings. *Health Education Research, 18,* 237-256.

Eccles, J.S., and Barber, B.L. (1999). Student council, volunteering, basketball, or marching band: What kind of extracurricular involvement matters? *Journal of Youth and Adolescence, 6*(3), 281-294.

Eggert, L.L., Thompson, E.A., Herting, J.R., and Nicholas, L.J. (1994). A prevention research program: Reconnecting at-risk youth. *Issues in Mental Health Nursing, 15,* 107-135.

Eigen, L. (1991). *Alcohol practices, policies, and potentials of American colleges and universities.* An OSAP White Paper. Rockville, MD: Office for Substance Abuse Prevention.

Elder, R.W., and Shults, R.A. (2002, December). Involvement by young drivers in fatal alcohol-related motor-vehicle crashes—United States, 1982-2001. *Morbidity and Mortality Weekly Report, 51*(48), 1089-1091.

Ellickson, P.L., Bell, R.M., and Harrison, E.R. (1993). Changing adolescent propensities to use drugs: Results from Project ALERT. *Health Education Quarterly, 20,* 227-242.

Elster, A.B., and Kuznets, N.J. (1994). *American Medical Association guidelines for adolescent preventive services.* Baltimore: Williams and Wilkins.

Engelberts, A.C., De Jonge, G.A., and Kostense, P.J. (1991). An analysis of trends in the incidence of sudden infant death in the Netherlands 1969 to 1989. *Journal of Pediatrics and Child Health, 27*(6), 329-333.

Ennett, S.T., and Bauman, K.E. (1991). Mediators in the relationship between parental and peer characteristics and beer drinking by early adolescents. *Journal of Applied Social Psychology, 21*(20), 1699-1711.

Entertainment Software Review Board. (2003). *ESRB game ratings, game rating and descriptor guide.* Available: http://www.esrb.com/esrbratings_guide.asp [August, 2003].

Everett, S.A., Schnuth, R.L., and Tribble, J.L. (1998). Tobacco and alcohol use in top-grossing American films. *Journal of Community Health, 23,* 317-324.

Fagan, J., and Zimring, F. (Eds.). (2000). *The changing borders of juvenile justice: Transfer of adolescents to the criminal court.* Chicago: John D. and Catherine T. Macarthur Foundation Series on Mental Health and Development, University of Chicago Press.

Fawcett, S.B., Lewis, R.K., Paine-Andrews, A., Francisco, V.T., Richter, K.P., Williams, E.L., and Copple, B. (1997). Evaluating community coalitions for prevention of substance abuse: The case of Project Freedom. *Health Education and Behavior, 24,* 812-828.

Feldman, S.S., and Rosenthal, D.A. (1990). The acculturation of autonomy expectations in Chinese high schoolers residing in two Western nations: Effects of length of residence. *International Journal of Psychology, 25,* 259-281.

Fendrich, M., and Johnson, T.P. (2001). Examining prevalence differences in three national surveys of youth: Impact of consent procedures, mode, and editing rules. *Journal of Drug Issues, 31*(3), 615-642.

Ferguson, S.A., Fields, M., and Voas, R.B. (2000, May). *Enforcement of zero tolerance laws in the United States.* Paper presented at the 15th International Conference on Alcohol, Drugs, and Traffic Safety, Stockholm, Sweden.

Finken, L.L., Jacobs, J.E., and Laguna, K. (1998). The role of age, experience, and situational factors in the drinking and driving decisions of college students. *Journal of Youth and Adolescence, 27,* 493-511.

Fischhoff, B., Parker, A.M., de Bruin, W., Downs, J., Palmgren, C., Dawes, R., and Manski, C. (2000). Teen expectations for significant life events. *Public Opinion Quarterly, 64,* 189-205.

Fletcher, A.C., Darling, N.E., Steinberg, L., and Dornbusch, S. (1995). The company they keep: Relation of adolescents' adjustment and behavior to their friends' perceptions of authoritative parenting in the social network. *Developmental Psychology, 31,* 300-310.

Fletcher, L.A., Toomey, T.L., Wagenaar, A.C., Short, B., and Willenbring, M.L. (2000). Alcohol home delivery services: A source of alcohol for underage drinkers. *Journal of Studies on Alcohol, 61,* 81-84.

Flewelling, R.L., Paschall, M.J., and Ringwalt, C. (2004). The epidemiology of underage drinking in the United States: An overview. In National Research Council and Institute of Medicine, *Reducing underage drinking: A collective responsibility, background papers.* [CD-ROM]. Committee on Developing a Strategy to Reduce and Prevent Underage Drinking, Division of Behavioral and Social Sciences and Education. Washington, DC: The National Academies Press.

Flores-Ortiz, Y.G. (1994). The role of cultural and gender values in alcohol use patterns among Chicana/Latina high school and university students: Implications for AIDS prevention. *International Journal of the Addictions, 29*(9), 1149-1171.

Flynn, B.S., Worden, J.K., Secker-Walker, R.H., Pirie, P.L., Badger, G.J., Carpenter, J.H., and Geller, B.M. (1994). Mass media and school interventions for cigarette smoking prevention: Effects two years after completion. *American Journal of Public Health, 84*(7), 1148-1150.

Ford, C.A., Millstein, S.G., Halpern-Felsher, B.L., and Irwin, C.E., Jr. (1997). Influence of physician confidentiality assurances on adolescents' willingness to disclose information and seek future health care: A randomized controlled trial. *Journal of the American Medical Association, 278,* 1029-1034.

Forster, J.L., McGovern, P.G., Wagenaar, A.C., Wolfson, M., Perry, C.L., and Anstine, P.S. (1994). The ability of young people to purchase alcohol without age identification in northeastern Minnesota, USA. *Addiction, 89,* 699-705.

Forster, J.L., Murray, D.M., Wolfson, M., and Wagenaar, A.C. (1995). Commercial availability of alcohol to young people: Results of alcohol purchase attempts. *Preventive Medicine, 24,* 342-347.

Foster, S.E., Vaughan, R.D., Foster, W.H., and Califano, J.A. (2003). Alcohol consumption and expenditures for underage drinking and adult excessive drinking. *Journal of the American Medical Association, 26*(8), 989-995.

Fowler, F.J., Jr., and Stringfellow, V.L. (2001). Learning from experience: Estimating teen use of alcohol, cigarettes, and marijuana from three survey protocols. *Journal of Drug Issues, 31*, 643-664.

Garfield, C.F., Chung, P.J., and Rathouz, P.J. (2003). Alcohol advertising in magazines and adolescent readership. *Journal of the American Medical Association, 289*(18), 2424-2429.

Gebhardt, T., Kaphingst, K., and DeJong, W. (2000). A campus-community coalition to control alcohol-related problems off campus: An environmental management case study. *Journal of American College Health, 48*(5), 211-215.

Giancola, P.R., and Mezzich, A.C. (2000). Neuropsychological deficits in female adolescents with a substance use disorder: Better accounted for by conduct disorder? *Journal of Studies on Alcohol, 61*(6), 809-817.

Gliksman, L., McKenzie, D., Single, E., Douglas, R., Brunet, S., and Moffatt, K. (1993). Role of alcohol providers in prevention: An evaluation of a server intervention programme. *Addiction, 88*, 1195-1203.

Goldberg, J.H., Halpern-Felsher, B.L., and Millstein, S.G. (2002). Beyond invulnerability: The importance of benefits in adolescents' decision to drink alcohol. *Health Psychology, 21*, 477-484.

Goldman, M.S., Brown, S.A., Christiansen, B.A., and Smith, G.T. (1991). Alcoholism and memory: Broadening the scope of alcohol-expectancy research. *Psychological Bulletin, 110*, 137-146.

Gorman, D.M., and Speer, P.W. (1997). Concentration of liquor outlets in an economically disadvantaged city in the Northeastern United States. *Substance Use and Misuse, 32*(14), 2033-2046.

Gottfredson, D.C., and Wilson, D.B. (2003). Characteristics of effective school-based substance abuse prevention. *Prevention Science, 4*(1), 23-38.

Grant, B.F., and Dawson, D.F. (1997). Age of onset of alcohol use and its association with DSM IV alcohol abuse and dependence: Results from the national longitudinal alcohol epidemiologic survey. *Journal of Substance Abuse, 9*, 103-110.

Greenberger, E., and Steinberg, L. (1986). *When teenagers work: The psychological and social costs of adolescent employment.* New York: Basic Books.

Grube, J.W. (1995). Television alcohol portrayals, alcohol advertising, and alcohol expectancies among children and adolescents. In S.E. Martin (Ed.), *The effects of mass media on use and abuse of alcohol.* Bethesda, MD: National Institute on Alcohol Abuse and Alcoholism.

Grube, J.W. (1997). Preventing sales of alcohol to minors: Results from a community trial. *Addiction, 92*(Suppl. 2), S251-S260.

Grube, J.W. (2001). *Comparison of drinking rates and problems: European countries and the United States.* Calverton, MD: Pacific Institute for Research and Evaluation, Office of Juvenile Justice Enforcing the Underage Drinking Laws Program.

Grube, J.W. (2004). Alcohol in the media: Drinking portrayals, alcohol advertising, and alcohol consumption among youth. In National Research Council and Institute of Medicine, *Reducing underage drinking: A collective responsibility, background papers.* [CD-ROM]. Committee on Developing a Strategy to Reduce and Prevent Underage Drinking, Division of Behavioral and Social Sciences and Education. Washington, DC: The National Academies Press.

Grube, J.W., and Nygaard, P. (2001). Adolescent drinking and alcohol policy. *Contemporary Drug Problems, 28*, 87-131.

Grube, J.W., Chen, M., Madden, P., and Morgan, M. (1995). Predicting adolescent drinking from alcohol expectancy values: A comparison of additive, interactive, and nonlinear models. *Journal of Applied Social Psychology, 25*(10), 839-857.

Grube, J.W., and Wallack, L. (1994). Television beer advertising and drinking knowledge, beliefs, and intentions among schoolchildren. *American Journal of Public Health, 84*, 254-259.

Gruber, E., DiClemente, R.J., Anderson, M.M., and Lodico, M. (1996). Early drinking onset and its association with alcohol use and problem behavior in late adolescence. *Preventive Medicine, 25*, 293-300.

Grunbaum, J.A., Kann, L., Kinchen, S.A., Williams, B., Ross, J.G., Lowry, R., and Kolbe, L. (2002, June). Youth risk behavior surveillance, United States, 2001. *Morbidity and Mortality Weekly Report, 51*(SS04), 1-64.

Hackbarth, D.P., Schnopp-Wyatt, D., Katz, D., Williams, J., Silvestri, B., and Pfleger, M. (2001). Collaborative research and action to control the geographic placement of outdoor advertising of alcohol and tobacco products in Chicago. *Public Health Reports, 116*(6), 558-567.

Hafemeister, T.L., and Jackson, S.L. (2004). Effectiveness of sanctions and law enforcement practices targeted at underage drinking not involving operation of a motor vehicle. In National Research Council and Institute of Medicine, *Reducing underage drinking: A collective responsibility, background papers*. [CD-ROM]. Committee on Developing a Strategy to Reduce and Prevent Underage Drinking, Division of Behavioral and Social Sciences and Education. Washington, DC: The National Academies Press.

Haines, M., and Spear, S. (1996). Changing the perception of the norm: A strategy to decrease binge drinking among college students. *Journal of American College Health, 45*, 134-140.

Hallfors, D., Cho, H., Livert, D., and Kadushin, C. (2002). Fighting back against substance abuse: Are community coalitions winning? *American Journal of Preventive Medicine, 23*(4), 237-245.

Halpern-Felsher, B.L., and Cauffman, E. (2001). Costs and benefits of a decision: Decision making competence in adolescents and adults. *Journal of Applied Developmental Psychology, 22*, 257-273.

Halpern-Felsher, B.L., Connell, J.P., Spencer, M.B., Aber, J.L., Duncan, G.P., Clifford, E., Crichlow, W.E., Usinger, P.A., Cole, S.P., Allen, L., and Seidman, E. (1997). Neighborhood and family factors predicting educational risk and attainment in African American and white children and adolescents. In J. Brooks-Gunn, G. Duncan, and J.L. Aber (Eds.), *Neighborhood poverty volume I: Context and consequences for children* (pp. 146-173). New York: Russell Sage Foundation.

Halpern-Felsher, B.L., Ozer, E.M., Millstein, S.G., Wibbelsman, C.J., Fuster, C.D., Elster, A.B., and Irwin, C.E. (2000). Preventive services in a health maintenance organization: How well do pediatricians screen and educate adolescent patients? *Archives of Pediatrics and Adolescent Medicine, 154*, 173-179.

Hansen, W., and Dusenbury, L. (2004). Alcohol use and misuse prevention strategies with minors. In National Research Council and Institute of Medicine, *Reducing underage drinking: A collective responsibility, background papers*. [CD-ROM]. Committee on Developing a Strategy to Reduce and Prevent Underage Drinking, Division of Behavioral and Social Sciences and Education. Washington, DC: The National Academies Press.

Hansen, W., and Graham, J.W. (1991). Preventing alcohol, marijuana, and cigarette use among adolescents: Peer resistance training versus establishing conservative norms. *Preventive Medicine, 20*, 414-430.

Hanson, D.J. (1990). The drinking age should be lowered. In R.C. Engs (Ed.), *Controversies in the addictions field: Volume 1* (pp. 85-95). Baltimore, MD: American Council on Alcoholism.

Hardesty, P.H., and Kirby, K.M. (1995). Relation between family religiousness and drug use within adolescent peer groups. *Journal of Social Behavior and Personality, 10*(2), 421-430.

Harford, T.C. (1984). Situational factors in drinking: A developmental perspective on drinking contexts. In P.M. Miller and T.D. Nirenburg (Eds.), *Prevention of alcohol abuse* (pp. 119-156). New York: Plenum Press.

Harford, T.C., Wechsler, H., and Muthen, B.O. (2002). The impact of current residence and high school drinking on alcohol problems among college students. *Journal of Studies on Alcohol, 63*(3), 271-279.

Harrington, N.T., and Leitenberg, H. (1994). Relationship between alcohol consumption and victim behaviors immediately preceding sexual aggression by an acquaintance. *Violence and Victims, 9*(4), 315-324.

Harrison, L.D. (2001). Understanding the differences in youth drug prevalence rates produced by the MTF, NHSDA, and YRBS studies. *Journal of Drug Issues, 31*(3), 665-694.

Harrison, P.A., Fulkerson, J.A., and Park, E. (2000). Relative importance of social versus commercial sources in youth access to tobacco, alcohol, and other drugs. *Preventive Medicine, 31*, 39-48.

Harter, S., Marold, D.B., Whitesell, N.R., and Cobbs, G. (1996). A model of the effects of perceived parent and peer support on adolescent false self behavior. *Child Development, 67*, 360-374.

Harwood, H.J., Fountain, D., and Livermore, G. (1998). *The economic cost of alcohol and drug abuse in the United States, 1992*. Rockville, MD: National Institute on Drug Abuse and National Institute on Alcohol Abuse and Alcoholism.

Hawkins, J.D., Catalano, R.F., Kosterman, R., Abbott, R., and Hill, K.G. (1999). Preventing adolescent health-risk behaviors by strengthening protection during childhood. *Archives of Pediatric Adolescent Medicine, 153*, 226-234.

Hawkins, J.D., Catalano, R.F., and Miller, J.Y. (1992). Risk and protective factors for alcohol and other drug problems in adolescence and early adulthood: Implications for substance-abuse prevention. *Psychological Bulletin, 112*(1), 64-105.

Hawthorne, G., Garrard, J., and Dunt, D.R. (1995). The Trojan Horse: Life education's drug education program, does it have public health benefit. *Addiction, 90*(2), 205-215.

Hays, R.D., and Ellickson, P.L. (1996). What is adolescent alcohol misuse in the United States according to the experts? *Alcohol and Alcoholism, 31*(3), 297-303.

Herd, D. (1993). Contesting culture: Alcohol-related identity movements in contemporary African-American communities. *Contemporary Drug Problems, 20*, 739-758.

Herd, D. (2003). Changes in the prevalence of alcohol use in rap song lyrics, 1979-1997. Unpublished.

Hibell, B., Andersson, B., Ahlström, S., Balakireva, O., Bjarnason, T., Kokkevi, A., and Morgan, M. (2000). *The 1999 ESPAD report: Alcohol and other drug use among students in 30 European countries*. Stockholm: Swedish Council for Information on Alcohol and Other Drugs.

Higher Education Center. (1998). *Planning campus events* (HEC 712). Newton, MA: The Higher Education Center for Alcohol and Other Drug Prevention.

Hingson, R.W., Heeren, T., and Winter, M. (1994). Effects of lower legal blood alcohol limits for young and adult drivers. *Alcohol, Drugs and Driving, 10*, 243-252.

Hingson, R.W., Heeren, T., Zakocs, R.C., Kopstein, A., and Wechsler, H. (2002). Magnitude of alcohol-related mortality and morbidity among U.S. college students ages 18-24. *Journal of Studies on Alcohol, 63*(2), 136-144.

Hingson, R.W., and Howland, J. (2002). Comprehensive community interventions to promote health: Implications for college-age drinking problems. *Journal of Studies on Alcohol, Suppl. 14*, 226-240.

Hingson, R.W., Howland, J., and Levenson, S. (1988a). Effects of legislative reform to reduce drunken driving and alcohol-related traffic fatalities. *Public Health Reports, 103*(6), 659-667.

Hingson, R.W., Howland, J., Morelock, S., and Heeren, T. (1988b). Legal interventions to reduce drunken driving and related fatalities among youthful drivers. *Alcohol, Drugs and Driving, 4,* 87-98.

Hingson, R.W., and Kenkel, D. (2004). Social, health, and economic consequences of underage drinking. In National Research Council and Institute of Medicine, *Reducing underage drinking: A collective responsibility, background papers.* [CD-ROM]. Committee on Developing a Strategy to Reduce and Prevent Underage Drinking, Division of Behavioral and Social Sciences and Education. Washington, DC: The National Academies Press.

Hingson, R.W., McGovern, T., Howland, J. Heeren, T., Winter, M., and Zakocs, R. (1996). Reducing alcohol-impaired driving in Massachusetts: The Saving Lives Program. *American Journal of Public Health, 86*(6), 791-797.

Holder, H.D. (1994). Alcohol availability and accessibility as part of the puzzle: Thoughts on alcohol problems and young people. In R. Zucker, G. Boyd, and J. Howard (Eds.), *The development of alcohol problems: Exploring the biopsychosocial matrix of risk* (pp. 249-254). (NIAAA Research Monograph #26). Rockville, MD: National Institute on Alcohol Abuse and Alcoholism.

Holder, H.D. (2004). Supply side approaches to reducing underage drinking: An assessment of the scientific evidence. In National Research Council and Institute of Medicine, *Reducing underage drinking: A collective responsibility, background papers.* [CD-ROM]. Committee on Developing a Strategy to Reduce and Prevent Underage Drinking, Division of Behavioral and Social Sciences and Education. Washington, DC: The National Academies Press.

Holder, H.D., Gruenewald, P.J., Ponicki, W.R., Grube, J.W., Saltz, R.F., Voas, R.B., Reynolds, R., Davis, J., Sanchez, L., Gaumont, G., Roeper, P., and Treno, A.J. (2000). Effect of community-based interventions on high-risk drinking and alcohol-related injuries. *Journal of the American Medical Association, 284*(18), 2341-2347.

Holder, H.D., Janes, K., Mosher, J., Saltz, R.F., Spurr, S., and Wagenaar, A.C. (1993). Alcoholic beverage server liability and the reduction of alcohol-involved problems. *Journal of Studies on Alcohol, 54,* 23-36.

Holder, H.D., Saltz, R.F., Grube, J.W., Treno, A.J., Reynolds, R.I., Voas, R.B., and Gruenewald, P.J. (1997a). Summing up: Lessons from a comprehensive community prevention trial to reduce alcohol-involved trauma. *Addiction, 92*(Suppl. 2), S293-S301.

Holder, H.D., Saltz, R.F., Grube, J.W., Voas, R.B., Gruenewald, P.J., and Treno, A.J. (1997b). A community prevention trial to reduce alcohol-involved accidental injury and death: Overview. *Addiction, 92*(Suppl. 2), S155-S172.

Holder, H.D., and Treno, A.J. (1997). Media advocacy in community prevention: News as a means to enhance policy change. *Addiction, 92*(Suppl. 2), S189-S199.

Holder, H.D., and Wagenaar, A.C. (1994). Mandated server training and reduced alcohol-involved traffic crashes: A time series analysis of the Oregon experience. *Accident Analysis and Prevention, 26,* 89-97.

Hornik, R., Maklan, D., Cadell, D., Prado, A., Barmada, C., Jacobsohn, L., Orwin, R., Sridharan, S., Zador, P., Southwell, B., Zanutto, E., Baskin, R., Chu, A., Morin, C., Taylor, K., and Steele, D. (2002, May). *Evaluation of the National Youth Anti-Drug Media Campaign: Fourth semi-annual report of findings: Executive summary.* Bethesda, MD: National Institutes of Health, National Institute on Drug Abuse.

Hu, T.W., Sung, H.Y., and Keeler, T.E. (1995). Reducing cigarette consumption in California: Tobacco taxes vs. an anti-smoking media campaign. *American Journal of Public Health, 85,* 1218-1222.

Humphrey, J., and Friedman, J. (1986). The onset of drinking and intoxication among university students. *Journal of Studies on Alcohol, 47*, 455-458.

Hurst, P.M., and Wright, P.G. (1981). Deterrence at last: The Ministry of Transport's alcohol blitzes. In L. Goldberg (Ed.), *Alcohol, drugs and traffic safety, Volume III*. Stockholm: Almqvist and Wiksell International.

Institute of Medicine. (1994a). *Growing up tobacco-free: Preventing nicotine dependence in children and youths*. In B. Lynch and R. Bonnie (Eds.), Committee on Preventing Nicotine Addiction in Children and Youths. Washington, DC: National Academy Press.

Institute of Medicine. (1994b). In P.J. Mrazek and R.J. Haggerty (Eds.), *Reducing risks for mental disorders: Frontiers for prevention intervention*. Committee on Prevention of Mental Health Disorders. Washington, DC: National Academy Press.

Institute of Medicine. (2002). *Speaking of health: Assessing health communication strategies for diverse populations*. Committee on Communication for Behavior Change in the 21st Century: Improving the Health of Diverse Populations, Board on Neuroscience and Behavioral Health. Washington, DC: The National Academies Press.

Institute of Medicine and National Research Council. (2001). *Adolescent risk and vulnerability: Summary of a workshop*. In B. Fischhoff, E.O. Nightingale, and J.G. Iannotta (Eds.), Board on Children, Youth, and Families. Washington, DC: National Academy Press.

International Center for Alcohol Policies. (2002). *Drinking age limits*. (ICAP Reports 4), revised. Washington, DC: International Center for Alcohol Policies.

Jaccard, J., and Turrisi, R. (1987). Cognitive processes and individual differences in judgments relevant to drunk driving. *Journal of Personality and Social Psychology, 53*, 135-145.

Jacobs, J.E. (2004). Perceptions of risk and social judgments: Biases and motivational factors. In National Research Council and Institute of Medicine, *Reducing underage drinking: A collective responsibility, background papers*. [CD-ROM]. Committee on Developing a Strategy to Reduce and Prevent Underage Drinking, Division of Behavioral and Social Sciences and Education. Washington, DC: The National Academies Press.

Jacobs, J.E. (2000). *Everyone else is doing it: Relations between bias in base rate estimates and involvement in problem behaviors*. Paper presented at the Society for Research on Adolescence, Chicago, IL.

Jacobs, J.E., and Ganzel, A.K. (1994). Decision making in adolescence: Are we asking the wrong question? In M.L. Maehr and P.R. Pintrich (Eds.), *Advances in achievement and motivation* (Vol. 8) (pp. 1-31). Greenwich, CT: JAI Press.

Jacobs, J.E., Greenwald, J.P., and Osgood, D.W. (1995). Developmental differences in base rate estimates of social behaviors and attitudes. *Social Development, 4*, 165-181.

Jacobs, J.E., and Klaczynski, P.A. (2002). The development of judgment and decision making during childhood and adolescence. *Current Directions in Psychological Science, 11*, 145-149.

Jainchill, N., Bhattacharya, G., and Yagelka, J. (1995). Therapeutic communities for adolescents. *NIDA Research Monograph, 156*, 190-217.

Jenson, J.M., Howard, M.O., and Yaffe, J. (1995). Treatment of adolescent substance abusers: Issues for practice and research. *Social Work in Health Care, 21*, 1-18.

Jernigan, D., and O'Hara, J. (2004). Alcohol advertising and promotion. In National Research Council and Institute of Medicine, *Reducing underage drinking: A collective responsibility, background papers*. [CD-ROM]. Committee on Developing a Strategy to Reduce and Prevent Underage Drinking, Division of Behavioral and Social Sciences and Education. Washington, DC: The National Academies Press.

Jernigan, D., and Wright, P.A. (1994). *Making news, changing policy: Case studies of media advocacy on alcohol and tobacco issues*. Rockville, MD: University Research Corporation, Marin Institute, Center for Substance Abuse Prevention.

Jernigan, D., and Wright, P.A. (1996). Media advocacy: Lessons from community experiences. *Journal of Public Health Policy, 17*(3), 306-329.

Jessor R., and Jessor S. (1980). A social-psychological framework for studying drug use. *NIDA Research Monograph, 30,* 102-109.

Johannessen, K., Collins, C., Mills-Novoa, B., and Glider, P. (1999). *A practical guide to alcohol abuse prevention: A campus case study in implementing social norms and environmental management approaches.* Tucson, AZ: Campus Health Services, University of Arizona.

Johannessen, K., Glider, P., Collins, C., Hueston, H., and DeJong, W. (2001). Preventing alcohol-related problems at the University of Arizona's homecoming: An environmental management case study. *American Journal of Drug and Alcohol Abuse, 27*(3), 587-597.

Johnson, V., and Pandina, R.J. (1993). A longitudinal examination of the relationships among stress, coping strategies, and problems associated with alcohol use. *Alcoholism: Clinical and Experimental Research, 17,* 696-702.

Johnston, L.D., O'Malley, P.M., and Bachman, J.G. (2002). *Monitoring the Future national results on adolescent drug use: Overview of key findings, 2001.* (NIH Publication No. 02-5105). Bethesda, MD: National Institute on Drug Abuse.

Johnston, L.D., O'Malley, P.M., and Bachman, J.G. (2003). *Monitoring the Future national results on adolescent drug use: Overview of key findings, 2002.* (NIH Publication No. 03-5374). Bethesda, MD: National Institute on Drug Abuse.

Johnston, L.D., O'Malley, P.M., Bachman, J.G., and Schulenberg, J.E. (1999). *Cigarette brands smoked by American teens: One brand predominates; three account for nearly all of teen smoking.* Ann Arbor, MI: University of Michigan News and Information Services.

Jones, B.T., Corbin, W., and Fromme, K. (2001). A review of expectancy theory and alcohol consumption. *Addiction, 96*(1), 427-436.

Jones, N., Pieper, C., and Robertson, L. (1992). The effect of the legal drinking age on fatal injuries of adolescents and young adults. *American Journal of Public Health, 82,* 112-114.

Jones-Webb, R., Toomey, T.L., Short, B., Murray, D.M., Wagenaar, A., and Wolfson, M. (1997). Relationships among alcohol availability, drinking location, alcohol consumption, and drinking problems in adolescents. *Substance Use and Misuse, 32,* 1261-1285.

Kallgren, C.A., Reno, R.R., and Cialdini, R.B. (2000). A focus theory of normative conduct: When norms do and do not affect behavior. *Personality and Social Psychology Bulletin, 26,* 1002-1012.

Kaminer, Y., and Bukstein, O. (1989). Adolescent chemical use and dependency: Current issues in epidemiology, treatment and prevention. *Acta Psychiatr Scand, 79,* 415-424.

Kandel, D.B. (1978). Homophily, selection, and socialization in adolescent friendships. *American Journal of Sociology, 84,* 427-436.

Kandel, D.B., and Logan, J.A. (1984). Patterns of drug use from adolescence to young adulthood: I. Periods of risk for initiation, continued use, and discontinuation. *American Journal of Public Health, 74*(7), 660-666.

Kellogg. (1999). *Binge drinking on college campuses.* Washington, DC: Office of Educational Research and Improvement.

Kelly, J.J., Slater, M.D., and Karan, D. (2002). Image advertisements' influence on adolescents' perceptions of the desirability of beer and cigarettes. *Journal of Public Policy and Marketing, 21*(2), 295-304.

Kenkel, D.S. (1993). Drinking, driving and deterrence: The effectiveness and social costs of alternative policies. *Journal of Law and Economics, 36*(2), 877-914.

Kenkel, D.S. (2000). Effects of changes in alcohol prices and taxes. In National Institute on Alcohol Abuse and Alcoholism, *10th special report to the U.S. Congress on alcohol and health* (pp. 341-354). Bethesda, MD: Author.

Kenny, M.E., and Donaldson, G.A. (1991). Contributions of parental attachment and family structure to the social and psychological functioning of first-year college students. *Journal of Counseling Psychology, 38,* 479-486.

Kessler, R.C., Crum, R.M., Warner, L.A., and Nelson, C.B. (1997). Lifetime co-occurrence of DSM-III-R alcohol abuse and dependence with other psychiatric disorders in the National Comorbidity Survey. *Archives of General Psychiatry, 54*(4), 313-321.

Kett, J. (1977). *Rites of passage: Adolescence in America 1790 to the present.* New York: Basic Books.

Kiley, J. (1998). *Pressing on: Citizen action and the Oakland alcohol outlet ordinance.* San Rafael, CA: Marin Institute.

Klepp, K.I., Schmid, L.A., and Murray, D.M. (1996). Effects of the increased minimum drinking age law on drinking and driving behavior among adolescents. *Addiction Research, 4,* 237-244.

Knight, J.R., Wechsler, H., Kuo, M., Seibring, M., Weitzman, E.R., and Schuckit, M.A. (2002). Alcohol abuse and dependence among U.S. college students. *Journal of Studies on Alcohol, 63*(3), 263-270.

Komro, K.A., Hu, F.B., and Flay, B.R. A public health perspective on urban adolescents. In H.J. Walberg, O. Reyes, and R.P. Weissberg (Eds.), *Children and youth: Interdisciplinary perspectives* (pp. 253-298). Thousand Oaks, CA: Sage.

Komro, K.A., Perry, C.L., Veblen-Mortenson, S., and Williams, C.L. (1994). Peer participation in Project Northland: A community-wide alcohol use prevention project. *Journal of School Health, 64,* 318-322.

Kruglanski, A.W. (1989). The psychology of being right: The problem of accuracy in social perception and cognition. *Psychological Bulletin, 106,* 395-409.

Kuther, T.L. (2002). Rational decision perspectives on alcohol consumption by youth: Revising the theory of planned behavior. *Addictive Behaviors, 27*(1), 35-47.

Lacey, J.H., Jones, R.K., and Smith, R.G. (1999). *Evaluation of checkpoint Tennessee: Tennessee's statewide sobriety checkpoint program.* Washington, DC: National Highway Traffic Safety Administration.

Lang, E., Stockwell, T., Rydon, P., and Beel, A. (1996). Use of pseudo-patrons to assess compliance with laws regarding underage drinking. *Australian and New Zealand Journal of Public Health, 20,* 296-300.

Lang, E., Stockwell, T., Rydon, P., and Beel, A. (1998). Can training bar staff in responsible serving practices reduce alcohol-related harm? *Drug and Alcohol Review, 17,* 39-50.

Langley, J.D, Wagenaar, A.C., and Begg, D.J. (1996). An evaluation of the New Zealand graduated driver licensing system. *Accident Analysis and Prevention, 28,* 139-146.

Lantz, P.M. (2004). Youth smoking prevention policy: Lessons learned and continuing challenges. In National Research Council and Institute of Medicine, *Reducing underage drinking: A collective responsibility, background papers.* [CD-ROM]. Committee on Developing a Strategy to Reduce and Prevent Underage Drinking, Division of Behavioral and Social Sciences and Education. Washington, DC: The National Academies Press.

Larimer, M.E., and Cronce, J.M. (2002). Identification, prevention and treatment: A review of individual-focused strategies to reduce problematic alcohol consumption by college students. *Journal of Studies on Alcohol, 14,* 148-163.

Larson, R., and Kleiber, D. (1990). Free-time activities as factors in adolescent adjustment. In P. Tolan and B. Choler (Eds.), *Handbook of clinical research and practice with adolescents.* New York: Oxford University Press.

Lastovicka, J.L. (1995). Methodological interpretation of the experimental and survey research evidence concerning alcohol adverting effects. In S.E. Martin (Ed.), *The effects of the mass media on the use and abuse of alcohol* (pp. 69-81). Bethesda, MD: National Institute on Alcohol Abuse and Alcoholism.

LaVeist, T.A., and Wallace, J.M. (2000). Health risk and inequitable distribution of liquor stores in African American neighborhoods. *Social Science and Medicine, 51*(4), 613-617.

Lee, C.Y., and Halpern-Felsher, B.L. (2001). Parenting of adolescents. In *Parenthood in America: An Encyclopedia.* Santa Barbara, CA: ABC-CLIO.

Lee, J.A., Jones-Webb, R.J., Short, B.J., and Wagenaar, A.C. (1997). Drinking location and risk of alcohol-impaired driving among high school students. *Addictive Behaviors, 22,* 387-393.

Lee, M. (1998). *Drowning in alcohol: Retail outlet density, economic decline, and revitalization in South L.A.* San Rafael, CA: Marin Institute.

Leigh, B.C. (1989). Confirmatory factor analysis of alcohol expectancy scales. *Journal of Studies on Alcohol, 50,* 268-277.

Lerner, R.M. (1995). *America's youth in crisis.* Thousand Oaks, CA: Sage.

Lerner, R.M., and Miller, J.R. (1993). Integrating human development research and intervention for America's children: The Michigan State University model. *Journal of Applied Developmental Psychology, 14,* 347-364.

Levy, D.T., Miller, T.R., Stewart, K., Spicer, R., and Cox, K. (1999, July). *Underage drinking: Immediate consequences and their costs.* Pacific Institute for Research and Evaluation, working paper, unpublished.

Lewis, R.K., Paine-Andrews, A., Fawcett, S.B., Francisco, V.T., Richter, K.P., Copple, B., and Copple, J.E. (1996). Evaluating the effects of a community coalition's efforts to reduce illegal sales of alcohol and tobacco products to minors. *Journal of Community Health, 21,* 429-436.

Light, J.M., Grube, J.W., Madden, P.A., and Gover, J. (2003). Adolescent alcohol use and suicidal ideation: A nonrecursive model. *Addictive Behaviors, 28,* 705-724.

Little, B., and Bishop, M. (1998). Minor drinkers/major consequences: Enforcement strategies for underage alcoholic beverage law violators. *FBI Law Enforcement Bulletin, 67*(6), 1-4.

Lustig, J.L., Ozer, E.M., Adams, S.H., Wibbelsman, C.J., Fuster, C.D., Bonar, R.W., and Irwin, C.E. (2001). Improving the delivery of adolescent clinical preventive services through skills-based training. *Pediatrics, 107,* 1100-1107.

Manger, T.H., Hawkins, J.D., Haggerty, K.P., and Catalano, R.F. (1992). Mobilizing communities to reduce risks for drug abuse: Lessons on using research to guide prevention practice. *Journal of Primary Prevention, 13*(1), 3-22.

Mann, R.E., Stoduto, G., Anglin, L., Pavic, B., Fallon, F., Lauzon, R., and Amitay, O.A. (1997). Graduated licensing in Ontario: Impact of the 0 BAL provision on adolescents' drinking-driving. In C. Mercier-Guyon (Ed.), *Alcohol, drugs, and traffic safety: Volume 3* (pp. 1055-1060). Annecy, France: Centre d'Etudes et de Recherches en Médecine du Trafic.

Manning, W.G., Keeler, E.B., Newhouse, J.P., Sloss, E.M., and Wasserman, J. (1989). The taxes of sin: Do smokers and drinkers pay their way? *Journal of the American Medical Association, 261,* 1604-1609.

Mansergh, G., Rohrbach, L., Montgomery, S.B., Pentz, M.A., and Johnson, C.A. (1996). Evaluation of community coalitions for alcohol and other drug prevention: A comparison of researcher and community-initiated models. *Journal of Community Psychology, 24,* 118-135.

Marlatt, G.A., Baer, J.S., Kivlahan, D.R., Dimeff, L.A., Larimer, M.E., Quigley, L.A., Somers, J.M., and Williams, E. (1998). Screening and brief intervention for high-risk college student drinkers: Results from a 2-year follow-up assessment. *Journal of Consulting and Clinical Psychology, 66(4)*, 604-615.

Marlatt, G.A., Baer, J.S., and Larimer, M.E. (1995). Preventing alcohol abuse in college students: A harm-reduction approach. In G.M. Boyd, J. Howard, and R. Zucker (Eds.), *Alcohol problems among adolescents: Current directions in prevention research* (pp. 147-172). Hillsdale, NJ: Lawrence Erlbaum.

Martin, C.A., Kelly, T.H., Rayens, M.K., Brogli, B.R., Brenzel, A., Smith, W.J., and Omar, H.A. (2002). Sensation seeking, puberty, and nicotine, alcohol, and marijuana use in adolescence. *Journal of the American Academy of Child and Adolescent Psychiatry, 41(12)*, 1495-1502.

Mathios, A., Avery, R., Bisogni, C., and Shanahan, J. (1998). Alcohol portrayal on prime-time television: Manifest and latent messages. *Journal of Studies on Alcohol, 59*, 305-310.

McGue, M., Sharma, A., and Benson, P. (1996). Parent and sibling influences on adolescent alcohol use and misuse: Evidence from a U.S. adoption cohort. *Journal of Studies on Alcohol, 57(1)*, 8-18.

McGuire, A. (1992). The art (and necessity) of coalition building: The California alcohol tax initiative. In A.B. Bergman (Ed.), *Political approaches to injury control at the state level* (pp. 37-45). Seattle: University of Washington Press.

McKay, J.R., Pettinati, H.M., Morrison, R., Feeley, M., Mulvaney, F.D., and Gallop, R. (2002). Relation of depression diagnoses to 2-year outcomes in cocaine-dependent patients in a randomized continuing care study. *Psychology of Addictive Behaviors, 16(3)*, 225-235.

McMorris, B., and Uggen, C. (2000). Alcohol and employment in the transition to adulthood. *Journal of Health and Social Behavior, 41*, 276-294.

Milby, J.B. (1981). *Addictive behavior and its treatment.* New York: Springer.

Miller, P.M., Smith, G.T., and Goldman, M.S. (1990). Emergence of alcohol expectancies in childhood: A possible critical period. *Journal of Studies on Alcohol, 51*, 343-349.

Miller, T.R., and Blincoe, L.J. (1994). Incidence and cost of alcohol-involved crashes in the United States. *Accident Analysis and Prevention, 26(5)*, 583-591.

Miller, W.R. (1998). Researching the spiritual dimensions of alcohol and other drug problems. *Addiction, 93(7)*, 979-990.

Miller, W.R., Zweben, A., DiClemente, C.C., and Rychtarik, R., (1992). *Motivational enhancement therapy manual: A clinical research guide for therapists treating individuals with alcohol abuse and dependence.* DHHS Publication No. (ADM) 92-1984. Rockville, MD: National Institute on Alcohol Abuse and Alcoholism.

Mills, J., and Bogenschneider, K. (2001). Can communities assess support for preventing adolescent alcohol and other drug use? Reliability and validity of a community assessment inventory. *Family Relations, 50(4)*, 355-375.

Millstein, S.G., and Halpern-Felsher, B.L. (2002). Judgments about risk and perceived invulnerability in adolescents and young adults. *Journal of Research on Adolescence, 12*, 399-422.

Millstein, S.G., and Marcell, A.V. (2003). Screening and counseling for adolescent alcohol use among primary care physicians in the United States. *Pediatrics, 111(1)*, 114-122.

Moffitt, T.E. (1993). Life-course-persistent and adolescence-limited antisocial behavior: A developmental taxonomy. *Psychological Review, 100*, 654-701.

Montemayor, R. (1982). The relationship between parent, adolescents, conflict, and the amount of time adolescents spend alone and with parents and peers. *Child Development, 53*, 1512-1519.

Monti, P.M., Colby, S.M., Barnett, N.P., Spirito, A., Rohsenow, D.J., Myers, M., Woolard, R., and Lewander, W. (1999). Brief intervention for harm reduction with alcohol-positive older adolescents in a hospital emergency department. *Journal of Consulting and Clinical Psychology, 67*(6), 989-994.

Mortimer, J.T., Finch, M., Shanahan, M., and Ryn, S. (1992). Work experience, mental health, and behavioral adjustment in adolescence. *Journal of Research on Adolescence, 2,* 24-57.

Mortimer, J.T., and Johnson, M.K. (1998). New perspectives on adolescent work and the transition to adulthood. In R. Jessor (Ed.), *New perspectives on adolescent risk behavior.* New York: Cambridge University Press.

Mosher, J. (1979). Dram shop law and the prevention of alcohol-related problems. *Journal of Studies on Alcohol, 40,* 773-798.

Mosher, J. and other contributors. (2002). *Liquor liability law.* Newark, NJ: Lexis Nexis.

Mosher, J.F., and Works, R.M. (1994). *Confronting Sacramento: State preemption, community control, and alcohol-outlet blight in two inner-city communities.* San Rafael, CA: Marin Institute.

Moskowitz, J.M. (1989). The primary prevention of alcohol problems: A critical review of the research literature. *Journal of Studies on Alcohol, 50*(1), 54-88.

Mothers Against Drunk Driving. (2002a). *It's time to get MADD all over again: Resuscitating the nation's efforts to prevent impaired driving.* A report from the MADD Impaired Driving Summit, June.

Mothers Against Drunk Driving. (2002b). *MADD online: Rating the states' 2002 report card.* Available: http://www.madd.org/activism/0,1056,5545,00.html [August 2003].

Motion Picture Association of America. (2003). Movie ratings, how it works. Available: http://www.mpaa.org/movieratings/about/content4.htm [August 2003].

Mullen, P.D., and Katayama, C.K. (1985). Heath promotion in private practice: An analysis. *Family Community Health, 8*(1), 79-87.

Murray, J.P., Jr. (1991). Youthful drinking and driving: Policy implications from mass media research. *Advances in Consumer Research, 18,* 120-122.

National Center on Addiction and Substance Abuse. (1994). *Rethinking rites of passage: Substance abuse on America's campuses.* New York: Columbia University.

National Center on Addiction and Substance Abuse. (2002). *Teen tipplers: America's underage drinking epidemic.* New York: Columbia University.

National Center on Addiction and Substance Abuse. (2003). *The economic value of underage drinking and adult excessive drinking to the alcohol industry: A CASA white paper.* New York: Columbia University.

National Highway Traffic Safety Administration. (1998). *Traffic safety facts 1998—Overview.* (DOT HS 808 956). Washington, DC: U.S. Department of Transportation.

National Highway Traffic Safety Administration. (2002a). *Traffic safety facts 2001—Alcohol.* (DOT HS 809 470). Washington, DC: U.S. Department of Transportation.

National Highway Traffic Safety Administration. (2002b). *Youth fatal crash and alcohol facts 2000.* (DOT HS 809 406). Washington, DC: U.S. Department of Transportation.

National Household Survey on Drug Abuse. (2001). *Results from the 2001 National Household Survey on Drug Abuse: Volume I. Summary of national findings.* (Office of Applied Studies, NHSDA Series H-17, DHHS Publication No. SMA 02-3758). Rockville, MD: Substance Abuse and Mental Health Services Administration.

National Household Survey on Drug Abuse. (2002, April 11). *Binge drinking among underage persons.* Rockville, MD: Author.

National Institute on Alcohol Abuse and Alcoholism. (1990, October). *Alcohol alert no. 10 PH 290: Alcohol and women.* Bethesda, MD: Author.

National Institute on Alcohol Abuse and Alcoholism. (1994, January). *Alcohol alert no. 23 PH 347: Alcohol and minorities.* Bethesda, MD: Author.

National Institute on Alcohol Abuse and Alcoholism. (1997, July). *Alcohol alert no. 37: Youth drinking: Risk factors and consequences.* Bethesda, MD: Author.

National Institute on Alcohol Abuse and Alcoholism. (2002). *A call to action: Changing the culture of drinking at U.S. colleges.* (NIH Publication No. 02-5010). Bethesda, MD: Author.

National Institute on Drug Abuse Community Epidemiology Work Group. (1999, December). *Epidemiologic trends in drug abuse, advance report.* Bethesda, MD: National Institute on Drug Abuse.

National Research Council. (2001). *Informing America's policy on illegal drugs: What we don't know keeps hurting us.* C.F. Manski, J.V. Pepper, and C.V. Petrie (Eds.), Committee on Data and Research for Policy on Illegal Drugs, Committee on Law and Justice and Committee on National Statistics. Washington, DC: National Academy Press.

National Research Council and Institute of Medicine (1994). *Under the influence? Drugs and the American workforce.* J. Normand, R.O. Lempert, and C.P. O'Brien (Eds.), Committee on Drug Use in the Workplace. Washington, DC: National Academy Press.

National Research Council and Institute of Medicine (2004). *Reducing underage drinking: A collective responsibility, background papers.* [CD-ROM]. Committee on Developing a Strategy to Reduce and Prevent Underage Drinking, Division of Behavioral and Social Sciences and Education. Washington, DC: The National Academies Press.

National Women's Health Information Center. (2002). *Women of color health data book. 2nd edition.* Bethesda, MD: Office of the Director, National Institutes of Health.

Nienstedt, B. (1990). The policy effects of a DWI law and a publicity campaign. In R. Surette (Ed.), *Mass media and criminal justice policy: Recent research and social effects* (pp. 193-203). Springfield, IL: C.C. Thomas.

Nisbett, R., and Wilson, T. (1977). Telling more than we can know: Verbal reports on mental processes. *Psychological Review, 84,* 231-259.

Novins, D.K., Spicer, P., Beals, J., and Manson, S.M. (2004). Preventing underage drinking in American Indian and Alaska Native communities: Contexts, epidemiology, and culture. In National Research Council and Institute of Medicine, *Reducing underage drinking: A collective responsibility, background papers.* [CD-ROM]. Committee on Developing a Strategy to Reduce and Prevent Underage Drinking, Division of Behavioral and Social Sciences and Education. Washington, DC: The National Academies Press.

Nucci, L., Guerra, N., and Lee, J. (1991). Adolescent judgments of the personal, prudential, and normative aspects of drug usage. *Developmental Psychology, 27,* 841-848.

Nye, C., Zucker, R., and Fitzgerald, H. (1995). Early intervention in the path to alcohol problems through conduct problems: Treatment involvement and child behavior change. *Journal of Consulting and Clinical Psychology, 63,* 831-840.

Oei, T.P., Fergusson, S., and Lee, N.K. (1998). The differential role of alcohol expectancies and drinking refusal self-efficacy in problem and nonproblem drinkers. *Journal of Studies on Alcohol, 59*(6), 704-711.

Office of National Drug Control Policy. (2001). *The economic costs of drug abuse in the United States: 1992-1998.* Publication No. NCJ-19-636. Washington, DC: Executive Office of the President.

Office of National Drug Control Policy. (2003, February). *National drug control strategy: FY 2004 budget summary.* Washington, DC: Executive Office of the President.

Ohsfeldt, R.L., and Morrisey, M.A. (1997). Beer taxes, workers' compensation, and industrial injury. *Review of Economics and Statistics, 79*(1), 155-160.

Olds, R.S., and Thombs, D.L. (2001). The relationship of adolescent perceptions of peer norms and parent involvement to cigarette and alcohol use. *Journal of School Health, 71*(6), 223-228.

O'Malley, P.M., and Johnston, L.D. (1999). Drinking and driving among American high school seniors: 1984-1997. *American Journal of Public Health, 89,* 678-684.

O'Malley, P.M., and Wagenaar, A.C. (1991). Effects of minimum drinking age laws on alcohol use, related behaviors and traffic crash involvement among Americans youth: 1976-1987. *Journal of Studies on Alcohol, 52,* 478-491.

Osgood, D.W. (1998). Hanging out with the gang: Routine activities, gang membership, and problem behavior. Poster session presented at the meeting for the Society for Research on Adolescence, San Diego.

Osgood, D.W., Wilson, J.K., O'Malley, P.M., Bachman, J.G., and Johnson, L.D. (1996). Routine activities and individual deviant behavior. *American Sociological Review, 61*(4), 635-655.

Ozer, E.M., Adams, S.H., Lustig, J.L., Millstein, S.G., Camfield, K., El-Diwany, S., Volpe, S., and Irwin, C.E. (2001). Can it be done? Implementing adolescent clinical preventive services. *Health Services Research, 36,* 150-165.

Ozer, E., Adams, S., Lustig, J., Millstein, S., Wibbelsman, C., Babb, J., Doyle, T., Redmond, N., and Irwin, C.E. (2003). The effect of preventive services on adolescent behavior. *Pediatric Research, 53,* 265A.

Pacific Institute for Research and Evaluation. (1999, October). *Costs of underage drinking* (updated edition). Report prepared for Office of Juvenile Justice and Delinquency Prevention, Office of Justice Programs, U.S. Department of Justice.

Pacula, R.L. (1998). Does increasing the beer tax reduce marijuana consumption? *Journal of Health Economics, 17*(5), 557-586.

Paglia, A., and Room, R. (1999). Preventing substance use problems among youth: A literature review and recommendations. *Journal of Primary Prevention, 20*(1), 3-50.

Palmer, C.J., Lohman, G., Gehring, D.D., Carlson, S., and Garrett, O. (2001). Parental notification: A new strategy to reduce alcohol abuse on campus. *NASPA Journal, 38*(3), 372-385.

Palmgreen, P., Donohew, L., Lorch, E.P., Hoyle, R.H., and Stephenson, M.T. (2001, February). Television campaigns and adolescent marijuana use: Tests of sensation seeking targeting. *American Journal of Public Health, 91*(2), 292-296.

Pandina, R.J., and Johnson, V. (1989). Familial drinking history as a predictor of alcohol and drug consumption among adolescent children. *Journal of Studies on Alcohol, 50,* 245-253.

Pandina, R.J., and Johnson, V. (1990). Serious alcohol and drug problems among adolescents with a family history of alcoholism. *Journal of Studies on Alcohol, 51,* 278-282.

Park, P. (1967). Dimensions of drinking among male college students. *Social Problems, 14*(4), 473-482.

Parke, P.D., and Ladd, G.W. (1992). *Family-peer relationships: Modes of linkages.* Hillsdale, NJ: Lawrence Erlbaum.

Parker, R.N., and Rebhun, L.A. (1995). *Alcohol and homicide: A deadly combination of two American traditions.* Albany: State University of New York Press.

Pentz, M.A., Dwyer, J.H., MacKinnon, D.P., Flay, B.R., Hansen, W.B., Wang, E.Y.I., and Johnson, C.A. (1989). A multicommunity trial for primary prevention of adolescent drug abuse: Effects on drug use prevalence. *Journal of the American Medical Association, 261*(22), 3259-3266.

Perkins, H.W. (2002). Social norms and the prevention of alcohol misuse in collegiate contexts. *Journal of Studies on Alcohol, 14,* 164-172.

Perkins, H.W., and Berkowitz, A.D. (1986). Perceiving the community norms of alcohol use among students: Some research implications for campus alcohol education programming. *International Journal of Addiction, 21,* 961-976.

Perkins, R.A., Jenkins, S.E., and McCullough, M.B. (1980). A look at drinking on a university campus. *College Student Journal, 14*(3), 222-229.

Perry, C.L., and Kelder, S.H. (1992). Prevention. In J.W. Langenbucher (Ed.), *Review of addictions: Research and treatment, volume 2* (pp. 453-472). New York: Pergamon Press.

Perry, C.L., Williams, C.L., Veblen-Mortenson, S., Toomey, T., Komro, K., Anstine, P.S., Wagenaar, A.C., and Wolfson, M. (1996). Project Northland: Outcomes of a communitywide alcohol use prevention program during early adolescence. *American Journal of Public Health, 86*(7), 956-965.

Perry, C.L., Williams, C.L., Komro, K.A., Veblen-Mortenson, S., Forster, J.L., Bernstein-Lachter, R., Pratt, L.K., Dudovitz, B., Munson, K.A., Farbakhsh, K., Finnegan, J., and McGovern, P. (2000). Project Northland high school interventions: Community action to reduce adolescent alcohol use. *Health Education and Behavior, 27*(1), 29-49.

Perry, C.L., Williams, C.L., Komro, K.A., Vebeln-Mortensen, S., Stigler, M.H., Munson, K.A., Farbadhsh, K., Jones, R.M., and Forster, J.L. (2002). Project Northland: Long-term outcomes of community action to reduce adolescent alcohol use. *Health Education Research Theory and Practice, 17*(1), 117-123.

Peters, C. (2002). Ohio college initiative to reduce high risk drinking: Evaluation report. Columbus, OH: Office of Criminal Justice Services.

Peterson, P.L., Hawkins, J.D., Abbott, R.D., and Catalano, R.F. (1994). Disentangling the effects of parent drinking, family management, and parental alcohol norms on current drinking by Black and White adolescents. *Journal of Research on Adolescence, 4*, 203-228.

Pickens, R.W., and Fletcher, W.W. (1991). Overview of treatment issues. *NIDA Research Monograph, 106*, 1-19.

Pierce, J., Emery, S., and Gilpin, E. (2002). The California Tobacco Control Program: A long term health communication project. In R. Hornik (Ed.), *Public health communication: Evidence for behavior change.* Mahwah, NJ: Lawrence Erlbaum.

Powell, A., and Willingham, M. (n.d.). *Strategies for reducing third party transactions of alcohol to underage youth.* Calverton, MD: OJJDP Underage Drinking Enforcement Training Center. Available: http://www.udetc.org/documents/Reducing%203rd%20 Party.pdf [August, 2003].

Prendergast, L. (1994). Substance use and abuse among college students: A review of the recent literature. *Journal of American College Health, 43*, 99-113.

Prentice, D.A., and Miller, D.T. (1993). Pluralistic ignorance and alcohol use on campus: Some consequences of misperceiving the social norm. *Journal of Personality and Social Psychology, 64*, 243-256.

President's Commission on Model State Drug Laws (1993). *Drug-free families, schools, and workplaces (Model Underage Alcohol Consumption Reduction Act).* Washington, DC: The White House.

Presidents Leadership Group. (1997). *Be vocal, be visible, be visionary: Recommendations for college and university presidents on alcohol and other drug prevention.* Washington, DC: The Higher Education Center for Alcohol and Other Drug Prevention.

Presley, C.A., Meilman, P.W., and Leichliter, J.S. (2002). College factors that influence drinking. *Journal of Studies on Alcohol, 14*, 82-90.

Preusser, D.F., and Williams, A.F. (1992). Sales of alcohol to underage purchasers in three New York counties and Washington DC. *Journal of Public Health Policy, 13*, 306-317.

Preusser, D.F., Ferguson, S.A., Williams, A.F., and Farmer, C.M. (1995). *Underage access to alcohol: Sources of alcohol and use of false identification.* Arlington, VA: Insurance Institute for Highway Safety.

Prinstein, M.J., Fetter, M.D., and La Greca, A.M. (1996, March). Can you judge adolescents by the company they keep? Peer group membership, substance use, and risk-taking behaviors. Paper presented at the meeting of the Society for Research on Adolescence, Boston, MA.

Pruitt, B.E., Kingery, P.M., Mirzaee, E., Heuberger, G., and Hurley, R.S. (1991). Peer influence and drug use among adolescents in rural areas. *Journal of Drug Education, 21*, 1-11.

Quadrel, M.J., Fischhoff, B., and Davis, W. (1993). Adolescent (in)vulnerability. *American Psychologist, 48*(2), 102-116.

Reifman, A., Barnes, G.M., Dintcheff, B.A., Farrell, M.P., and Uhteg, L. (1998). Parental and peer influences on the onset of heavier drinking among adolescents. *Journal of Studies on Alcohol, 59*(3), 311-317.

Rice, K.G. (1992). Separation-individuation and adjustment to college: A longitudinal study. *Journal of Counseling Psychology, 39*, 203-213.

Robert Wood Johnson Foundation. (1993). *Substance abuse: The nation's number one health problem. Key indicators for policy.* Princeton, NJ: Author.

Roberts, D.F., Foehr, U.G., Rideout, V.J., and Brodie, M. (1999a). *Kids and media @ the new millennium.* Palo Alto, CA: Kaiser Family Foundation.

Roberts, D.F., Henriksen, L., and Christensen, P.G. (1999b). *Substance use in popular movies and music.* Washington, DC: Office of National Drug Control Policy.

Roccella, E.J. (2002). The contributions of public health education toward reduction of cardiovascular disease mortality: Experiences from the National High Blood Pressure Education Program. In R. Hornik (Ed.), *Public health communication: Evidence for behavior change* (pp. 73-84). Mahwah, NJ: Lawrence Erlbaum.

Rohrbach, L.A., Johnson, C.A., Mansergh, G., Fishkin, S.A., and Neumann, F.B. (1997). Alcohol-related outcomes of the day one community partnership. *Evaluation and Program Planning, 20*(3), 315-322.

Room, R. (1989). *Community action and alcohol problems: Some historical perspectives.* Berkeley, CA: Alcohol Research Group.

Room, R. (2004). Drinking and coming of age in a cross-cultural perspective. In National Research Council and Institute of Medicine, *Reducing underage drinking: A collective responsibility, background papers.* [CD-ROM]. Committee on Developing a Strategy to Reduce and Prevent Underage Drinking, Division of Behavioral and Social Sciences and Education. Washington, DC: The National Academies Press.

Room, R., Jernigan, D., Carlini-Marlatt, B., Gurege, O., Mäkelä, K., Marshall, M., Medina-Mora, M.E., Monteiro, M., Parry, C., Partanen, J. Riley, L., and Saxena, S. (2002). *Alcohol in developing societies: A public health approach.* Helsinki: Hakapaino Oy: Finnish Foundation for Alcohol Studies in collaboration with World Health Organization.

Rootman, I., and Moser, J. (1985). *Community response to alcohol-related problems: A World Health Organization project.* (DHHS Publication No. ADM 85-1371). Washington, DC: U.S. Government Printing Office.

Roper Center at University of Connecticut. (1987, September). Public opinion online, accession # 0025861, question 001, Gallup Poll. Available: http://www.ropercenter.uconn.edu/ipoll.html [February, 2003].

Roper Center at University of Connecticut. (1988, September). Public opinion online, accession # 0150315, question 005, Gallup Poll. Available: http://www.ropercenter.uconn.edu/ipoll.html [February, 2003].

Roper Center at the University of Connecticut. (2003a). Public opinion online, accession #0412701, Question 031. Available: http://www.ropercenter.uconn.edu/ipoll.html [February, 2003].

Roper Center at the University of Connecticut. (2003b). Public opinion online, accession #0412675, CASA National Underage Drinking Survey. Available: http://www.ropercenter.uconn.edu/ipoll.html [February, 2003].

Rose, G. (1985). Sick individuals and sick populations. *International Journal of Epidemiology, 14,* 32-38.

Ross, H.L. (1982). *Deterring the drinking driver.* Lexington, MA: Lexington.

Ruhm, C.J. (1996). Alcohol policies and highway vehicle fatalities. *Journal of Health Economics, 15,* 435-454.

Saffer, H. (1997). Alcohol advertising and motor vehicle fatalities. *Review of Economics and Statistics, 79,* 431-442.

Saffer, H., and Grossman, M. (1987). Beer taxes, the legal drinking age, and youth motor vehicle fatalities. *Journal of Legal Studies, 16,* 351-374.

Saltz, R.F. (1987). Roles of bars and restaurants in preventing alcohol-impaired driving: An evaluation of server intervention. *Evaluation and Health Professions, 10,* 5-27.

Saltz, R.F. (1989). Research needs and opportunities in server intervention programs. *Health Education Quarterly, 16,* 429-438.

Saltz, R.F. (1997). Prevention where alcohol is sold and consumed: Server intervention and responsible beverage service. In M. Plant, E. Single, and T. Stockwell (Eds.), *Alcohol: Minimizing the harm. What works?* (pp. 72-84). New York: Free Association.

Saltz, R.F., and Stanghetta, P. (1997). A community-wide responsible beverage service program in three communities: Early findings. *Addiction, 92*(Suppl. 2), S237-S249.

Schoen, C., Davis, K., Collins, K.S., Greenberg, L., Des Roches, C., and Abrams, M. (1997, November). *The Commonwealth Fund survey of the health of adolescent girls.* New York: Commonwealth Fund.

Schroeder, C., and Prentice, D. (1998). Exposing pluralistic ignorance to reduce alcohol use among college students. *Journal of Applied Social Psychology, 28,* 2150-2180.

Schulenberg, J., O'Malley, P., Bachman, J., Wadsworth, K., and Johnston, L. (1996). Getting drunk and growing up: Trajectories of frequent binge drinking during the transition to young adulthood. *Journal of Studies on Alcohol, 57,* 289-304.

Schwartz, R.H., Farrow, J.A., Banks, B., and Giesel, A.E. (1998). Use of false ID cards and other deceptive methods to purchase alcoholic beverages during high school. *Journal of Addictive Diseases, 17,* 25-34.

Seevak, A. (1997, December). *Oakland shows the way: The coalition on alcohol outlet issues and media advocacy as a tool for policy change.* Berkeley: Berkeley Media Studies.

Sher, K.J., Bartholow, B.D., and Nanda, S. (2001). Short- and long-term effects of fraternity and sorority membership on heavy drinking: A social norms perspective. *Psychology of Addictive Behaviors, 15*(1), 42-51.

Shope, J.T., Molnar, L.J., Elliott, M.R., and Waller, P.F. (2001). Graduated driver licensing in Michigan: Early impact on motor vehicle crashes among 16-year-old drivers. *Journal of the American Medical Association, 286,* 1593-1598.

Siegel, M. (2002). The effectiveness of state-level tobacco control interventions: A review of program implementation and behavioral outcomes. *Annual Review of Public Health, 23,* 45-71.

Siegel, M., and Biener, L. (2000). The impact of an antismoking media campaign on progression to established smoking: Results of a longitudinal youth study. *American Journal of Public Health, 90*(3), 380-386.

Sieving, R.E. (1997). Process of parental influence on alcohol use among young adolescents. *Dissertation Abstracts International, 57*(8), 5006-B.

Sieving, R.E., Perry, C.L., and Williams, C.L. (2000). Do friendships change behaviors, or do behaviors change friendships? Examining paths of influence in young adolescents' alcohol use. *Journal of Adolescent Health, 26*(1), 27-35.

Slater, M.D., Rouner, D., Domenech-Rodriguez, M.M., Beauvais, F., Murphy, K., and Van Leuven, J. (1997). Adolescent responses to TV beer ads and sports content/context: Gender and ethnic differences. *Journalism and Mass Communication Quarterly, 74,* 108-122.

Sloan, F.A., Reilly, B.A., and Schenzler, C. (1994). Effects of prices, civil and criminal sanctions, and law enforcement on alcohol-related mortality. *Journal of Studies on Alcohol, 55,* 454-465.

Sloan, F.A., Stout, E.M., Whetten-Goldstein, K., and Liang, L. (2000). *Drinkers, drivers, and bartenders: Balancing private choices and public accountability.* Chicago: University of Chicago Press.

Slovic, P. (2000). What does it mean to know a cumulative risk? Adolescents' perceptions of short-term and long-term consequences of smoking. *Journal of Behavioral Decision Making, 13*(2), 259-266.

Sly, D.F., Hopkins, R.S., Trapido, E., and Ray, S. (2001). Influence of a counter-advertising media campaign on initiation of smoking: The Florida truth campaign. *American Journal of Public Health, 91*(2), 233-238.

Small, S.A., Silverburg, S.B., and Kerns, D.T.I. (1993). Adolescents' perceptions of the costs and benefits of engaging in health-compromising behaviors. *Journal of Youth and Adolescence, 22*(1), 73-87.

Smart, R.G. (1988). Does alcohol advertising affect overall consumption? A review of empirical studies. *Journal of Studies on Alcohol, 49*(4), 314-323.

Smith, D.I. (1986). Effect of low proscribed blood alcohol levels (BALs) on traffic accidents among newly licensed drivers. *Medical Science and the Law, 26,* 144-148.

Smith, G., Goldman, M., Greenbaum, P., and Christiansen, B. (1995). Expectancy for social facilitation from drinking: The divergent paths of high-expectancy and low-expectancy adolescents. *Journal of Abnormal Psychology, 104*(1), 32-40.

Smith, M. (1989). Students, suds, and summonses: Strategies for coping with campus alcohol abuse. *Journal of College Student Development, 30*(2), 118-122.

Snow, R.W., and Landrum, J.W. (1986). Drinking locations and frequency of drunkenness among Mississippi DUI offenders. *American Journal of Drug and Alcohol Abuse, 12*(4), 389-402.

Snyder, L.B., and Hamilton, M.A. (2002). A meta-analysis of U.S. health campaign effects on behavior: Emphasize enforcement, exposure and new information and beware the secular trend. In R. Hornik (Ed.), *Public health communication: Evidence for behavior change* (pp. 357-384). Mahwah, NJ: Lawrence Erlbaum.

Spear, L.P. (2002). The adolescent brain and the college drinker: Biological basis of propensity to use and misuse alcohol. *Journal on Studying Alcohol Suppl. 14,* 71-81.

Spoth, R.L., Redmond, C., and Shin, C. (2001). Randomized trial of brief family interventions for general populations: Adolescent substance use outcomes 4 years following baseline. *Journal of Consulting and Clinical Psychology, 69*(4), 627-642.

Stacy, A.W., Widaman, K.F., and Marlatt, G.A. (1990). Expectancy models of alcohol use. *Journal of Personality and Social Psychology, 58,* 918-928.

Steinberg, L., and Cauffman, E. (1996). Maturity of judgment in adolescence: Psychosocial factors in adolescent decision making. *Law and Human Behavior, 20,* 249-272.

Steinberg, L., Fegley, S., and Dornbusch, S.M. (1993). Negative impact of part-time work on adolescent adjustment: Evidence from a longitudinal study. *Developmental Psychology, 29,* 171-180.

Steinberg, L.D., Fletcher, A., and Darling, N. (1994). Parental monitoring and peer influences on adolescent substance use. *Pediatrics, 93,* 1060-1064.

Stewart, L., and Casswell, S. (1993). Media advocacy for alcohol policy support: Results from the New Zealand Community Action Project. *Health Promotion International, 8*(3), 167-175.

Stice, E., Barrera, M., and Chassin, L. (1998). Prospective differential prediction of adolescent alcohol use and problem use: Examining the mechanisms of effect. *Journal of Abnormal Psychology, 107*(4), 616-628.

Stout, E.M., Sloan, F.A., Liang, L., and Davies, H.H. (2000). Reducing harmful alcohol-related behaviors: Effective regulatory methods. *Journal of Studies on Alcohol, 61,* 402-412.

Strategic Marketing Services. (2002). *Your teen and alcohol, Do you really know?* Portland, ME: Maine Office of Substance Abuse. Available: http://www.maineparents.net [March 3, 2003].

Streicker, J. (Ed.). (2000). *Case histories in alcohol policy.* San Francisco, CA: Trauma Foundation.

Strunge, H. (1998). Danish experiences of national campaigns on alcohol 1990-1996. *Drugs: Education, Prevention and Policy, 5*(1), 73-79.

Strunin, L., and Hingson, R. (1992). Alcohol, drugs, and adolescent sexual behavior. *International Journal of the Addictions, 27*(2), 129-146.

Stuster, J.W., and Blowers, P.A. (1995). *Experimental evaluation of sobriety checkpoint programs.* Washington, DC: National Highway Traffic Safety Administration.

Substance Abuse and Mental Health Services Administration. (2000). *Substance abuse treatment in adult and juvenile correctional facilities: Findings from the uniform facilities data set 1977 survey of correctional facilities.* (Drug and Alcohol Services Information System Series S-9). Rockville, MD: Author, Office of Applied Studies.

Substance Abuse and Mental Health Services Administration. (2001). *Summary of findings from the 2000 National Household Survey on Drug Abuse.* (NHSDA Series H-13, DHHS Publication No. SMA 01-3549). Rockville, MD: Author.

Substance Abuse and Mental Health Services Administration. (2002, April 11). *Binge drinking among underage persons.* Rockville, MD: Author.

Substance Abuse and Mental Health Services Administration. (2002, September 13). *Low rates of alcohol use among Asian youths.* Rockville, MD: Author.

Substance Abuse and Mental Health Services Administration. (2003, April 13). *Alcohol use.* Rockville, MD: Author

Swendsen, J.D., Conway, K.P., Rounsaville, B.J., and Merikangas, K.R. (2002). Are personality traits familial risk factors for substance use disorders? Results of a controlled family study. *American Journal of Psychiatry, 159*(10), 1760-1766.

Swisher, J.D., and Hoffman, A. (1975). Information: The irrelevant variable in drug education. In B.W. Corder, R.A. Smith, and J.D. Swisher (Eds.), *Drug abuse prevention: Perspectives and approaches for educators.* Dubuque, IA: William C. Brown.

Tapert, S.F., and Brown, S.A. (1999). Neuropsychological correlates of adolescent substance abuse: Four-year outcomes. *Journal of the International Neuropsychological Society, 5,* 481-493.

Tapert, S.F., Brown, G., Meloy, M., Dager, A., Cheung, E., and Brown, S. (2001). MRI measurement of brain function in alcohol use disordered adolescents. *Alcoholism: Clinical and Experimental Research, 25,* 80A.

Tay, R. (2000). Methodological issues in evaluation models: The New Zealand Road Safety Advertising Campaign revisited. *Road and Transportation Research, 10*(2), 29-39.

Taylor, T.K., and Biglan, A. (1998). Behavioral parenting skills programs: A review of the literature for clinicians. *Clinical Child and Family Psychology Review, 1,* 41-60.

Thompson, K., and Yokota, F. (2001). Depiction of alcohol, tobacco, and other substances in G-rated animated feature films. *Pediatrics, 107,* 1369-1374.

Thorson, E. (1995). Studies on the effects of alcohol advertising: Two underexplored aspects. In S.E. Martin (Ed.), *The effects of the mass media on use and abuse of alcohol.* Bethesda, MD: National Institute on Alcohol Abuse and Alcoholism.

Tobler, N.S. (1992). Drug prevention programs that can work: Research findings. *Journal of Addictive Diseases, 11*(3), 1-28.

Tobler, N.S., Roona, M.R., Ochshorn, P., Marshall, D.G., Streke, A.V., and Stackpole, K.M. (2000). School-based adolescent drug prevention programs: 1998 meta-analysis. *The Journal of Primary Prevention, 20*, 275-336.

Tobler, N.S., and Stratton, H.H. (1997). Effectiveness of school-based drug prevention programs: A meta-analysis of research. *Journal of Primary Prevention, 18*, 71-128.

Toomey, T.L., and Wagenaar, A.C. (1999). Policy options for prevention: The case of alcohol. *Journal of Public Health Policy, 20*, 193-212.

Toomey, T.L., Wagenaar, A.C., Gehan, J.P., Kilian, G., Murray, D.M., and Perry, C.L. (2001). Project ARM: Alcohol Risk Management to prevent sales to underage and intoxicated patrons. *Health Education and Behavior, 28*, 186-199.

Tyler, T.R. (1992). *Why people obey the law.* New Haven: Yale University Press.

Tyler, T.R., and Huo, Y.J. (2002). *Trust in the law: Encouraging public cooperation with the police and courts.* New York: Russell Sage Foundation.

Ulmer, R.G., Ferguson, S.A., Williams, A.F., and Preusser, D.F. (2000). *Teenage crash reduction associated with delayed licensure in Connecticut.* Arlington, VA: Insurance Institute for Highway Safety.

U.S. Federal Trade Commission. (1999, September). *Self-regulation in the alcohol industry: A review of industry efforts to avoid promoting alcohol to underage consumers.* Washington, DC: Author.

U.S. Federal Trade Commission. (2000, September). *Marketing violent entertainment to children: A review of self-regulation and industry practices in the motion picture, music recording and electronic game industries. A report of the Federal Trade Commission.* Washington, DC: Author.

U.S. Federal Trade Commission. (2001, December). *Marketing violent entertainment to children: A one-year follow-up review of industry practices in the motion picture, music recording and electronic game industries. A report to Congress.* Washington, DC: Author.

U.S. Federal Trade Commission. (2002, June). *Marketing violent entertainment to children: A twenty-one month follow-up review of industry practices in the motion picture, music recording and electronic game industries. A report to Congress.* Washington, DC: Author.

U.S. General Accounting Office. (1987). *Drinking-age laws: An evaluation synthesis of their impact on highway safety.* GAO/PEMD-87-10. Washington, DC: Author.

U.S. General Accounting Office. (2001, May). *Underage drinking: Information on federal funds targeted at prevention.* GAO-01-503. Washington, DC: Author.

U.S. Navy. (n.d.). PREVENT: Personal Responsibility and Values: Education and Training; Knowledge to Action. Available: http://www.preventonline.org [February, 2003].

Vicary, J.R., Snyder, A.R., and Henry, K.L. (2000). The effects of family variables and personal competencies on the initiation of alcohol use by rural seventh grade students. *Adolescent and Family Health, 1*(1), 11-20.

Voas, R.B., Holder, H.D., and Gruenewald, P.J. (1997). The effect of drinking and driving interventions on alcohol-involved traffic crashes within a comprehensive community trial. *Addiction, 92*(Suppl. 2), 221-236.

Voas, R.B., Lange, J.E., and Tippetts, A.E. (1998). Enforcement of the zero tolerance law in California: A missed opportunity? In *42nd Annual Proceedings of the Association for the Advancement of Automotive Medicine* (pp. 369-383). Des Plaines, IL: Association for the Advancement of Automotive Medicine.

Voas, R.B., Tippetts, A.S., and Fell, J. (1999, September). *United States limits drinking by youth under age 21: Does this reduce fatal crash involvements?* Paper presented at the annual meeting of the Association for the Advancement of Automotive Medicine, Barcelona, Spain.

Wagenaar, A.C. (1981). Effects of an increase in the legal minimum drinking age. *Journal of Health Policy, 2*, 206-225.

Wagenaar, A.C. (1986). Preventing highway crashes by raising the legal minimum age for drinking: The Michigan experience 6 years later. *Journal of Safety Research, 17*, 101-109.

Wagenaar, A.C., Finnegan, J.R., Wolfson, M., Anstine, P.S., Williams, C.L., and Perry, C.L. (1993). Where and how adolescents obtain alcoholic beverages. *Public Health Reports, 108*(4), 459-464.

Wagenaar, A.C., Gehan, J.P., Jones-Webb, R., Toomey, T.L., and Forster, J. (1999). Communities mobilizing for change on alcohol: Lessons and results from a 15-community randomized trial. *Journal of Community Psychology, 27*, 315-326.

Wagenaar, A.C., Harwood, E., and Bernat, D. (2002). *The Robert Wood Johnson Foundation 2001 youth access to alcohol survey: Summary report.* Minneapolis: University of Minnesota, Alcohol Epidemiology Program.

Wagenaar, A.C., and Holder, H.D. (1991). Effects of an alcohol beverage server liability law on traffic crash injuries. *Alcoholism: Clinical and Experimental Research, 15*, 942-947.

Wagenaar, A.C., and Maybee, R.G. (1986). Legal minimum drinking age in Texas: Effects of an increase from 18 to 19. *Journal of Safety Research, 17*, 165-178.

Wagenaar, A.C., Murray, D.M., Gehan, J.P., Wolfson, M., Forster, J.L., Toomery, T.L., Perry, C.L., and Jones-Webb, R. (2000a). Communities mobilizing for change on alcohol: Outcomes from a randomized community trial. *Journal of Studies on Alcohol, 61*, 85-94.

Wagenaar, A.C., Murray, D.M., and Toomey, T.L. (2000b). Communities mobilizing for change on alcohol (CMCA): Effects of a randomized trial on arrests and traffic crashes. *Addiction, 95*(2), 209-217.

Wagenaar, A.C., O'Malley, P.M., and LaFond, C. (2001). Very low legal BAC limits for young drivers: Effects on drinking, driving, and driving-after-drinking behaviors in 30 states. *American Journal of Public Health, 91*, 801-804.

Wagenaar, A.C., and Perry, C.L. (1994). Community strategies for the reduction of youth drinking: Theory and application. *Journal of Research on Adolescence, 4*, 319–345.

Wagenaar, A.C., and Toomey, T.L. (2002). Effects of minimum drinking age laws: Review and analyses of the literature from 1960 to 2000. *Journal of Studies on Alcohol, 14*, 206-225.

Wagenaar, A.C., Toomey, T.L., Murray, D.M., Short, B.J., Wolfson, M., and Jones-Webb, R. (1996). Sources of alcohol for underage drinkers. *Journal of Studies on Alcohol, 57*, 325-333.

Wagenaar, A.C., and Wolfson, M. (1994). Enforcement of the legal minimum drinking age in the United States. *Journal of Public Health Policy, 15*, 37-53.

Wagenaar, A.C., and Wolfson, M. (1995). Deterring sales and provision of alcohol to minors: A study of enforcement in 295 counties in four states. *Public Health Reports, 110*, 419-427.

Walker, S., Grube, J., Chen, M.J., Light, J. and Treno, A. (2001, June). *Driving under the influence and riding with drinking drivers: The importance of ethnicity, gender and drinking context.* Presented at the annual meeting of the Research Society on Alcoholism, Montréal, Canada.

Wallack, L. (1992). Editorial: Warning: The alcohol industry is not your friend. *British Journal of Addiction, 87*, 175-177.

Wallack, L. (1993). Editorial reply: Some proposals for the alcohol industry. *Addiction, 88,* 167-178.

Wallack, L. (2000). The role of mass media in creating social capital: A new direction for public health. In B.D. Smedley and S.L. Syme (Eds.), *Promoting health: Intervention strategies from social and behavioral research* (pp. 337-365). Committee on Capitalizing on Social Science and Behavioral Research to Improve the Public's Health, Division of Health Promotion and Disease Prevention, Institute of Medicine. Washington, DC: National Academy Press.

Wallack, L., and Barrows, D. (1982). Evaluating primary prevention: The California "Winners" Alcohol Program. *International Quarterly of Community Health Education, 3*(4), 307-335.

Wallack, L., Dorman, L., Jernigan, D., and Themba, M. (1996). *Media advocacy and public health: Power for prevention.* Thousand Oaks, CA: Sage.

Wallack, S. (1979). *The California Prevention Demonstration Program evaluation: Description, methods, and findings.* Berkeley: University of California, Social Research Group, School of Public Health.

Warner, K.E. (1981). Cigarette smoking in the 1970's: The impact of the antismoking campaign on consumption. *Science, 211*(4483), 729-731.

Webb, J.A., and Baer, P.R. (1995). Influence of family disharmony and parental alcohol-use on adolescent social skills, self-efficacy, and alcohol-use. *Addictive Behaviors, 20*(1), 127-135.

Webster, R.A., Hunter, M., and Keats, J.A. (1994). Personality and sociodemographic influences on adolescents substance use: A path-analysis. *International Journal of the Addictions, 29*(7), 941-956.

Wechsler, H. (1996). Alcohol and the American college campus: A report from the Harvard School of Public Health. *Change, 28*(4), 20-25.

Wechsler, H., and Wuethrich, B. (2002). *Dying to drink: Confronting binge drinking on college campuses.* New York: Rodale, Inc.

Wechsler, H., Davenport, A., Dowdall, G.W., Moeykens, B., and Castillo, S. (1994). Health and behavioral consequences of binge drinking in college: A national survey of students at 140 campuses. *Journal of the American Medical Association, 272*(21), 1672-1677.

Wechsler, H., Moeykens, B., Davenport, A., Castillo, S., and Hansen, J. (1995). The adverse impact of heavy episodic drinkers on other college students. *Journal of Studies on Alcohol, 56,* 628-634.

Wechsler, H., Molnar, B.E., Davenport, A., and Baer, J. (1999). College alcohol use: A full or empty glass? *Journal of American College Health, 47*(6), 247-252.

Wechsler, H., Lee, J.E., Kuo, M., and Lee, H. (2000). College binge drinking in the 1990's: A continuing problem, results of the Harvard School of Public Health 1999 College Alcohol Study. *Journal of American College Health, 48*(5), 199-210.

Wechsler, H., Lee, J.E., Gledhill-Hoyt, J., and Nelson, T.F. (2001a). Alcohol use and problems at colleges banning alcohol: Results of a national survey. *Journal of Studies on Alcohol, 62*(2), 133-141.

Wechsler, H., Lee, J.E., Nelson, T.F., and Kuo, M. (2001b). Underage college students' drinking behavior, access to alcohol, and the influence of deterrence policies: Findings from the Harvard School of Public Health College Alcohol Study. *Journal of American College Health, 50*(2), 223-236.

Wechsler, H., Lee, J.E., Nelson, T.F., and Lee, H. (2001c). Drinking levels, alcohol problems and secondhand effects in substance-free college residences: Results of a national study. *Journal of Studies on Alcohol, 62*(1), 23-31.

Wechsler H., Lee, J.E., Kuo, M., Seibring, M., Nelson, T.F., and Lee, H.P. (2002). Trends in college binge drinking during a period of increased prevention efforts: Findings from four Harvard School of Public Health study surveys, 1993-2001. *Journal of American College Health*, 50(5), 203-217.

Weinberg, N.Z., Dielman, T.E., Mandell, W., and Shope, J.T. (1994). Parental drinking and gender factors in the prediction of early adolescent alcohol-use. *International Journal of the Addictions*, 29(1), 89-104.

Weitzman, E.R., Folkman, A., Folkman, K.L., and Wechsler, H. (2003a). The relationship of alcohol outlet density to heavy and frequent drinking and drinking-related problems among college students at eight universities. *Health and Place*, 9(1), 1-6.

Weitzman, E.R., Nelson, T.F., and Wechsler, H. (2003b). Taking up binge drinking in college: The influences of person, social group, and environment. *Journal of Adolescent Health*, 32(1), 26-35.

Werch, C.E., Pappas, D.M., Carlson, J.M., DiClemente, C.C., Chally, P.S., and Snider, J.A. (2000). Results of a social norm intervention to prevent binge drinking among first-year residential college students. *Journal of American College Health*, 49(2), 85-92.

Werner, M.F. (1995). Principles of brief intervention for adolescent alcohol, tobacco, and other drug use. *Pediatric Clinical of North America*, 42, 335-349.

Whetten-Goldstein, K., Sloan, F.A., Stout, E., and Liang, L. (2000). Civil liability, criminal law, and other policies and alcohol-related motor vehicle fatalities in the United States: 1984-1995. *Accident Analysis and Prevention*, 32, 723-733.

White, A.M., Ghia, A.J., Levin, E.D., and Swartzwelder, H.S. (2000). Binge pattern ethanol exposure in adolescent and adult rats: differential impact on subsequent responsiveness to ethanol. *Alcoholism, Clinical and Experimental Research*, 24(8), 1251-1256.

Williams, A.F., Wells, J.K., and Reinfurt, D.W. (1996). Increasing seat belt use in North Carolina. *Journal of Safety Research*, 27(1), 33-41.

Williams, C.L., and Perry, C.L. (1998). Lessons from project Northland: Preventing alcohol problems during adolescence. *Alcohol Health and Research World*, 22(2), 107-116.

Williams, C.L., Perry, C.L., Farbakhsh, K., and Veblen-Mortenson, S. (1999). Project Northland: Comprehensive alcohol use prevention for young adolescents, their parents, schools, peers and communities. *Journal of Studies on Alcohol*, 13, 112-124.

Williams, J., Chaloupka, F.J., and Wechsler, H. (2002). Higher alcohol prices and student drinking. *National Bureau of Economic Research*, 50(5), 223-236.

Willinger, M., Ko, C.W., Hoffman, H.J., Kessler, R.C., and Corwin, M.J. (2000). Factors associated with caregivers' choice of infant sleep position, 1994 to 198: The National Infant Sleep Position Study. *Journal of the American Medical Association*, 283(16), 2135-2142.

Willingham, M. (n.d.). *Reducing alcohol sales to underage purchasers A practical guide to compliance investigations*. Calverton, MD: OJJDP Underage Drinking Enforcement Training Center.

Wine Institute. (2003). *Code of advertising standards*. Available: http://www.wineinstitute.org/ [June, 2003].

Winsten, J.A. (1994). Promoting designated drivers: The Harvard Alcohol Project. *American Journal of Preventive Medicine*, 10(Suppl. 3), 11-14.

Wintre, M.G., and Sugar, L.A. (2000). Parenting, personality and the university transition. *Journal of College Student Development*, 41, 202-214.

Wolfson, M., Altman, D., DuRant, R., Shrestha, A., Patterson, T.E., Williams, A., Hensberry, R., Zaccaro, D., Foley, K., Champion, H., Preisser, J., Vitale, J., and Garner, G. (2003). Impact evaluation: Impact of a large nonrandomized community trial on enforcement of underage drinking laws and underage drinking. In *National Evaluation of the Enforcing Underage Drinking Laws Program: Year 3 Report* (Chapter 3). Winston-Salem, NC: Wake Forest University School of Medicine, Department of Public Health Sciences.

Wolfson, M., Toomey, T.L., Forster, J.L., Wagenaar, A.C., McGovern, P.G., and Perry, C.L. (1996a). Characteristics, policies and practices of alcohol outlets and sales to underage persons. *Journal of Studies on Alcohol, 57*, 670-674.

Wolfson, M., Toomey, T.L., Murray, D.M., Forster, J.L., Short, B.J., and Wagenaar, A.C. (1996b). Alcohol outlet policies and practices concerning sales to underage people. *Addiction, 91*, 589-602.

Wolfson, M., Wagenaar, A.C., and Hornseth, G.W. (1995). Law officer's views on enforcement of the minimum drinking age: A four-state study. *Public Health Reports, 110*, 428-438.

Wood, M.D., Nagoshi, C.T., and Dennis, D.A. (1992). Alcohol norms and expectations as predictors of alcohol use and problems in a college student sample. *American Journal of Drug and Alcohol Abuse, 18*(4), 461-476.

Wright, P.A. (n.d.). *Organizing for change: Confronting alcohol, tobacco, and other drug issues at the grassroots levels.* Center for Substance Abuse Prevention. Rockville, MD: University Research Corporation.

Wyllie, A., Zhang, J.F., and Casswell, S. (1998a). Responses to televised alcohol advertisements associated with drinking behavior of 10–17-year-olds. *Addiction, 93*(5), 361–371.

Wyllie, A., Zhang, J.F., and Casswell, S. (1998b). Positive responses to televised beer advertisements associated with drinking and problems reported by 18 to 29 year olds. *Addiction, 93*(5), 749-760.

Yu, J., Varone, R., and Shacket, R.W. (1997). *Fifteen-year review of drinking age laws: Preliminary findings of the 1996 New York State Youth Alcohol Survey.* New York: Office of Alcoholism and Substance Abuse.

Ziemelis, A. (1998, January). *Drug prevention in higher education: Efforts, evidence, and promising directions.* Paper presented at the Higher Education Center for Alcohol and Other Drug Prevention Annual Meeting, Charleston, SC.

Zimring, F.E. (1982). *The changing legal world of adolescence.* New York: Free Press.

Zuckerman, M. (1979). *Sensation seeking: Beyond the optimal level of arousal.* Hillsdale, NJ: Lawrence Erlbaum.

Zwerling, C., and Jones, M.P. (1999). Evaluation of the effectiveness of low blood alcohol concentration laws for younger drivers. *American Journal of Preventive Medicine, 16*(Suppl. 1), 76-80.

Appendix A

Statement of Task

The Board on Children, Youth, and Families of the National Research Council and the Institute of Medicine will form a new committee to review existing federal, state and nongovernmental programs, including media-based programs, designed to change the attitudes and health behaviors of youth. The review will include programs that focus directly on behavior change as well as those designed to change underage drinking behavior through reduction of adolescent access to alcohol (such as through increased excise taxation, aggressive enforcement of age and identification checks, and restriction of alcohol on college campuses). The committee shall produce a consensus panel report based on this review. The report will provide a cost-effective strategy to prevent and reduce underage drinking, including: an outline and implementation plan, message points that will be effective in changing the attitudes and health behaviors of youth concerning underage drinking, target audience identification, goals and objectives, and the estimated costs of development and implementation.

The committee will meet several times during the course of this study. It will begin by developing a general approach to conducting this project, including the identification of criteria for selection of appropriate programs for review. The committee will plan and oversee a public forum to obtain input from all relevant stakeholders and will hear presentations from a variety of experts regarding various aspects of substance abuse prevention and youth behavior change. These presentations may be accompanied by additional independent analyses or commissioned work that addresses various components of the overall committee charge.

The committee will produce a consensus report that will be widely disseminated to interested stakeholders.

Appendix B

Agenda and Participants
October 10-11, 2002
Public Workshop

Agenda

Thursday, October 10, 2002

11:00 a.m.   **Welcome and Purpose of the Workshop**

Richard J. Bonnie, Committee and Workshop Chair
University of Virginia Law School

11:15   **Underage Drinking: The Scope and Consequences of the Problem**

Epidemiology of Underage Drinking
Robert Flewelling, Pacific Institute for Research and Evaluation

Health Consequences
Sandra Brown, University of California, San Diego

Social Costs and Consequences
Ralph Hingson, Boston University School of Public Health

12:00 p.m.   Open Discussion

12:30   LUNCH

1:15 **Risk Factors, Risk Perception, and Youth Decision Making**

Risk and Protective Factors and Cognitive Development
Bonnie Halpern-Felsher, University of California,
San Francisco

Risk Perception and Decision Making
Janis Jacobs, Pennsylvania State University

Respondent: Robert Pandina, Rutgers

2:00 Open Discussion

2:30 **The Special Case of the Military**

Kenneth Hoffman, United States Army Medical Corps

2:45 Open Discussion

3:00 **Media and Advertising**

Media-Based Interventions
Charles Atkin, Michigan State University

Industry Marketing and Advertising Strategies
James O'Hara, Center on Alcohol Marketing and
Youth

The Effect of Advertising on Youth
Joel Grube, Prevention Research Center

4:00 Open Discussion

4:30 **Alcohol Use and Misuse Prevention Strategies for Minors**

William Hansen and Linda Dusenbury,
Tanglewood Research Inc.

5:00 Open Discussion

5:30 Adjourn

Friday, October 11, 2002

8:00 a.m.   Continental Breakfast

8:30   Welcome and Brief Recap

             Richard J. Bonnie

8:45   **The Special Case of College Drinking**

             A Call To Action
             Ralph Hingson, Boston University School of Public
             Health

             Respondent: Daniel Trujillo, Massachusetts Institute
             of Technology

9:15   Open Discussion

9:45   BREAK

10:00   **Drinking and Coming of Age in a Cross-Cultural
             Perspective**

             Robin Room, Center for Social Research on
             Alcohol and Drugs
             Stockholm University

10:30   Open Discussion

11:00   **Environmental Approaches**

             Supply-Side Approaches
             Harold Holder, Prevention Research Center

             The Effect of Pricing
             Frank Chaloupka, University of Illinois at Chicago

11:30   Open Discussion

12:00 p.m.   LUNCH

1:00   **Lessons Learned from Youth Smoking Prevention**

            Paula Lantz, University of Michigan School of Public
Health

1:30   Discussion

2:00   Closing Remarks

2:30   Workshop Adjourns

OTHER PARTICIPANTS

Kimberly Ball, The Century Council
Jeff Becker, Beer Institute
Gayle Boyd, National Institute on Alcohol Abuse and Alcoholism
John Calfree, American Enterprise Institute
Shannon Campagna, National Beer Wholesalers Association
Sharon Cantelon, Office of Juvenile Justice and Delinquency Prevention
Joan Corboy, Remove Intoxicated Drivers
Johnneta Davis-Joyce, Pacific Institute for Research and Evaluation
Arthur DeCelle, Beer Institute
Gary Decker, The Century Council
Andy Dobson, National Beer Wholesalers Association
Gwyndolyn Ensley, Department of Health and Human Services
Susan Ferguson, Insurance Institute for Highway Safety
James Frank, National Highway Traffic Safety Administration
David French, Mothers Against Drunk Driving
D. St. George, Center for Substance Abuse and Prevention
Monica Gourovitz, Distilled Spirits Council of the U.S.
Pat Green, The CDM Group
Susan Haney, Beer Institute
Roberta Hochberg, Leadership to Keep Children Alcohol Free
Kelly Kahn, National Institute on Alcohol Abuse and Alcoholism
Geoffrey Laredo, National Institute on Alcohol Abuse and Alcoholism
Laurie Knight, National Beer Wholesalers Association
Stephanie Manning, Mothers Against Drunk Driving
Mina McDaniel, Greer, Margolis, Mitchell, Burns, and Associates
Michael Miguel, representative of Congressman Dan Miller
Kimberly Miller, Center for Science in the Public Interest
Thomas Murphy, Department of Justice
Cheryl Neverman, National Highway Traffic Safety Administration
Patricia Powell, National Institute on Alcohol Abuse and Alcoholism

Craig Purser, National Beer Wholesalers Association
Amber Reed, Beer Institute
Rebecca Reeve, Governor's Institute on Alcohol and Substance Abuse
Cynthia Simms, National Capital Coalition to Prevent Underage Drinking
Joe Stanton, Beer Institute
Erik Strickland, Mothers Against Drunk Driving
Leslie Snyder, association not known
Will Taliaferro, Greer, Margolis, Mitchell, Burns, and Associates
Kyndel Turvaville, Beacon Consulting Group
Judith Vicary, Pennsylvania State University
Allan Williams, Insurance Institute for Highway Safety
Steve Wing, Substance Abuse and Mental Health Services Administration
Donald Zeigler, American Medical Association

Appendix C

Agenda and Participants, November 18, 2002 Open Committee Meeting and Public Forum

Agenda

This meeting is being held to gather information to help the committee conduct its study. This committee will examine the information and material obtained during this, and other public meetings, in an effort to inform its work. Although opinions may be stated and lively discussion may ensue, no conclusions are being drawn at this time; no recommendations will be made. In fact, the committee will deliberate thoroughly before writing its draft report. Moreover, once the draft report is written, it must go through a rigorous review by experts who are anonymous to the committee, and the committee then must respond to this review with appropriate revisions that adequately satisfy the Academy's Report Review committee and the chair of the NRC before it is considered an NRC report. Therefore, observers who draw conclusions about the committee's work based on today's discussions will be doing so prematurely.

Furthermore, individual committee members often engage in discussion and questioning for the specific purpose of probing an issue and sharpening an argument. The comments of any given committee member may not necessarily reflect the position he or she may actually hold on the subject under discussion, to say nothing of that person's future position as it may evolve in the course of the project. Any inference about an individuals position regarding findings or recommendations in the final report are therefore also premature.

11:30 a.m.   Cultural/Community Panel:
              Presentation of Working Papers

              Matthew Taylor, University of Wisconsin-La Crosse
              Felipe Castro, Arizona State University
              Douglas Novins, University of Colorado,
              Health Sciences Center

12:30 p.m.   LUNCH (on your own)

1:15   **Research on Youth Perspectives**

              Jeff Arnett, University of Maryland

1:45   **The Role of Sanctions in Underage Drinking**

              Thomas Hafemeister, University of Virginia

2:15   BREAK

2:30   Public Forum, Speakers

              Wesley Perkins (Hobart and William Smith Colleges)
              Jeff Linkenbach (Montana State University)
              John Nelson (American Medical Association)
              Jeff Becker (Beer Institute)
              Adam Chafetz (Health Commission)
              Chris Curtis (Virginia Dept. of Alcoholic Beverage
                 Control)
              Justin Saint Cyr (Youth Activist)
              William Georges (The Century Council)
              Monica Gourovitz (Distilled Spirits Council of the U.S.)
              Kimberly Miller (Center for Science in the Public
                 Interest)
              Wendy Hamilton (Mothers Against Drunk Driving)
              David Mitchell (Greer, Margolis, Mitchell, Burns, and
                 Associates)
              Murphy Painter (Louisiana Office of Alcohol and
                 Tobacco Control)
              Jasmine Pickner (Student Activist)
              Theresa Racicot (Leadership to Keep Children Alcohol
                 Free)
              David Rehr (National Beer Wholesalers Association)

Gary Stapleton (Student Activist-Students Against Drunk
   Driving)
Penny Wells (Students Against Drunk Driving)

5:30/6:00   Adjourn

OTHER PARTICIPANTS

Gayle Boyd, National Institute on Alcohol Abuse and Alcoholism
Shannon Campagna, National Beer Wholesalers Association
Joan Corboy, Remove Intoxicated Drivers
Jacquelyn D'Addams, Greer, Margolis, Mitchell, Burns, and Associates
Johnneta Davis-Joyce, Pacific Institute for Research and Evaluation
Arthur DeCelle, Beer Institute
Andy Dobson, National Beer Wholesalers Association
Susan Ferguson, Insurance Institute for Highway Safety
James Frank, National Highway Traffic Safety Administration
Stacy Harbison, Arent, Fox, Kintner, Plotkin, and Kahn
Shelly Jackson, National Institute of Justice, Washington, DC
Michael Johnson, Wine and Spirits Association of America
Laurie Knight, National Beer Wholesalers Association
Jennifer Loukissas, National Institute on Alcohol Abuse and Alcoholism
Stephanie Manning, Mothers Against Drunk Driving
Suzanne Medgycsi-Mistchang, Institute on Alcohol Abuse and Alcoholism
Thomas Murphy, Department of Justice
Geoffrey Laredo, National Institute on Alcohol Abuse and Alcoholism
Omlie Lynne, Distilled Spirits Council of the U.S.
Craig Purser, National Beer Wholesalers Association
Rebecca Reeve, Governor's Institute on Alcohol and Substance Abuse
Marcia Silcox, Silcox Communications
Erik Strickland, Mothers Against Drunk Driving
Will Taliaferro, Greer, Margolis, Mitchell, Burns, and Associates
Meena Vagnier, Community Anti-Drug Coalitions of America
LaTonya Wesley, American Psychological Association
Allan Williams, Insurance Institute for Highway Safety
Steve Wing, Substance Abuse and Mental Health Services Administration
Alison Whitesides, National Restaurant Association

Appendix D

Other Public Contributors

The committee commissioned numerous papers to synthesize the scientific literature and inform the committee's deliberations. Some of the papers had multiple authors, although only the lead author presented the papers to the committee at their meetings (see Appendixes B and C). The work of all of the authors is appreciated; they are all listed below under paper authors.

Multiple other organizations or individuals provided written information to the committee or responded to specific requests for information from the committee. Those individuals are listed below as other contributors. Individuals listed in earlier appendixes are not repeated here.

PAPER AUTHORS

Charles Atkin, Michigan State University
Janette Beals, Health Sciences Center, University of Colorado
Michael Biehl, University of California, San Francisco
Rosalind Brannigan, Drug Strategies, Washington DC
Sandra Brown, University of California, San Diego
Felipe Gonzalez Castro, Arizona State University
Frank Chaloupka, University of Illinois at Chicago
Linda Dusenbury, Tanglewood Research Inc., Greensboro, NC
Mathea Falco, Drug Strategies, Washington DC
Robert Flewelling, Pacific Institute for Research and Evaluation, Chapel Hill, NC

Julie Garfinkle, Arizona State University
Thomas Hafemeister, School of Medicine, University of Virginia
Ralph Hingson, Boston University, MA
Kenneth Hoffman, TRICARE Management, Falls Church, VA
Harold Holder, Prevention Research Center, Berkeley, CA
Shelly Jackson, National Institute of Justice, Washington DC
David Jernigan, Georgetown University, Washington DC
Donald Kenkel, Cornell University
Paula Lantz, University of Michigan
Spero Manson, Health Sciences Center, University of Colorado
Douglas Novins, Health Sciences Center, University of Colorado
James O'Hara, Georgetown University, Washington DC
Mallie Paschall, Prevention Research Center, Berkeley, CA
Chris Ringwalt, Pacific Institute for Research and Evaluation,
    Chapel Hill, NC
Robin Room, Stockholm University, Sweden
Paul Spicer, Health Sciences Center, University of Colorado
Susan Tapert, University of California, San Diego
Matthew Taylor, University of Wisconsin, La Crosse

OTHER CONTRIBUTORS

Genevieve Ames, Prevention Research Center, Berkeley, CA
Sarah Becker, Beacon Consulting Group
Mary Lou Bell, The Bell Group
Richard Blau, Holland and Knight LLP
Rosina Bowman
Verda Bradley, Department of Mental Health, Los Angeles
Dennis Brezina, Aluminum Anonymous Inc.
Paul Brounstein, Substance Abuse and Mental Health Services
    Administration, Rockville, MD
Kristin Buck, Mothers Against Drunk Driving
Raul Caetano, School of Public Health, University of Texas
Tom Colthurst, University of California, San Diego
Royer F. Cook, The ISA Group, Alexandria, VA
Suzanne Cosgrove, Health Communications Inc.
Peter Cressy, Distilled Spirits Council of the United States
Johnnetta Davis, Pacific Institute for Research and Evaluation,
    Calverton, MD
T. Delaney, Social Law Library
Barbara Deloian, National Association of Pediatric Nurse Practitioners
Juanita Duggan, Wine and Spirits Wholesalers of America Inc.
Kate Emanuel, The Advertising Council

Richard Erlich, Superior Court, Alaska
Wei Fang, Governor's Institute on Alcohol and Substance Abuse
Charles Fichette, Law Student, University of Virginia
Brian Flynn, University of Vermont
Susan Foster, The National Center on Addiction and Substance Abuse at
    Columbia University
Michael R. Frone, Research Institute on Addictions, New York State
    University
Stan Glantz, Institute for Health Policy Studies, University of California,
    San Francisco
Marcus Grant, International Center for Alcohol Policies
Thomas K. Greenfield, Alcohol Research Group, Public Health Institute,
    Berkeley, CA
George Hacker, Alcohol Policies Project
Greg Hamilton, Texas Alcoholic Beverage Control
Florence Hilliard, University of Wisconsin-Madison
Francis Holt, Spectrum Health Systems Inc.
Shirley Igo, National PTA
Art Jaeger, Consumer Federation of America
Lloyd Johnston, Institute for Social Research, University of Michigan
Ammie Kesse, Substance Abuse and Mental Health Services
    Administration
Nicole King, The Center on Alcohol Marketing and Youth
Jeff Kushner, St. Louis City Drug Court
Leonard Lamkin, American Medical Association
Geoffrey Laredo, National Institute on Alcohol Abuse and Alcoholism
Stephanie Mennen, Mothers Against Drunk Driving
Ted Miller, Pacific Institute for Research and Evaluation, Calverton, MD
James Mosher, Prevention Research Center, Berkeley, CA
Bernard Murphy, Pacific Institute for Research and Evaluation,
    Calverton, MD
Stacia Murphy, National Council on Alcoholism and Drug Dependence
Robert O'Neil, School of Law, University of Virginia
Nydia Ortiz-Pons, Ponce School of Medicine
Janeen Osborne, Division of Workplace Development
David Reotz, Liquor Enforcement Division, CO
Susan Rieves-Austin, Blue Ridge Behavioral Healthcare
Steven Schmidt, Bureau of Alcohol Education
Jim Sgueo, National Alcohol Beverage Control Association
Ellen Shields-Fletcher, Department of Justice, Office of Juvenile Justice
    and Delinquency Prevention, Washington DC
Deb Simkin, American Academy of Child and Adolescent Psychiatry

Michael Slater, Colorado State University
Alexander Wagenaar, School of Public Health, University of Minnesota
Eric Wagner, Florida International University
Larry Wallack, School of Community Health, Portland State University, OR
Stephen Wing, Substance Abuse and Mental Health Services
    Administration
Mark Wolfson, School of Medicine, Wake Forest University, Winston-
    Salem, NC
James Wright, Department of Transportation, National Highway Traffic
    Safety Administration, Washington DC
Li-Tzy Wu, Center for Risk Behavior and Mental Health Research,
    Research Triangle Park, NC

Appendix E

Biographical Sketches of Committee Members and Staff

Richard J. Bonnie (*Chair*) is John S. Battle professor of law and professor of psychiatric medicine at the University of Virginia and director of the university's Institute of Law, Psychiatry, and Public Policy. He writes and teaches in the fields of criminal law and procedure, mental health law, bioethics, and public health law. Active in public service throughout his academic career, he served as associate director of the National Commission on Marijuana and Drug Abuse (1971-1973); as a member of the National Advisory Council on Drug Abuse (1975-1980); as chair of Virginia's State Human Rights Committee, responsible for protecting rights of persons with mental disabilities (1979-1985); and as adviser for the American Bar Association's Criminal Justice Mental Health Standards Project (1981-1988). He was a member of the John D. and Catherine T. MacArthur Foundation Research Network on Mental Health and the Law (1988-1996), and is currently on the MacArthur Research Network on Mandated Community Treatment. He is a member of the Institute of Medicine.

Marilyn Aguirre-Molina is a professor of population and family health at the Mailman School of Public Health at Columbia University. Previously, she served as the executive vice president of the California Endowment and as a senior program officer at the Robert Wood Johnson Foundation. Her work focuses on program development and applied research that address policy and public health approaches to the prevention of health problems among young people (alcohol and tobacco use), particularly among ethnic and racial minority populations. She is a member of various national boards and committees that focus on public health issues, including the National Advisory Council of the National Institute on Alcohol Abuse and Alcoholism and the Subcommittee on College Drinking at the National Institutes of Health. In addition to her interest in health promotion for youth, she has worked extensively on Latino health policy issues. Her most recent book is *Latina Health in the U.S.: A Public Health Reader*.

Philip J. Cook is the ITT/Terry Sanford distinguished professor of public policy studies, professor of economics, and professor of sociology at Duke University. His research has focused on the costs and consequences of the widespread availability of guns, the prevention of alcohol-related problems through restrictions on alcohol availability, the efficacy of minimum-purchase-age laws in preventing fatal crashes, and the causes and consequences of the growing inequality of earnings. He is a member of the Institute of Medicine.

Judith A. Cushing is president and chief executive officer of the Oregon Partnership, a statewide nonprofit organization dedicated to substance abuse prevention and treatment referral services. Previously, she served as project coordinator of the Oregon Office of Alcohol and Drug Abuse Programs' Oregon Together Project responsible for all aspects of strategy implementation using the risk and protective factor model for 75 community coalitions throughout Oregon. That project became the national model for Communities That Care, a research-based model for community based prevention and mobilization. She is a lecturer, adviser, and consultant to national, state, and community organizations, including the White House Office of National Drug Control Policy, the Substance Abuse and Mental Health Services Administration, and the National Institute on Alcohol Abuse and Alcoholism. A member of national advisory boards at the Drug Enforcement Administration and Community Anti-Drug Coalitions of America, she also serves on the executive board of the National Family Partnership. She is a 1994 fellow of the Join Together National Leadership Fellows Program.

Joel W. Grube is director of the Prevention Research Center of the Pacific Institute for Research and Evaluation. Previously, he was coordinator of the Public Opinion Laboratory (1977-1978) and assistant director of the Social Research Center at Washington State University (1978-1981); senior research officer at the Economic and Social Research Institute in Dublin, Ireland (1981-1983); and a postdoctoral research fellow in alcohol studies at the School of Public Health of the University of California, Berkeley (1985-1986). His research focuses on social-psychological and environmental influences, including advertising and the media, on drinking and other problem behaviors among adolescents and young adults. His current research projects include a longitudinal study of the effects of alcohol outlet density on underage drinking and drinking problems, a longitudinal study on the effects of alcohol advertising on the drinking beliefs and behaviors of children and adolescents, and a longitudinal study on the effects of exposure to sexuality in the media on adolescents' sexual risk taking.

Bonnie L. Halpern-Felsher is an associate professor in the Division of Adolescent Medicine, Department of Pediatrics at the University of California, San Francisco (UCSF). She is also a faculty member at UCSF's Psychology and Medicine Postdoctoral Program, the Center for Health and Community, and the Comprehensive Cancer Center. She is a developmental psychologist whose research has focused on health-related decision making, perceptions of risk and vulnerability, and health communication. She has also conducted research on the relationships among parenting practices, peer relationships, adolescents' self-perceptions, and risky behavior. She has served as a consultant to a number of community-level adolescent health promotion programs and has been an active member on several national campaigns to understand and reduce adolescent risk behavior.

William B. Hansen has been president of Tanglewood Research since 1993. He received an honors B.A. degree from the University of Utah and M.S. and Ph.D. degrees in social psychology from the University of Houston. He has served on the faculty at UCLA (1978-1984), the University of Southern California (1980-1989), and Bowman Gray School of Medicine (1989-1996). A widely recognized expert in alcohol and drug prevention, he has written numerous curricula for school and community-based prevention, including Project SMART, Project STAR, and All Stars. He has authored more than 80 articles in scientific journals on research and evaluation methods, prevention theory, and strategies for successful prevention practice. The goal of his research has been to identify and evaluate evidence-based approaches to prevention that can achieve reductions in the onset of use and that can be applied in everyday settings. He has been the principal investigator on major studies to test norm setting and refusal skills strategies for preventing the onset of alcohol use and the development of alcohol problems among young adolescents, the basis of common alcohol and drug abuse education efforts, and projects designed to translate knowledge about prevention into practice. He has been an adviser to the U.S. Office of Technology Assessment, the U.S. Department of Education, the National Institute on Drug Abuse, the Center for Substance Abuse Prevention, numerous state agencies, numerous foundations, the United Nations, the Swiss, Spanish, Mexican, and Portuguese Departments of Health, and the U.S. Information Agency.

Denise Herd is associate professor of behavioral sciences in the Division of Health and Social Behavior of the School of Public Health at the University of California, Berkeley. Her research focuses on drinking and drug use patterns and problems, images of alcohol and violence in rap music, activism regarding local alcohol policy in African American communities, and social movements. She contributed to *Alcohol Use Among Ethnic Minorities* from the National Institute of Alcohol Abuse and Alcoholism, and she has received funding from the National Institutes of Health and the Robert Wood Johnson Foundation for a study on community mobilization regarding alcohol policy issues. She received an award through the Innovators Combating Substance Abuse Program at the Robert Wood Johnson Foundation.

Robert Hornik is Wilbur Schramm professor of communication and health policy at the Annenberg School for Communication at the University of Pennsylvania. He has a wide range of experience in mass-media communication evaluations, including breastfeeding promotion, AIDS education, immunization and child survival projects, and anti-drug and domestic violence media campaigns at the community, national, and international levels. He has been a consultant and member of various committees of the World Health Organization (WHO), including its Care-Seeking Project Technical Advisory Committee, and to the White House Office of National Drug Control Policy, the United States Agency for International Development, the United Nations Children's Fund, the Centers for Disease Control and Prevention, and the World Bank. He won the Andreasen Scholar Award in social marketing, and the Fisher Mentorship Award from the International Communication Association. He is the scientific director for the evaluation of the Office of National Drug Control Policy's National Youth Anti-Drug Media Campaign.

Janis Jacobs is professor of human development and family studies, professor of psychology, and vice provost for Undergraduate Education and International Programs at Pennsylvania State University. Her research and writing focus on the development of social cognitive processes during childhood and adolescence. One major area of study focuses on the formation of judgment biases in real-world decisions, emphasizing developmental trends during childhood and adolescence, and the role of social influences on judgment and decision making. Her second major area of study also involves social cognition, but is focused on gender differences in achievement motivation, self-perceptions of achievement, and parents' influence on achievement. She has worked on two longitudinal survey studies, one in which the self-perceptions, achievement attitudes, and choices of a group of individuals were tracked between ages 6 and 18, and the other in which the self-perceptions and achievement choices of a group were tracked between ages 12 and 28. In her role as vice provost, she has been involved in the university's efforts to prevent underage and binge drinking.

Mark H. Moore is the Guggenheim Professor of criminal justice policy and management and director of the Hauser Center for Non-Profit Organizations at the Kennedy School of Government at Harvard University. He was the founding chairman of the Kennedy School's Committee on Executive Programs and served in that role for over a decade. He is also the faculty chair of the school's Program in Criminal Justice Policy and Management. His research interests are in public management and leadership, in criminal justice policy and management, and in the intersection of the two. In the intersection of public management and criminal justice, he has written (with others) *From Children to Citizens: Vol. I., The Mandate for Juvenile Justice and Beyond 911: A New Era for Policing.*

Mary Ellen O'Connell is a senior program officer with the Board on Children, Youth, and Families. She is the study director for the Committee on Developing a Strategy to Reduce and Prevent Underage Drinking and the Committee on Evaluation of Children's Health: Measures of Risk, Protective and Promotional Factors for Assessing Child Health in the Community. Mary Ellen also developed two standalone workshops for the board on welfare reform and children and gun violence. She came to the board from the U.S. Department of Health and Human Services (HHS), where she spent 8 years in the Office of the Assistant Secretary for Planning and Evaluation (ASPE), most recently as director of State and Local Initiatives. During her tenure in ASPE, Mary Ellen focused on data, research, and policy related to homelessness and community-based health decision making. Prior to HHS, Mary Ellen worked at the U.S. Department of Housing and Urban Development on homeless policy and program design issues. She also was a member of an R.O.W. Sciences' team conducting the national evaluation of an NIAAA research demonstration project and worked for several years at the department of public welfare in the Commonwealth of Massachusetts as the director of field services. Mary Ellen received her bachelor's degree with distinction from Cornell University and a master's degree in the management of human services from the Heller School at Brandeis University.

Daniel A. Trujillo is the associate dean for Community Development and Substance Abuse programs at the Massachusetts Institute of Technology. He also serves as a center associate for the U.S. Department of Education's Higher Education Center for Alcohol and Other Drug Prevention. His major areas of research have focused on environmental and individual strategies for alcohol and other drug prevention and intervention. Previously, while at the University of Missouri-Columbia, the State University of New York-Albany, and the Massachusetts Institute of Technology, he directed the development, implementation, and evaluation of social norm marketing campaigns targeting alcohol use, sexual behavior, and health protective behavior; the development of university-community coalitions to work with city and state agencies and local tavern owners to end alcohol advertising and promotions on campus, to end drink specials offered in local licensed establishments, and to increase the enforcement of underage drinking laws; and the revision, implementation, and evaluation of policy and sanction initiatives, including the use of parental notification. He is currently working with the Massachusetts Department of Public Health on the implementation and evaluation of a statewide coalition project to address underage and problem drinking.

Index